The Women's Health Companion to Maternal-Child Nursing Care

Optimizing Outcomes for Mothers, Children, & Families

The Women's Health Companion to Maternal-Child Nursing Care

Optimizing Outcomes for Mothers, Children, & Families

Shelton M. Hisley, PhD, RNC, WHNP-BC

Assistant Professor of Nursing (Retired)
University of North Carolina at Wilmington
Wilmington, North Carolina

F.A. Davis Company • Philadelphia

F.A. Davis Company
1915 Arch Street
Philadelphia, PA 19103
www.fadavis.com

Printed in the United States of America

Last digit indicates print number: 10 9 8 7 6 5 4 3

Publisher: Lisa B. Deitch
Director of Content Development: Darlene D. Pedersen
Project Editor: Jamie Elfrank
Design & Illustration Coordinator: Carolyn O'Brien

As new scientific information becomes available through basic and clinical research, recommended treatments and drug therapies undergo changes. The author(s) and publisher have done everything possible to make this book accurate, up to date, and in accord with accepted standards at the time of publication. The author(s), editors, and publisher are not responsible for errors or omissions or for consequences from application of the book, and make no warranty, expressed or implied, in regard to the contents of the book. Any practice described in this book should be applied by the reader in accordance with professional standards of care used in regard to the unique circumstances that may apply in each situation. The reader is advised always to check product information (package inserts) for changes and new information regarding dose and contraindications before administering any drug. Caution is especially urged when using new or infrequently ordered drugs.

Library of Congress Cataloging-in-Publication Data
Hisley, Shelton M.
The women's health companion to maternal-child nursing care: optimizing outcomes for mothers, children, and families/Shelton M. Hisley.
 p. ; cm.
 Includes bibliographical references and index.
 ISBN-13: 978-0-8036-2814-4
 1. Maternity nursing--Textbooks. I. Hisley, Shelton M. II. Title.
 [DNLM: 1. Maternal-Child Nursing--methods. 2. Cultural Diversity. 3.
 Evidence-Based Nursing--methods. 4. Holistic Nursing--methods. WY 157.3
 W263m 2009]
RG951.W37 2009
618.2'0231--dc22

                                             2008051815

Health Promotion Approach to the Women's Health Content

The broad directives set forth in the Healthy People 2010 national initiative are central in the development and delivery of contemporary medical and nursing education. Today's emphasis on health care has shifted from an illness-focused model to a preventive model grounded in the shared goals of health promotion, health protection, and preventive services for all individuals. Consistent with this model, nursing education today embraces a wellness-centered approach that emphasizes health promotion and maintenance. The women's health information offered in the *Women's Health Companion to*

Maternal-Child Nursing Care: Optimizing Outcomes for Mothers, Children, & Families is framed in a health promotion context designed to appeal to nursing educators and students alike. Constructed to compliment and enhance the parent text *Maternal-Child Nursing Care: Optimizing Outcomes for Mothers, Children, & Families, the Women's Health Companion* is presented in a similar style with special features that parallel those found in the basic book and emphasize the nurse's role in health promotion and community-based care. This information is designed to allow students to increase their understanding about strategies for promoting women's health and enhance their expertise in caring for women of all ages in a variety of settings.

Table of Contents

Promoting Reproductive Health Through an Understanding of Sexually Transmitted Diseases   73

Promoting Reproductive Health Through an Understanding of Cervical Cytology Screening, Human Papillomavirus, and Cervical Cancer   90

Promoting Menopausal Health   113

Promoting Mental Health and Physical Safety Through an Understanding of Intimate Partner Violence

Shelton M. Hisley, PhD, RNC, WHNP-BC

 I Got Flowers Today

I got flowers today.
It wasn't my birthday or any other special day.
We had our first argument last night, and he said a lot of cruel things that really hurt me.
I know he is sorry and didn't mean the things he said.
Because he sent me flowers today.

I got flowers today.
It wasn't our anniversary or any other special day.
Last night he threw me into a wall and started to choke me.
It seemed like a nightmare.
I couldn't believe it was real.
I woke up this morning sore and bruised all over.
I know he must be sorry.
Because he sent me flowers today.

I got flowers today,
And it wasn't Mother's Day or any other special day.
Last night he beat me up again.
And it was much worse than all the other times.
If I leave him, what will I do?
What about money?
I'm afraid of him and scared to leave.
But I know he must be sorry.
Because he sent me flowers today.

I got flowers today.
Today was a very special day.
It was the day of my funeral.
Last night he finally killed me.
He beat me to death.
If only I had gathered enough courage and strength to leave him,
I would not have gotten flowers…today.

—Paulette Kelly

LEARNING TARGETS *At the completion of this chapter the student will be able to:*

◆ Define the term *intimate partner violence.*

◆ Describe the different types of intimate partner violence.

◆ Identify a national health goal related to intimate partner violence and discuss how nurses may be instrumental in helping the nation to achieve this goal.

◆ Discuss characteristics of the three phases typically included in a cycle of violence and describe how partners generally react during each phase.

◆ Explain how to conduct intimate partner violence screening and assessments.

◆ Describe the nurse's role in planning and providing care for victims of intimate partner violence.

Introduction

This chapter focuses on violence against women and the nurse's role in promoting mental health and physical safety for victims of intimate partner violence. Formerly termed *domestic violence* (DV), *intimate partner violence* (IPV) is considered a more modern term that recognizes that in contemporary society, intimate partners do not always share the same household. IPV is a significant public health problem that causes physical and emotional trauma for women, men, and children and leads to a myriad of health problems for the victims. Individuals who have been abused may be subjected to unnecessary diagnostic testing for various chronic problems that may be related to physical and emotional abuse. Although the physical manifestations of abuse may be treated by the health-care professional, it is incumbent upon the nurse to also address the underlying causes of the injuries and empower the victim with safety information and other appropriate resources (Krieger, 2008; Mahoney, 2006).

Nurses have long been at the forefront of research in the area of violence against women. Early investigations by Campbell (1986), Parker and McFarlane (1991), and McFarlane and colleagues (1991) helped to raise awareness about this significant public health problem (Williams, Brackley, Hibler, & Prater, 2008). Nurses who care for women and are advocates for the prevention of abuse are perfectly situated to screen patients and educate others on the importance of screening (Moran, 2008).

An important *Healthy People 2010* national goal clearly underscores the magnitude of intimate partner violence: *Reduce physical abuse directed at women by male partners to no more than 27 per 1,000 couples from a current baseline of 30 per 1,000 couples.* Nurses can be instrumental in helping the nation to achieve this goal by routinely assessing women and their families to identify those at risk, assisting with counseling or initiating referrals for professional care, and maintaining contact to ensure that appropriate follow-up mechanisms are in place (Family Violence Prevention Fund, 2008a; U.S. Department of Health and Human Services [USDHHS], 2000).

Definition, Incidence, and Impact on Individuals and Society

Intimate partner violence (IPV) is defined as physical, sexual, or psychological harm or social isolation perpetrated by a current or former partner (adult or adolescent), in an intimate or dating relationship. The violence can occur between members of heterosexual or homosexual couples and does not require sexual intimacy. The abuser's actions are intended to instill fear and to intimidate and control the victim (Davila, 2006; Family Violence Prevention Fund, 2008a; Stinson & Robinson, 2006; Ward & Wood, 2009; Yonaka, Yoder, Darrow, & Sherck, 2007).

Viewed as a potentially preventable public health problem, IPV affected more than 32 million individuals in the United States between 1993 and 2005. Around the world, at least one in every three women has been beaten, coerced into sex, or otherwise abused during her lifetime. Intimate partner violence is the most common form of violence directed against women, and according to the World Health Organization (WHO), one out of every six women has been a victim of IPV. In many situations, women are victimized more than once by the same partner. In this country, it is estimated that approximately 5.3 million women experience IPV each year, and women have a one in four chance of becoming a victim of IPV at some point during their lifetime. During 2001, more than half a million American women (588,490 women) were victims of nonfatal violence at the hands of an intimate partner. In 2005, IPV resulted in 1,510 deaths; of these deaths, 22% were males and 78% were females (Centers for Disease Control and Prevention [CDC], 2009; Moran, 2008; Tjaden & Thoennes, 2000a; WHO, 2005; Williams et al., 2008).

 Nursing Insight— IPV: Appreciating the scope of the problem

In 2007, the Bureau of Justice Statistics of the U.S. Department of Justice published "Intimate Partner Violence in the United States," a report that showed that, sadly, statistics on IPV have not changed much over the past few years. "Domestic homicides against women rose from 1,155 murders in 2004 to 1,181 in 2005. That means that, on average, in 2005 more than three women a day were murdered by their husbands or boyfriends in the United States" (Family Violence Prevention Fund, 2007). Findings from a study conducted by the CDC (2003) showed that there are approximately 2 million injuries to women from IPV each year, and nearly one in four women report experiencing violence by a current or former spouse or boyfriend during some time in her life (Family Violence Prevention Fund, 2008b).

A man with a history of violence often brings violence into the family. The abuser's expressions of violent behavior usually erupt early in the courtship and grow progressively worse. Violence is used to handle conflicts, and the abuser exerts power to elicit a pervasive feeling of powerlessness in those around him. Male abusers frequently have a history of early and prolonged exposure to family violence as children, and alcohol is often associated with the violent behavior (Blereau, 2009; Bull, 2009; Krieger, 2008).

According to the U.S. Department of Justice (2007), female victims are substantially more likely than male victims to be killed by an intimate partner. In fact, male abusers kill their female partners four times more often than female abusers kill males involved in IPV. From 1976 to 2004, most homicides involved spouses, although in recent years the number of deaths by boyfriends and girlfriends has increased. More than two-thirds of spouse and ex-spouse victims of IPV were killed by firearms between 1976 and 2004. Interestingly, during this time period, female abusers were more likely to kill their partners with knives than were any other group of intimates (Krieger, 2008; Rennison, 2003).

Intimate partner violence reaches across all strata of society and affects persons regardless of economic status, ethnic background, educational level, or religious status. The economic toll of the violence is substantial. It is estimated that the costs of IPV, physical assault, and stalking exceed $5.8 billion per year. Of this amount, $4.1 billion is directly related to physical and mental health services (CDC, 2003; Moran, 2008; Tjaden & Thoennes, 2000a; U.S. Department of Justice, 2007; Ward & Wood, 2009; Yonaka et al, 2007). Individuals affected by IPV experience a productivity loss of 8 million days of paid work (the equivalent of 32,000 full-time jobs) and approximately 5.6 million days of unpaid household work each year (CDC, 2003).

 Ethnocultural Considerations— Intimate partner violence

According to Tjaden and Thoennes (2000b), in the United States, the groups found to have the highest prevalence of IPV are American Indian and Alaskan Native women and men, African American women, and Hispanic women. Glass (2005) reported that Latinas are known to under-use traditional intervention services such as domestic violence shelters, health-care services, and law enforcement agencies because of a lack of health insurance, language and cultural barriers, and a general distrust of formal systems. Caucasian women report less IPV than do non-Caucasians, and Asian women report significantly less IPV than do other racial groups. Peedicayil and colleagues (2004) conducted a study of 9,938 women in India and reported a 13% prevalence rate of moderate to severe violence—including slapping, beating, kicking, and use of a weapon—during pregnancy. It is important for nurses to remember that violence may be underreported as a result of cultural norms. Although cultures may differ in their perceptions and definitions of abuse, the act of inflicting harm to another is against the law.

Those who perpetrate the abuse may refuse to allow their victims to work or attend school. Women who are abused are more likely to be unemployed, suffer from health problems, and receive public assistance than are women who are not victims of abuse. Those with severe and persistent mental illness are more likely to be involved in controlling and violent relationships. In the workplace, an additional burden is frequently placed on coworkers to compensate for the IPV victim's repeated absenteeism. Another indicator of the substantial economic burden of abuse is reflected in the millions of tax dollars channeled into supporting programs created to assist IPV victims (Krieger, 2008; Moracco et al., 2004).

 Nursing Insight— Accuracy issues with reported IPV statistics

Accuracy in regard to IPV statistics is difficult to determine. It is estimated that only 20% to 50% of the assaults are actually reported to the police (National Domestic Violence Hotline, 2008). According to Tjaden and Thoennes (2000a), only 25% of all physical assaults against women, and fewer assaults against men, are reported to police. Coker and colleagues (2002) estimated that 29% of all women and 22% of all men will experience physical, sexual, or psychological abuse at some point in their lifetime. Victims of abuse may be reluctant to report personal violence because of fear or embarrassment or because those from whom they sought help did not directly ask about abuse.

According to Johnson and Leone (2005), victims of repeated violence over time sustain more serious injuries than do victims of one-time abuse incidents. Young women and economically challenged individuals are affected more often by IPV than any other population (Heise & Garcia-Moreno, 2002). Economic hardship is known to exacerbate IPV. Financial stress may lead to more frequent and violent abuse: Out-of-work husbands and boyfriends spend more time at home and thus have more opportunities to abuse their partners, and women are less likely to leave abusive situations for fear that they will not be able to support themselves (Blereau, 2009; Johnson & Leone, 2005).

Approximately 50% of children living in homes of intimate partner violence are also victimized. Children living in households affected by maternal abuse are 57 times more likely to suffer personal harm and are at greater risk for psychiatric disorders, developmental problems, school failure, violence against others, and low self-esteem. Those who perpetrate IPV create instability within their families while causing untold physical and psychological damage (Bull, 2009; Krieger, 2008; Parkinson, Adams, & Emerling, 2001).

Nursing Insight— Recognizing social factors in violent behavior

Violent behavior in intimate relationships is often rooted in multiple social factors. For example, the perpetrators and victims of family violence may learn about violent behavior by either witnessing or experiencing it firsthand. Other social factors include poverty and oppression, low income, unemployment, difficulty in maintaining interpersonal ties, marital instability and disruption, and single-parent families (Hamolia, 2005).

The CDC National Center for Injury Prevention and Control (2003) and other researchers list multiple factors that place an individual at risk for committing intimate partner abuse and for being a victim of intimate partner abuse (Tables 1-1 and 1-2).

 Now Can You— **Discuss certain facts about IPV?**

1. Define the term *intimate partner violence*?
2. Identify a national goal related to IPV and discuss how nurses can be instrumental in helping the nation to achieve this goal?
3. Explain why it is difficult to obtain accurate statistics about the prevalence of IPV?
4. List 10 risk factors for committing IPV and 10 risk factors for being a victim of IPV?

Types of Abuse

Abuse may occur in many forms, and victims may be repeatedly subjected to more than one type of abuse. Physical abuse is only one manifestation of intimate partner violence. Other types of abuse include sexual abuse, mental (emotional) abuse, social abuse, and economic abuse.

PHYSICAL ABUSE

Physical abuse may include spitting, kicking, punching, grabbing, slapping, or strangulation. The abused woman may be seen in the health clinic, doctor's office, or emergency department with vague, chronic, nonspecific complaints, and often there is a history of overuse of health services or unexplainable injuries such as bruises and fractures. Nurses should be alert to the patient's chronic issues as possible symptoms of abuse. For example, the woman may seek treatment for headaches, anxiety, stress, insomnia, or fatigue. The IPV victim's appearance may vary: She may be disheveled, dirty, and distressed or neat, well groomed, and calm. Oftentimes, abused women are

Table 1-1 Risk Factors for Committing Intimate Partner Violence

Individual Factors	Relationship Factors
Young age	Marital conflict
Low self-esteem	Marital instability
Low income	Male dominance in the family
Low academic achievement	Poor family functioning
Aggressive or delinquent behavior as a child	Emotional dependence and insecurity
Alcohol or drug use	Belief in strict gender roles
Witnessing or experiencing childhood violence	Desire for power and control in relationships
Social isolation	Angry or hostile behavior toward a partner
Unemployment	

Table 1-2 Risk Factors for Being a Victim of Intimate Partner Violence

Individual Factors	Relationship Factors
History of child abuse	Marital conflict
History of physical abuse	Marital instability
History of sexual abuse	Male dominance in the family
Prior injury from the same partner	Poor family functioning
Having a verbally abusive partner	Partner history of alcohol or drug abuse
Economic stress, low income	
Tobacco, alcohol, and illicit drug use	
Depression or suicide attempts	
History of sexually transmitted infections	
Young age (less than 24 years, especially adolescents)	
Lack of high school diploma	
Unplanned pregnancies (often as a result of birth control sabotage)	

subjected to unnecessary diagnostic testing to determine the cause of the chronic conditions (Krieger, 2008; Mahoney, 2006; Ward & Wood, 2009).

 Optimizing Outcomes— **Recognizing signs of intimate partner violence**

By recognizing signs of IPV, nurses can be instrumental in helping to make an accurate diagnosis and in securing appropriate assistance for the abused woman. Specifically, the nurse should remain alert to the following indicators, which may be signs of IPV:

- Overuse of health services
- Vague, nonspecific complaints
- Repeated missed appointments
- Unexplained injuries
- Untreated serious injuries
- Significant delay between the injury and the presentation for care
- Injuries that do not match the patient's description of how they were incurred
- Evidence or a history of previous injuries
- Bilateral or multiple injuries in various stages of healing
- Intimate partner who refuses to leave the patient's side
- Intimate partner who insists on explaining how the injury was incurred (Blereau, 2009; Krieger, 2008)

Certain behavioral clues may point to abuse. For example, the intimate partner may refuse to leave the victim during the interview and physical assessment. The abuser may display extreme attentiveness toward the victim and attempt to describe to the care provider exactly how the injuries were sustained. The abuser may hover, dominate, and control the information given. The abuser may refuse to allow the victim to share private time with the health professional. The information about the circumstances surrounding the injury may not match the actual injuries. Frequently, victims suffer repeated injuries and delay medical treatment for serious injuries. Research conducted by Crandall and associates (2004) revealed that 93% of female IPV victims had made at least one previous injury visit to a health-care facility, and 44% of women murdered during an IPV episode had visited an emergency department within 2 years of being murdered (Krieger, 2008; Ward & Wood, 2009).

 Optimizing Outcomes— Recognizing physical patterns of IPV injury

Nurses should be aware that physical injuries inflicted during intimate partner violence are likely to appear in a central pattern on the face, chest, breasts, abdomen, and neck. The patient may complain of abdominal pain upon palpation, chest pain related to rib trauma, or musculoskeletal pain accompanied by redness and swelling. Bruises may be noted on the inner aspect of the arms and/or legs, along with injuries suggestive of a defensive-type posture, such as an injury to the ulnar aspect of the forearm (Ward & Wood, 2009).

Intimate partner violence frequently results in head, neck, and facial injuries. It is estimated that up to 90% of abused victims sustain head and neck injuries, and IPV is believed to account for between 34% and 73% of all facial injuries in women (Blereau, 2009).

Arosena and colleagues (2009) discovered that specific patterns of facial injury are more likely to be associated with IPV than with other sources of injury, such as motor vehicle crashes or even with assault by a stranger. The researchers reviewed the medical and dental records of 326 women with facial trauma treated by specialists at a university hospital. Their findings revealed that injuries around the eye or upper face were more likely to be associated with IPV, while mandible fractures were more likely to be caused by assault by an unknown assailant. Victims of IPV more often sustained zygomatic complex fractures, orbital blow-out fractures, and intracranial injuries than did other patients with facial trauma (Arosarena, Fritsch, Hsueh, Aynehchi, & Haug, 2009; Blereau, 2009).

 Nursing Insight— IPV and patterns of facial trauma

A woman's face is the most meaningful area on her person. According to an otolaryngologist who has extensively studied injuries inflicted during IPV, the pattern of facial trauma sustained is reflective of this fact. Thus, hitting in the face figures prominently in IPV. This particular pattern may be contrasted with that typically seen in the assault of a robber, for example, whose ultimate goal is primarily to disable the victim (Blereau, 2009; Lite, 2009).

Women who are strangled during IPV may or may not demonstrate physical evidence of an injury to the neck. Strack and McClane (1999) reported that visible evidence such as red marks, scratches, scrapes, bruises, or rope burns may be apparent in only 15% of strangulation cases. Nurses should be alert to patient complaints such as persistent throat pain, voice changes, or difficulty swallowing, which may be indicators of neck trauma sustained during an act of violence. Chin abrasions may be present—as the victim lowers the chin in an instinctive effort to protect the neck, the skin is scraped against the abuser's hands. Victims of strangulation attempts should be evaluated for possible damage (e.g., fracture) to the hyoid bone, a small horseshoe-shaped bone in the neck that supports the tongue. Although breathing difficulty may initially appear to be mild, damage to the hyoid bone or other underlying structures may result in fatal asphyxiation up to 36 or more hours after the assault (Krieger, 2008; Strack & McClane, 1999).

 Nursing Insight— Recognizing the unique problems of older women subjected to IPV

Women of all ages are at risk for IPV. When trying to leave an abuser, older women may face challenges such as feelings of shame and worries about money. However, abused women who are 55 years and older are confronted with still another challenge. Having grown up and gotten married during a time when IPV was often ignored, older women have suffered many years of abuse and, like other victims of IPV, frequently have problems with poor self-image and guilt. Older women who have been abused are also less likely to confide in anyone about the abuse, they may have health problems that keep them dependent on their abusive partner, feel committed to caring for their abusive and aging partners, and are fearful of being alone (American College of Obstetricians and Gynecologists [ACOG], 2008; USDHHS, 2009).

 Now Can You— Discuss physical injury associated with IPV?

1. Identify eight clinical red flags that may be indicative of IPV?
2. Describe behavioral characteristics of the abuser that may be indicative of IPV?
3. Explain what is meant by a "central pattern" of injury and why this is often observed in victims of IPV?

SEXUAL ABUSE

Sexual abuse may include the abuser's use of force to carry out sexual intercourse or other sexual activities against the victim's will. It may include forced participation in an early initiation of sexual activity; forced participation in sexual activity viewed to be humiliating or degrading; decreased condom use or otherwise unprotected sexual intercourse; having multiple sexual partners; and trading sex for food, money, drugs, or other items. Sexual abuse may increase the likelihood of exposure to sexually transmitted diseases (STDs), including HIV and AIDS. Recurrent vaginal infections and/or an unusually high number of STDs or frequent miscarriages can be warning signs of sexual abuse. Interestingly, sexual assaults committed by strangers are more likely to be reported than are rapes and sexual assaults committed by an intimate partner (CDC, 2003;

Family Violence Prevention Fund, 2008b; Krieger, 2008; Rennison, 2003; Ward & Wood, 2009).

Another manifestation of sexual abuse involves forcing undesired pregnancy or forcing pregnancies to rapidly occur after one another. Pregnancy constitutes an especially dangerous time for abused women. Physical violence during pregnancy has far-reaching effects for the infant as well as the mother. Battery during pregnancy is associated with a greater incidence of low-birth-weight neonates, preterm birth, and neonatal death. According to the Family Violence Prevention Fund (2008b), IPV accounts for 31% of the homicides among pregnant women and is the leading cause of traumatic death for pregnant and postpartum women in the United States (Krieger, 2008; Yost, Bloom, McIntire, & Leveno, 2005).

 Nursing Insight— *Maternal intimate partner violence: The sobering statistics*

Women who experience abuse in the year prior to and/or during a recent pregnancy are 40% to 60% more likely than nonabused women to suffer from high blood pressure, vaginal bleeding, severe nausea, and kidney or urinary tract infections during pregnancy. They are also more likely to require hospitalization during pregnancy and are 37% more likely to give birth to preterm infants. Neonates born to abused mothers are 17% more likely to be underweight at birth and are 30% more likely than other infants to require neonatal intensive care (Silverman, Decker, Reed, & Raj, 2006).

MENTAL (EMOTIONAL) ABUSE

Mental or emotional abuse includes acts such as coercion, making threats, and stalking. The abuser may verbally abuse the victim with criticism, insults, put-downs, or name calling. The perpetrator may use facial expressions or gestures to intimidate and instill fear. Other forms of emotional abuse include the perpetrator's use of threats of harm to children, family members, or pets. Not uncommonly, abusers destroy the victim's property, abuse their pets, or display weapons to force the victim into submission. The abuser may mislead children into viewing the victim as having "earned" the abuse by causing the perpetrator to become angry—in this situation, the children often blame the victim for the resulting violence. The perpetrator frequently places the blame on the victim—denying fault and instead claiming that any physical injury resulted from the victim's "clumsiness." Often, the victim's injuries are minimized and the abuser creates excuses for the abusive behavior. The perpetrator may also attempt to convince others that the victim is incompetent or guilty of fabrication and not to be believed or taken seriously (Krieger, 2008).

 Now Can You— **Discuss aspects of sexual and mental abuse?**

1. Identify four examples of sexual abuse?
2. Describe maternal and neonatal problems that may stem from abuse during pregnancy?
3. Identify three characteristics of mental abuse?

SOCIAL ABUSE

Social abuse may include the abuser isolating or limiting the victim's contact and time spent with family and friends; the abuser may also require the victim to obtain permission to leave the house. The victim may be forbidden from seeking outside employment or from attending school. The perpetrator may conduct "odometer checks" on the victim's car to confirm that the victim has not left home and in some situations, the victim is required to provide a detailed account of any time spent away from the abuser. The victim may be denied access to medical services. The abuser may prevent the victim from keeping medical or other appointments, thereby creating strain on relationships with health-care providers, employers, friends, and family members (Krieger, 2008; Plichta, 2004).

The abuser may harm the victim's reputation and intimidate the victim's family and friends. Not infrequently, a breakdown in the victim's interpersonal relationships occurs, removing an important source of emotional support for the victim. Social abuse may include the perpetrator stalking the victim. According to the CDC (2003), 1 million women and 371,000 men are stalked by IPV abusers. It has been estimated that only 50% of stalking activity against women is actually reported to the police. Stalking constitutes a serious threat, and the victim should be encouraged to report this behavior to the police (CDC, 2003; Krieger, 2008; Tjaden & Thoennes, 2002a).

ECONOMIC ABUSE

Economic abuse may include the abuser's controlling all aspects of the victim's finances, refusing to share money, forcing the victim to account for any money spent, and forbidding the victim from working outside of the home. For the perpetrator, these actions help to bring about the victim's emotional and financial dependency on the abuser. The abuser may force the victim to repeatedly miss work, place frequent telephone calls to the victim at the workplace, or show up at the workplace unannounced in an attempt to jeopardize the victim's work ethic and job security. According to the American Bar Association (2008), 70% of IPV victims are employed, and greater than 70% of them admit that their abusers harass them at work, either over the telephone or in person. Also, abusers cause more than 60% of their victims to be late or absent from work or both (American Bar Association, 2008; Krieger, 2008).

 Nursing Insight— *Use of the power and control wheel to enhance understanding*

The Power and Control Wheel (Figure 1-1) was developed by battered women in Duluth, Minnesota. The women, all victims of IPV, were attending women's education groups sponsored by the women's shelter. The Power and Control Wheel is meant to graphically illustrate the scope of men's abusive behaviors toward women.

The Equality Wheel (Figure 1-2), also developed by the Minnesota Domestic Abuse Intervention Project, was created to describe the changes needed for men who batter to move from being abusive to being part of a nonviolent partnership. Used together, the wheels provide a mechanism for identifying and exploring abuse and then making behavioral changes toward nonviolent behavior.

Figure 1-1 The Power and Control Wheel: A model of power and control issues that perpetuate battering. (Developed by the Duluth Domestic Abuse Intervention Project, Duluth, Minnesota.)

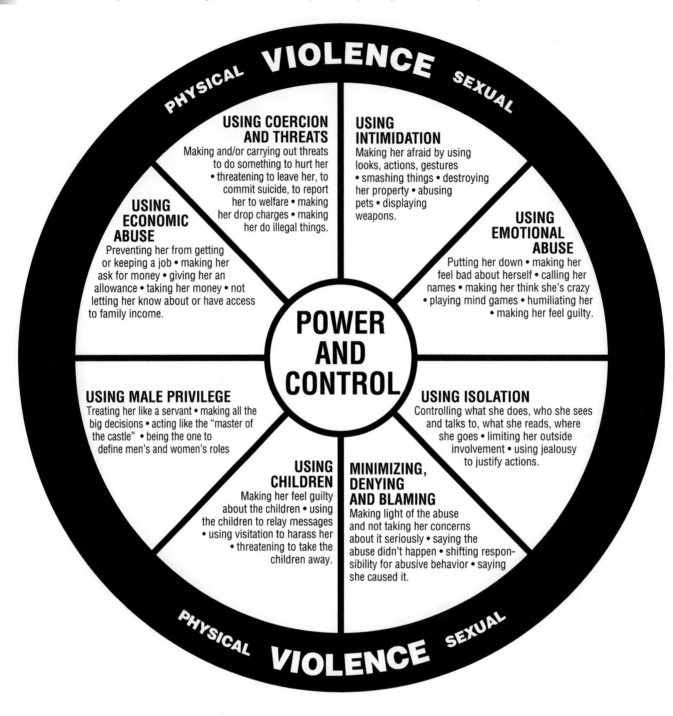

DOMESTIC ABUSE INTERVENTION PROJECT

202 East Superior Street
Duluth, Minnesota 55802
218-722-2781
www.duluth-model.org

Figure 1-2 The Equality Wheel: May be used in concert with the Power and Control Wheel to help individuals see alternate ways of being in relationships with women that are free of violence and controlling behavior. (Developed by the Duluth Domestic Abuse Intervention Project, Duluth, Minnesota.)

Optimizing Outcomes— **Recognizing vulnerable victims of abuse**

Nurses should be aware that certain vulnerable individuals might be more likely to be affected by IPV. Women with disabilities are vulnerable to physical, sexual, and mental abuse, neglect, and exploitation. The abuse may include withholding necessary assistive devices, care, or treatment. Immigrant and refugee women are at risk for violence and abuse because of isolation and manipulation by their partners, language and cultural differences, and a prevailing lack of awareness of their rights and legal and social resources (ACOG, 2007).

 Now Can You— **Discuss aspects of social and economic abuse?**

1. Describe three characteristics of social abuse?
2. Describe three characteristics of economic abuse?
3. Explain how the Power and Control Wheel and the Equality Wheel may be used to enhance understanding about male-directed abusive behavior toward women and offer behavioral strategies for the transition into a nonviolent, noncontrolling relationship?

Phases of Abuse

Three phases of abuse have been identified: (1) tension building; (2) acute violence; and (3) a tranquil, loving period of calm and remorse, sometimes termed the "honeymoon period." Although not all abusive relationships follow this cycle, many victims can readily recognize this pattern (Walker, 1979, 1984).

TENSION-BUILDING PHASE

The first phase is characterized as a period of increasing tension. During this time, the abuser demonstrates hostility and anger without culminating into violent outbursts. The victim senses the escalating behavior and attempts to placate the abuser. In many situations, the victim's behavior postpones rather than prevents the abuse. At some point, the victim realizes that she cannot control the violent behavior and withdraws to cope. This action only heightens the abuser's anger (Krieger, 2008; Walker, 1979, 1984).

VIOLENCE PHASE

In the second phase, the abuser discharges the pent-up tension. This phase may be triggered by an internal response in the abuser or by an external crisis. Over a period of hours or days, the abuser may engage in a number of violent acts, such as biting, slapping, punching, stomping, choking, pushing, burning, or mutilation. Most injuries are directed at the face, neck, chest, breasts, buttocks, and abdomen; the hands and forearms are often damaged as the victim attempts to protect herself. The abuser often makes the victim feel that she has angered the abuser and thus is responsible for the abuse. Frequently, the woman minimizes the extent of injury and is reluctant to seek medical care (Krieger, 2008; Walker, 1979, 1984).

THE HONEYMOON PHASE

During the third phase, the abuser feels remorse and apologizes profusely. He promises that the abuse will never happen again and may even believe that it will not. The abuser showers his victim with love and kindness, lulling her into forgiveness and a desire to continue the relationship. The victim desperately wants to believe her abuser and is renewed in her hope that he really will change. This phase provides the positive reinforcement for remaining in the relationship. The victim denies the reality that the abuse will recur. Unless there is some intervention at this point, this phase will end and the cycle of violence will be repeated (Krieger, 2008; Varcolis, Carson, & Shoemaker, 2006; Walker, 1979, 1984).

VICTIMS' REACTIONS TO THE PHASES OF ABUSE

Victims react in various ways to each of the three phases of abuse. During the first, or tension-building, phase, the woman uses denial as a defense mechanism. If the relationship is not terminated at this point, the abuse continues to escalate in frequency and violence, and the victim indirectly "gives permission" for the abuse to continue. During the second (violence) phase, the woman can no longer deny that the violence is occurring. Unfortunately, she is unable to stop the violence because she is fearful of provoking further violence. She resorts to the use of various coping mechanisms such as dutiful obedience and cooperation as she conforms to the abuser's wishes in a desperate effort to reduce the violence. This behavior has been termed "learned helplessness." Not surprisingly, the victim feels hopeless, powerless, and depressed and may have difficulty seeking help at this point because she is immobilized by a sense of guilt and does not believe that others may wish to help her.

 Nursing Insight— Gaining an understanding of the IPV victims' behavior/recovery phases

Kearney's (2001) seminal research was designed to gain insight into why IPV victims remain with or return to their abusers. Four phases of IPV victim recovery were identified:

Enduring love/relationship obligation: Characterized by a desire to love/be loved; belief that the relationship is "forever"; fearfulness of disclosure to family and friends; personal feelings of shame and guilt and self-blame for the abuse

The more I do, the worse I am: Characterized by attempts to meet the abuser's needs despite the fact that the abuse now occurs routinely; feelings of self-doubt, loss of personal identity; displaying of harmful behaviors (e.g., substance abuse, alcoholism, suicide attempts) to cope with the emotional strain or coping behaviors (e.g., extreme dieting or overeating) to gain some semblance of control over their lives (CDC, 2003)

I've had enough: Characterized by the realization that the relationship is abusive and will not be tolerated, but fear of the unknown and a lack of information about how to seek safe shelter—this point in the relationship is an opportune time for nurses to advocate for victims by providing support, education, and information about community resources

I was finding me: Characterized by the ability to live a life separate from the abuser; may need tools (e.g., economic resources) to remain independent; requires continued support and encouragement; ongoing self-discovery/recovery; moving from the role of "victim" to one of "survivor"

 Now Can You— **Discuss the phases of abuse?**

1. Identify the three phases of abuse and describe characteristics of each phase?
2. Explain how victims often react to each of the three phases of abuse?
3. Describe how Kearney's (2001) research provides insights into IPV victims' behavior and how this information is useful to nurses?

Intimate Partner Violence Screening, Documenting, and Reporting

SCREENING FOR IPV

In 2000, the American Nurses Association (ANA) published a position statement on violence against women. This important document advocates universal screening, routine assessment, and documentation of abuse for all victims in any health-care setting. Universal screening means that *all* patients are assessed for IPV, regardless of the presence or absence of any abuse indicators. Routine screening can facilitate early identification of IPV when signs and symptoms may not be readily apparent and timely referral for appropriate services that may prevent further injury (Ward & Wood, 2009; Wilson, Lane, & Gillespie, 2006). If the screening tool suggests that the patient may be at high risk for abuse, a more detailed assessment should be performed (Krieger, 2008).

 Nursing Insight— *Recognizing potential barriers to IPV screening*

Nurses must be aware of potential barriers to routine IPV screening in the clinical setting. Time constraints, a lack of awareness of IPV, a lack of instructions on how to inquire about abuse, language and cultural differences, and a practitioner's personal history of abuse are factors that may prevent health-care professionals from performing routine IPV screening (Yonaka et al., 2007). Chang and colleagues (2003) explored positive and negative consequences of IPV screening. Positive consequences included the following: a feeling that the practitioners cared, growing awareness that IPV is a problem, and a reduction in the victims' sense of social isolation. Negative consequences included feelings of being judged and being intruded upon, increasing anxiety, and disappointment in the practitioner's response (Williams et al., 2008).

In 2004, the U.S. Preventive Services Task Force (USPSTF) found insufficient evidence to recommend for or against routine screening of women for IPV. The Task Force noted that the potential harms (e.g., anxiety, fear of being stigmatized) of screening for IPV need to be documented in more rigorous studies. In addition, the USPSTF reported that no studies have determined the validity

 where research and practice meet: **Routine Screening for IPV**

Williams and colleagues (2008) conducted a pilot study designed to assess the IPV screening practices of advanced practice nurses and physicians. The participants completed a survey about routine IPV screening of female patients and whether they had received IPV-related education. Based on the findings, the researchers suggested that professional educational programs routinely include content on IPV screening, beliefs, practices, and barriers to screening and concluded that despite the USPSTF position against routine screening, practitioners should routinely screen for IPV to err on the side of patient safety.

of the screening tools designed to identify IPV. Although current evidence to support routine screening is insufficient, health-care settings may still provide a unique opportunity for IPV victims to confide in their care providers and to seek help. Despite a lack of confirmed efficacy, national consensus guidelines still recommend routine screening (Family Violence Prevention Fund, 2008b; Klevens & Saltzman, 2009; Williams et al., 2008).

❝ What to say ❞ — *Conducting the IPV interview*

After ensuring privacy, the nurse should maintain eye contact and begin with a statement such as "In this office, a part of our routine care is to ask about intimate partner violence." Then, proceed with open-ended questions such as, "How are things at home? Do you feel safe at home? Do you feel safe in your community?" If injuries are present, it is important to acknowledge them and ask how they occurred. If the patient's responses do not seem to match the mechanism of the injury, voice concern about the inconsistency, but don't push for details. Always promote trust and convey caring and let the patient know that violence is wrong and that no one deserves to be hurt. Demonstrating a nonjudgmental attitude and creating trust is an essential strategy in facilitating the patient's disclosure of abuse, especially in a busy clinical setting. Research suggests that IPV screening does not necessarily add significant time to a patient visit (Bull, 2009; Du Plat-Jones, 2006; Rhodes et al., 2007; Ward & Wood, 2009).

Once a patient discloses abuse, the nurse should facilitate an assessment to determine urgent safety needs and to guide the plan of care. If the patient is in immediate danger, an assessment for suicide and/or homicide may be indicated as well (Ward & Wood, 2009).

 Nursing Insight— *Finding the right words to facilitate understanding and disclosure of abuse*

Patients may not always use the word *abuse* when describing their intimate relationships. It is important to be aware of words that suggest that abuse is occurring. For example, the patient may confide that her partner "has a temper" or "gets angry easily." Using the same terms expressed by the patient may enhance her comfort in confiding about the full extent of the abuse (Krieger, 2008; Valente, 2002).

Across Care Settings: **Community resources share in supporting the victim of IPV**

When IPV is identified, nurses and other health-care professionals share the responsibility of offering referrals to confidential victim and social support resources within the community. Referrals should be made regardless of whether the woman chooses to report the abuse to law enforcement. In the ideal situation, all health-care providers should be a part of a coordinated community response to reduce domestic violence, a response in which shelters, hospitals, health-care providers, legal advocates, and law enforcement work together to improve safety and save lives (Association of Women's Health, Obstetric, and Neonatal Nurses, 2007; Krieger, 2008).

A number of screening tools have been developed to assess for intimate partner violence. These include the Woman Abuse Screening Tool (WAST) (Brown, Lent, Schmidt, & Sas, 2000), Abuse Risk Inventory, Conflict Tactics Scale (Yegadis, 1989), and the Danger Assessment Scale (Campbell, 1989). The Abuse Assessment Screen (Family Violence Prevention Fund, 2004) is a brief, easy-to-use validated tool that contains five simple questions along with a body map to provide visual reference for physical injury (see Figure 1-3). If the woman has disclosed IPV, the nurse must document that a risk assessment was completed (Family Violence Prevention Fund, 2004; Ward & Wood, 2009).

DOCUMENTING IPV

Accurate documentation is essential, as it provides a record of the abuse, facilitates communication among the various professionals who are dealing with the case, and provides a record of previous episodes of abuse. Since documentation provides evidence of abuse escalation, it can be beneficial in helping the patient to recognize and acknowledge the abuse (Ward & Wood, 2009).

 Be sure to— Obtain patient consent before IPV information disclosure

Nurses are aware that careful documentation of IPV-related information is essential in supporting the victim's assertions and charges. Proper documentation enables the woman to obtain protection and assistance, which may range from obtaining a restraining order to receiving victim compensation. However, nurses must remember that disclosure of confidential information may take place only with the explicit consent of the patient (Griffith, 2008; Rhodes et al., 2007; Ward & Woods, 2009).

In addition to obtaining the past health history, social history, and sexual history, the nurse documents subjective data related to the current IPV incident. Information recorded includes a description of the incident in the patient's own words. If the victim names the abuser, the name should be documented as well. All subjective information provided by the patient is recorded in quotation marks to indicate that the statements represent exactly what the patient said. It is important to record the time that the patient reports that the incident occurred, as well as the time that the patient's descriptive statements were made. The nurse also notes the date and location of the incident (Family Violence Prevention Fund, 2004; Ward & Wood, 2009).

The patient's general appearance and demeanor is recorded, and additional subjective information, such as reported threats and psychological abuse perpetrated by the abuser, is documented as well. Findings from the physical examination are carefully documented. Body maps are useful in accurately pinpointing the areas of injury, including the location, size, and age. Once the patient's signed consent has been obtained, photographs may be taken. Photographs provide an excellent visual record of the injuries. Additional information including the results of laboratory and diagnostic tests, radiography, and all referrals (e.g., other health-care professionals, local shelters) are recorded on the patient's health record (Ward & Wood, 2009).

 Optimizing Outcomes— With photographs of the injuries

A minimum of three photographs should be taken of each injury: a full body photograph of the victim to establish identity, an injury photo taken a medium distance from the body, and a close-up photo of each individual injury. All photographs are clearly labeled with the patient's name, date, time that they were taken, and the photographer's name. Ideally, a blue background, which shows the depth and defines the clarity of an injury, is used. Additional photographs can be taken at the follow-up visit (2 to 4 days) to provide additional documentation of the progression of the injuries (Family Violence Prevention Fund, 2004; Hamme, Moynihan, & Pagliaro, 2005; Pyrek, 2006; Ward & Wood, 2009).

REPORTING IPV

It is important for nurses to be knowledgeable about IPV reporting guidelines for their particular practice state. Proponents of mandatory IPV reporting describe the following benefits associated with mandatory IPV reporting:

Facilitates the prosecution of perpetrators
Helps to identify victims; promotes interventions
Improves data collection (Lewis-O'Connor, 2004; Ward & Wood, 2009)

 Be sure to— Be knowledgeable of state law regarding reporting of IPV

Nurses must be familiar with laws on the mandatory reporting of IPV; requirements vary from state to state. Currently, six states (California, Kentucky, New Mexico, Rhode Island, New Hampshire, and Colorado) have laws requiring comprehensive reporting of IPV obtained by either victim disclosure or suspicion of IPV. A synopsis of current state statutes and reporting guidelines is available at http://www.endabuse.org/userfiles/file/Consensus.pdf. The Association of Women's Health, Obstetric and Neonatal Nurses

1) Have you ever been emotionally or physically abused by your partner or someone important to you?

Yes ☐   No ☐

If yes by whom? _____

Total number of times _____

2) Within the last year, have you been hit, slapped, kicked or otherwise physically hurt by someone?

Yes ☐   No ☐

If yes by whom? _____

Total number of times _____

3) Since you've been pregnant, have you been hit, slapped, kicked, or otherwise physically hurt by someone?

Yes ☐   No ☐

If yes by whom? _____

Total number of times _____

4. Within the last year, has anyone forced you to have sexual activities?

Yes ☐   No ☐

If yes by whom? _____

Total number of times _____

5. Are you afraid of your partner or anyone you listed above?

Yes ☐   No ☐

MARK THE AREA OF INJURY ON A BODY MAP AND SCORE EACH INCIDENT ACCORDING TO THE FOLLOWING SCALE:

If any of the descriptions for the higher number apply, use the higher number.

1 = Threats of abuse including use of a weapon

2 = Slapping, pushing; no injuries and/or lasting pain

3 = Punching, kicking, bruises, cuts, and/or continuing pain

4 = Beating up, severe contusions, burns, broken bones

5 = Head injury, internal injury, permanent injury

6 = Use of weapon; wound from weapon

Figure 1-3 Abuse Assessment Screen. (Produced by the Family Violence Prevention Fund, 383 Rhode Island St., Ste. 304, San Francisco, CA, 94103-5133, (415) 252-8900, TTY: (800) 595-4889, www.endabuse.org.)

(AWHONN) supports health-care professionals reporting IPV with the informed consent of the abused woman. However, the organization recognizes that health-care providers must abide by state law (AWHONN, 2007).

However, it must be pointed out that mandatory reporting violates the framework on which the ethical codes of nursing are based. The ANA Code of Ethics for Nurses, provision 3, states, "the nurse promotes, advocates for, and strives to protect the health, safety, and rights of the patient" (ANA, 2005). Mandatory reporting of IPV may place victims in danger and violates the victim's right to make personal choices. Furthermore, mandatory reporting laws place the responsibility of the victim's safety on health-care professionals, who, in turn, must rely on law enforcement and the courts to provide safety for the victim. This process may not necessarily be a desirable alternative, considering that in many situations, the abuser is incarcerated for only a brief period of time (Smith, Rainey, Smith, Alamares, & Grogg, 2008; Ward & Wood, 2009).

 Now Can You— Discuss IPV screening, documenting, and reporting?

1. Explain the nurse's role in conducting screening for IPV?
2. Describe how to document IPV and identify when the patient's informed consent must be obtained?
3. Identify the IPV reporting requirements of your practice state?

Nursing Interventions

EDUCATION AND COUNSELING

Education and counseling constitutes an essential nursing role in IPV care. The nurse should inquire about violence and family conflict, listen to the woman's story, and provide information and referrals. Nurses should reassure their patients that they will provide help regardless of whether they choose to remain in the relationship. Nurses must assist victims of violence by informing them of available options and by providing support in making decisions. Allowing the woman to break the cycle of abuse restores her power and enables her to regain control of her life (Burge, Schneider, Ivy, & Catala, 2005; Coker et al., 2007; Ward & Wood, 2009). Nursing diagnoses may be related to physical injuries, emotional trauma, and the need for seeking help (see Box 1-1). In addition, abused women may be formally diagnosed as having posttraumatic stress disorder (PTSD) if their symptoms meet the explicit criteria outlined in the *Diagnostic and Statistical Manual of Mental Disorders* (American Psychiatric Association, 2000).

Nurses can educate their patients about strategies to protect themselves from harm in their home environment. When physical abuse appears to be imminent, women should be taught to remove themselves from the kitchen where there are weapons such as knives that may be used to inflict harm. Victims should also be taught to stay out of bathrooms, closets, or small spaces where the abuser can trap the victim. If possible, the woman should leave the home or go to a room with a door or window to escape or lock the abuser outside. Women should be encouraged to call 911 in an emergency and go to their health-care

---

Box 1-1 Examples of Nursing Diagnoses for Victims of IPV

- Powerlessness related to perception that it is impossible to leave the abusing partner
- Fear related to the ongoing threat of violence
- Social Isolation related to the need to conceal evidence of the abuse
- Ineffective Denial related to an inability to acknowledge that the partner is abusive
- Compromised Family Coping related to the dysfunctional relationship between self and the abusive partner
- Chronic, Situational Low Self-esteem related to the continuing physical and mental abuse
- Helplessness related to the ongoing exposure to physical, mental, sexual, social, and economic abuse
- Injury related to physical and emotional abuse
- Knowledge Deficit related to the cycle of violence
- Knowledge Deficit related to available resources

---

provider or nearest emergency room for care when their injuries require medical attention. Victims may go to a local women's shelter or crisis center for housing and counseling. It has been estimated that 50% of all homeless women and children in the United States are fleeing IPV. They may also call the National Domestic Violence Hotline (1-800-799-SAFE [7233]) for additional information and assistance. Women should also be encouraged to learn self-defense skills through enrollment in a course, if possible, and to seek education from an IPV program (American Bar Association, 2008; Family Violence Prevention Fund, 2008b; Krieger, 2008; National Domestic Violence Hotline, 2008).

The woman may also be encouraged to prepare a packed bag with essential items that will be needed if she needs to make a hasty escape from her abuser. Hiding the bag in a handy, safe place or leaving it with a neighbor helps to ensure that the "ready escape bag" will be available if needed. Necessary items include certain documents that will be needed to establish stability, such as housing and financial assistance (Krieger, 2008).

 Optimizing Outcomes— With a ready escape bag containing important items

Nurses can teach IPV victims how to assemble a ready escape bag to facilitate a hasty departure from an unsafe home situation. The bag should contain money, an extra set of car keys, birth certificates, lists of medications and doses, medical records (for self and children), passports, court papers, Social Security card, car title, insurance card, and immigration papers (Krieger, 2008; Ward & Wood, 2009).

It is important to ensure that the woman keeps all information about her safety plan stored in a safe place away from her abuser. Danger to the victim is heightened if the abuser believes that the victim may leave or report the abuse to the police (Family Violence Prevention Fund, 2004; Ward & Wood, 2009).

If the abuser has moved out of the home, the woman should be advised to change the locks on the doors and secure locks for the windows. She may ask neighbors to call the police if they observe the abuser at the victim's house, and the victim and neighbor(s) may develop a system of signals to alert the neighbor when to call the police. The nurse should counsel the woman to obtain an unlisted phone number, block caller ID, and use an answering machine to screen phone calls. Rather than use a personal home computer, it may be wise to use a friend's or library computer, as the abuser may be able to monitor the woman's computer activities or have access to the e-mail addresses of the victim's family members and friends. The woman should also be encouraged to change her online passwords and create a new e-mail account to avoid the abuser's harassment (Krieger, 2008). Additional safety strategies are listed in Box 1-2.

 Optimizing Outcomes— Using the ABCDEs to provide sensitive care for the IPV victim

Nurses should remember the "ABCDEs of Caring" (Campbell & Furniss, 2002) to provide appropriate, sensitive care for victims of IPV:

  A – Reassuring the woman that she is not **alone**
  B – Expressing the **belief** that violence directed against the woman is unacceptable and not her fault
  C – **Confidentiality** of the shared information will be maintained (explain the mandatory reporting laws of the practice state, when applicable)
  D – **Documentation** – descriptive documentation includes quoted statements, accurate descriptions of all injuries, and photographs (with the woman's written consent)
  E – **Education** about the cycle of violence and community and national resources
  S – **Safety**—always the most important component of the intervention, especially since one of the most dangerous times for the victim is when she decides to leave her abuser

TREATMENT AND FOLLOW-UP

In the clinic, office, or hospital setting, nurses should carefully document all injuries in great detail and use body maps to enhance clarification. Terms such as *strangulation* should be used in place of *choked*, which implies that a foreign object has been lodged in the patient's trachea or esophagus. By

definition, strangulation is an assault with malicious intent that causes harm to the victim. Treatment interventions and discharge information must be clearly noted on the chart, along with a description of all referrals and follow-up options that were provided to the patient. Nurses can offer immediate contact with an IPV counselor either in person or by phone, and referral to a mental health provider may also be appropriate (Krieger, 2008; Ward & Wood, 2009).

Nurses must ensure that an adequate referral system is in place for victims of IPV. A number of resources are available to assist nurses in providing appropriate, sensitive care in a timely manner and to take action against IPV perpetrators (Box 1-3). Establishing a professional relationship with the local domestic violence center empowers the nurse with a variety of resources to better help the victim of abuse (Ward & Wood, 2009).

IPV centers offer services that frequently include a 24-hour hotline, advocacy with community systems, and temporary shelter for victims who cannot return home because of safety concerns for themselves and their children. Advocacy with community systems includes referral for services such as legal aid, housing, mental health, substance abuse, and dental referral resources. In most situations, IPV centers also assist victims in accessing local and state government programs (Ward & Wood, 2009).

Nurses who deal with victims of IPV should also be familiar with the local sexual assault center. Women who have been sexually assaulted can benefit from the specialized services (e.g., individualized counseling, support

---

Box 1-3 Additional IPV Resources

Centers for Disease Control and Prevention
http://www.cdc.gov/ncipc/dvp/IPV/default.htm
DomesticViolence.org
http://www.domesticviolence.org/
Family Violence Prevention Fund
http://www.endabuse.org/
Medline Plus
http://www.nim.nih.gov/medlineplus/domesticviolence.html
National Center for Victims of Crime, Stalking Resource Center
1-800-394-2255
National Coalition Against Domestic Violence
http://www.ncadv.org/
National Domestic Violence Hotline
1-800-799-SAFE (1-800-787-3224 (TTY)
http://www.ndvh.org
National Teen Dating Abuse Helpline
1-866-331-9474
Rape, Abuse, and Incest National Network (RAINN)
1-800-656-HOPE (4673)
U.S. Department of Justice
http://www.ovw.usdoj.gov/domesticviolence.htm
WomensHealth.gov
http://www.4women.gov/violence/types/domestic.cfm
World Health Organization
http://www.who.int/entity/violence_injury-prevention/violence/world-report/factsheets/en/ipvfacts.pdf

---

Box 1-2 Safety Strategies for Victims of IPV

Nurses can teach women to do the following:
• Remain aware of surroundings at all times.
• Shop and bank at different places, especially if being stalked.
• Use different routes for driving to work, or try to receive rides from different persons.
• Obtain a protection order.
• Refrain from lunching alone.
• Cancel all joint credit card and bank accounts.
• Ask for workplace escorts to the car or public transportation.
• Determine whether an immediate danger exists; if so, go to a safe place and call 911 (Krieger, 2008).

groups) provided by these centers. Nurses can also advocate for IPV awareness and assistance by placing information about local resources in various public and private locations throughout the clinic or office (e.g., waiting area, bathroom, examination room) where patients can have ready access to them. Many clinics distribute business-size IPV cards that contain essential information such as strategies for self-protection and protection of children and the National Domestic Violence Hotline phone number. The business-size card is particularly useful as it can be easily concealed (Ward & Wood, 2009).

Nurses must also recognize the victim's need for legal information. For those with access to a computer, the Web site WomensLaw.org (http://www.womenslaw.org) contains an abundance of easy-to-understand information for women living with or escaping IPV. The Web site offers suggestions for obtaining restraining orders, court forms and other legal documents, and provides locations for various law enforcement offices (Ward & Wood, 2009). Women who have no access to a computer may receive assistance by dialing the toll-free phone number for the National Domestic Violence Hotline (1-800-799-SAFE).

Excellent IPV resources are available for nurses and other health-care professionals. The Minnesota Center Against Violence and Abuse (http://www.mincava.umn.edu) offers educational resources for training on violence of any type, including IPV, teen violence, and dating violence.

 Optimizing Outcomes— With an IPV tool designed especially for health-care professionals

The Minnesota Center Against Violence and Abuse Web site offers "A Medical Provider's Guide to Managing the Care of Domestic Violence Patients Within a Cultural Context," a training and reference guide for health-care professionals. This tool is designed to help reduce cultural, linguistic, and systemic barriers that keep IPV victims, particularly immigrant women and women of color, from reporting abuse to their care providers (Ward & Wood, 2009).

Once a patient leaves the health-care setting, a lack of personal contact does not mean that interventions cannot occur. McFarland and colleagues (2004) used telephone interviews to conduct a longitudinal study on abused women. After an initial personal contact with abused women to ask about inclusion in the study and to obtain informed consent, researchers contacted the women with either six intervention and four follow-up calls (experimental group) or four follow-up calls only (control group). During the phone calls, the interviewers asked women in the experimental group to answer yes or no to a series of safety-promoting behaviors. These behaviors included such actions as hiding money, hiding house and car keys, removing weapons from the house, asking neighbors to call police if violence begins, establishing a code with family and friends, and obtaining items such as birth certificates, important phone numbers, identification cards, and rent and utility receipts. The research findings indicated that women in the intervention group (those who received six additional phone calls) practiced more safety-promoting behaviors than did those in the control group and that the required nursing time was minimal. Such research findings are significant in supporting the important role that nurses and other members of the health-care team can have in helping victims of domestic violence take control of their environments and practice positive behaviors that can break the cycle of abuse.

 Now Can You— **Discuss the nurse's role when caring for victims of IPV?**

1. Formulate five nursing diagnoses that may be appropriate for victims of IPV?
2. Describe three ways that IPV victims can enhance personal safety at home and items that they should include in a "ready escape bag"?

summary points

♦ *Intimate partner violence* (IPV) is defined as physical, sexual, or psychological harm or social isolation perpetrated by a current or former partner in an intimate or dating relationship.

♦ The abuser's actions are intended to instill fear and to intimidate and control the victim.

♦ Intimate partner violence reaches across all strata of society and affects persons regardless of economic status, ethnic background, educational level, or religious status.

♦ Women who are abused are more likely to be unemployed, suffer from health problems, and receive public assistance than are women who are not victims of abuse.

♦ Routine screening can facilitate early identification of IPV when signs and symptoms may not be readily apparent.

♦ Accurate documentation of abuse is essential, and nurses must be knowledgeable about IPV reporting guidelines for their particular practice state.

♦ Nurses must assist victims of violence by informing them of available options and by providing support in making decisions.

review questions

Multiple Choice

1. Nurses should be alert to signs of IPV, which may include
   A. Overuse of health services
   B. Injuries consistent with the patient's explanation as to cause
   C. Consistency in keeping health-care appointments
   D. Reporting specific, descriptive complaints

2. Potential barriers to routine IPV screening in the clinical setting may include
   A. Having an awareness of IPV
   B. Sharing the patient's language and cultural values
   C. Understanding how to inquire about abuse
   D. Having a personal history of abuse

3. When physical abuse is imminent, a home safety strategy that the nurse can teach the patient is to
   A. Hide in the bathroom
   B. Seek shelter in a closet
   C. Remove herself from the kitchen
   D. Confront the abuser in an assertive way

4. The nurse can encourage the woman to develop a plan to facilitate safety from the abuser. A safety strategy is to
   A. Pack a ready escape bag containing essential items
   B. Leave a "good-bye" note for the abuser
   C. Maintain usual habits for banking and shopping
   D. Keep computer e-mail accounts and online passwords as originally set up

5. IPV is an abusive relationship characterized by the abuser's desire to have
   A. The victim's sympathy
   B. Power and control in the relationship
   C. A sense of intimacy
   D. Financial security

REFERENCES

American Bar Association. (2008). *Survey of recent statistics.* Commission on Domestic Violence. Retrieved January 31, 2010, from http://www.abanet.org/domviol/statistics.html

American College of Obstetricians and Gynecologists (ACOG). (2008). *Guidelines for women's health care. A resource manual* (3rd ed.). Washington, DC: Author.

American Nurses Association. (2000). *Violence against women* (Position statement). Retrieved January 30, 2010, from http://www.nursingworld.org/MainMenuCategories/HealthcareandPolicyIssues/ANAPositionStatements/social.aspx

American Nurses Association (ANA). (2005). *Code of ethics for nurses with interpretive statements.* Retrieved February 2, 2010, from http://nursingworld.org/MainMenuCategories/ThePracticeofProfessionalNursing/EthicsStandards/CodeofEthics.aspx

American Psychiatric Association. (2000). *Diagnostic and statistic manual of mental disorders* (4th ed., text revision). Washington, DC: American Psychiatric Association Press.

Arosarena, O. A., Fritsch, T. A., Hsueh, Y., Aynehchi, B., & Haug, R. (2009). Maxillofacial injuries and violence against women. *Archives of Facial Plastic Surgery, 11*(1), 48–52.

Association of Women's Health, Obstetric and Neonatal Nurses. (2007). *Mandatory reporting of intimate partner violence* (Position paper). Washington, DC: Author. Retrieved January 30, 2010, from https://www.awhonn.org/awhonn/content.do?name=05_HealthPolicyLegislation/5H_PositionStatements.htm

Blereau, R. P. (2009). Woman with multiple head and neck injuries. *Consultant, 49*(9), 565–568.

Brown, J., Lent, B., Schmidt, G., & Sas, G. (2000). Application of the Women Abuse Screening Tool (WAST) and WAST-Short in the family practice setting. *Journal of Family Practice, 49*(10), 896–903.

Bull, A. (2009). Screening for intimate partner violence: Offering the tissue box. *Journal for Nurse Practitioners, 5*(8), 620–621.

Burge, S. K., Schneider, F. D., Ivy, L., & Catala, S. (2005). Patients' advice to physicians about intervening in family conflict. *Annals of Family Medicine, 3*(3), 248–254.

Campbell, J. (1986). Nursing assessment for risk of homicide with battered women. *Advances in Nursing Science, 8*(4), 36–51.

Campbell, J. (1989). Women's responses to sexual abuse in intimate relationships. *Health Care for Women International, 10*(1), 335–340.

Campbell, J., & Furniss, K. (2002). *Violence against women: Identification, screening, and management of intimate partner violence.* Washington, DC: Association of Women's Health, Obstetric, and Neonatal Nurses.

Centers for Disease Control and Prevention (CDC), National Center for Injury Prevention and Control. (2003). *Costs of intimate partner violence against women in the United States.* Retrieved January 29, 2010, from http://www.cdc.gov/violenceprevention/pub/IPV_cost.html

Centers for Disease Control and Prevention (CDC). (2009). *Intimate partner violence: Fact sheet.* Retrieved January 29, 2010, from http://www.cdc.gov/violenceprevention/pdf/IPV_factsheet-a.pdf

Chang, J. C., Decker, M., Moracco, K. E., Martin, S. L., Petersen, R., & Frasier, P. Y. (2003). What happens when health care providers ask about intimate partner violence? A description of consequences from the perspectives of female survivors. *Journal of the American Medical Women's Association, 58*(2), 76–81.

Coker, A., Davis, K., Arias, Il, Desai, S., Sanderson, M., Brandt, H., & Smith, P. H. (2002). Physical and mental health effects of intimate partner violence for men and women. *American Journal of Preventive Medicine, 23*(4), 260–268.

Coker, A. L., Flerx, V. C., Smith, P. H., Whitaker, D. J., Fadden, M. K., & Williams, M. (2007). Partner violence screening in rural health care clinics. *American Journal of Public Health, 97*(7), 1319–1325.

Crandall, M., Nathens, A., Kernic, M., Holt, V., & Rivara, F. (2004). Predicting future injury among women in abusive relationships. *Journal of Trauma—Injury Infection and Critical Care, 56*(8), 906–912.

Davila, Y. (2006). Increasing nurses' knowledge and skills for enhanced response to intimate partner violence. *Journal of Continuing Education in Nursing, 37*(4), 171–177.

Du Plat-Jones, J. (2006). Domestic violence: The role of health professionals. *Nursing Standard, 21*(10), 44–48.

Family Violence Prevention Fund. (2004). *National consensus guidelines on identifying and responding to domestic violence victimization in health care settings.* Updated February 2004. Retrieved February 2, 2010, from http://www.endabuse.org/userfiles/file/Consensus.pdf

Family Violence Prevention Fund. (2007). *Justice Department releases '05 intimate partner violence data.* Retrieved January 29, 2010, from http://www.endabuse.org/content/features/detail/919/

Family Violence Prevention Fund. (2008a). *Intimate partner violence and Healthy People 2010 fact sheet.* Retrieved January 29, 2010, from http://www.endabuse.org/userfiles/file/Children_and_Families/ipv.pdf

Family Violence Prevention Fund. (2008b). *Survey finds health problems more common for victims of violence.* Retrieved January 29, 2010, from http://www.endabuse.org/content/news/detail/1070

Griffith, R. (2008). Patient confidentiality: Rights and duties of nurse prescribers. *Nurse Prescribing, 6*(3), 116–120.

Hamme, R., Moynihan, B., & Pagliaro, E. (2005). *Forensic nursing.* Sudbury, MA: Jones and Bartlett.

Hamolia, C. (2005). Preventing and managing aggressive behavior. In G. Stuart & M. Laraia (Eds.), *Principles and practice of psychiatric nursing* (8th ed.). St. Louis, MO: Mosby.

Heise, L., & Garcia-Moreno, C. (2002). Violence by intimate partners. In E. Krug, L. Dahlberg, & J. Mercy (Eds.), *World report on violence and health* (pp. 87–121). Geneva, Switzerland: World Health Organization.

Johnson, M., & Leone, J. (2005). The differential effects of intimate terrorism and situational couple violence. *Journal of Family Issues, 26*(8), 322–349.

Kearney, M. (2001). Enduring love: A formal theory of women's experience of domestic violence. *Research in Nursing and Health, 24*(3), 270–282.

Klevens, J., & Saltzman, L. E. (2009). The controversy on screening for intimate partner violence: A question of semantics? *Journal of Women's Health, 18*(2), 143–145.

Krieger, C. L. (2008). Intimate partner violence: A review for nurses. *Nursing for Women's Health, 12*(3), 226–234.

Lewis-O'Connor, A. (2004). Policy perspectives. "Dying to tell?" Do mandatory reporting laws benefit victims of domestic violence? *American Journal of Nursing, 104*(10), 75–76.

Lite, J. (2009). Domestic violence victims have distinct facial injuries, study says. *Scientific American 60-second science blog.* Retrieved January 29, 2010, from http://www.scientificamerican.com/blog/post.cfm?id=domestic-violence-victims-have-dist-2009-01-19

Mahoney, B. (2006). Reducing barriers against routine screening for intimate partner violence. *American Journal for Nurse Practitioners, 10*(10), 45–58.

McFarlane, J., Christoffel, K., Bateman, L., Miller, V., & Bullock, L. (1991). Assessing for abuse: Self-report versus nurse interview. *Public Health Nursing, 8*(4), 245–250.

McFarland, J., Malecha, A., Gist, J., Watson, K., Batten, E., Hall, I., & Smith, S. (2004). Original research: Increasing the safety promoting behaviors of abused women. *American Journal of Nursing, 104*(3), 40–51.

Moran, B. A. (2008). Intimate partner violence: The difference nurses can make. *Nursing for Women's Health, 12*(3), 194–196.

Moracco, K., Brown, C., Martin, S., Chang, J., Dulli, L., Loucks-Sorrell, M., Turner, T., Bou-Saada, I., & Starsoneck, L. (2005). Mental health issues among female clients of domestic violence programs in North Carolina. *Psychiatric Services, 55*(9), 1036–1040.

National Domestic Violence Hotline. (2008). *National domestic violence hotline.* Retrieved January 29, 2010, from: http://www.ndvh.org

Parker, B., & McFarlane, J. (1991). Nursing assessment of the battered pregnant woman. *American Journal of Maternal Child Nursing, 16*(6), 161–164.

Parkinson, G., Adams, R., & Emerling, F. (2001). Maternal domestic violence screening in an office-based pediatric practice. *Pediatrics, 108*(6), E43.

Peedicayil, A., Sadowski, L. S., Jeyaseelan, L., Shankar, V., Jain, D., Suresh, S., & Bangdiwala, S. I. (2004). Spousal physical violence against women during pregnancy. *British Journal of Obstetrics and Gynaecology, 111*(7), 682–687.

Plichta, S. (2004). Intimate partner violence and physical health consequences: Policy and practice implication. *Journal of Interpersonal Violence, 19*(6), 1296–1323.

Pyrek, K. (2006). *Forensic nursing.* New York: CRC Press.

Rennison, C. (2003). *Intimate partner violence, 1993–2001.* Washington, DC: U.S. Department of Justice, Bureau of Justice Statistics (Publication No. NCJ197838).

Rhodes, K. V., Frankel, R. M., Levinthal, N., Prenoveau, N., Bailey, J., & Levinson, W. (2007). "You're not a victim of domestic violence, are you?" Provider–patient communication about domestic violence. *Annals of Internal Medicine, 147*(9), 620–627.

Silverman, J. G., Decker, M. R., Reed, E., & Raj, A. (2006). Intimate partner violence victimization prior to and during pregnancy among women residing in 26 U.S. states: Associations with maternal and neonatal health. *American Journal of Obstetrics and Gynecology, 195*(1), 140–148.

Smith, J., Rainey, S., Smith, K., Alamares, C., & Grogg, D. (2008). Barriers to the mandatory reporting of domestic violence encountered by nursing professionals. *Journal of Trauma Nursing, 15*(1), 9–11.

Stinson, C., & Robinson, R. (2006). Intimate partner violence: Continuing education for registered nurses. *Journal of Continuing Education in Nursing, 37*(2), 58–64.

Strack, G. B., & McClane, G. (1999). *How to improve your investigation and prosecution of strangulation cases.* Austin, TX: National Center of Domestic and Sexual Violence. Retrieved January 30, 2010, from http://www.ncdsv.org/images/strangulation_article.pdf

Tjaden, P., & Thoennes, N. (2000a). *Full report of the prevalence, incidence, and consequences of violence against women: Findings from the National Violence Against Women Survey, 2000.* Retrieved January 29, 2010, from http://www.ncjrs.gov/pdffiles1/nij/183781.pdf

Tjaden, P., & Thoennes, N. (2000b). *Extent, nature and consequences of intimate partner violence: Findings from the National Violence Against Women Survey.* Washington, DC: National Institute of Justice and the Centers for Disease Control and Prevention.

U.S. Department of Health and Human Services. (2000). *Healthy People 2010.* Washington, DC: Author.

U.S. Department of Health and Human Services. National Women's Health Information Center. (2009). *Violence against women. Domestic and intimate partner violence.* Retrieved January 29, 2010, from http://www.womenshealth.gov/violence/types/domestic.cfm

U.S. Department of Justice, Bureau of Justice Statistics. (2007). *Criminal victimization.* Retrieved January 29, 2010, from http://bjs.ojp.usdoj.gov/index.cfm?ty=pbdetail&iid=1000

U.S. Preventive Services Task Force. (2004). Screening for family and intimate partner violence. *Annals of Internal Medicine, 140*(8), 382–386.

Valente, S. (2002). Evaluating intimate partner violence. *Journal of the American Academy of Nurse Practitioners, 14*(6), 505–516.

Varcolis, E., Carson, V., & Shoemaker, N. (2006). *Foundations of psychiatric mental health nursing: A clinical approach.* St. Louis, MO: Saunders Elsevier.

Walker, L. (1979). *The battered woman.* New York: Harper & Row.

Walker, L. (1984). *The battered woman syndrome* (Vol. 6). New York: Springer.

Ward, C., & Wood, A. (2009). Intimate partner violence: NP role in assessment. *American Journal for Nurse Practitioners, 13*(10), 9–15.

Williams, G. B., Brackley, M. H., Hibler, T. R., & Prater, S. J. (2008). Screening for intimate partner violence. *Women's Health Care: A Practical Journal for Nurse Practitioners, 7*(8), 10–26.

Wilson, J., Lane, E., & Gillespie, T. (2006). Identifying and responding to intimate partner violence in the health care setting. *Oklahoma Nurse, 51*(2), 28–33.

World Health Organization. (2005). *WHO multi-country study on women's health and domestic violence against women. Summary report of initial results on prevalence, health outcomes, and women's responses.* Geneva, Switzerland: Author.

Yonaka, L., Yoder, M., Darrow, J., & Sherck, J. (2007). Barriers to screening for domestic violence in the emergency department. *Journal of Continuing Education in Nursing, 38*(1), 37–45.

Yegadis, K. (1989). *Women's mental health in primary care.* Philadelphia: W. B. Saunders.

Yost, N., Bloom, S., McIntier, G., & Leveno, K. (2005). A prospective observational study of domestic violence during pregnancy. *Obstetrics and Gynecology, 106*(1), 61–65.

 For more information, go to http://davisplus.fadavis.com/

Promoting Reproductive Health Through an Understanding of Premenstrual Syndrome

Shelton M. Hisley, PhD, RNC, WHNP-BC

Live your life while you have it.
Life is a splendid gift—there is nothing small about it.

—Florence Nightingale

LEARNING TARGETS *At the completion of this chapter, the student will be able to:*

- Identify diagnostic criteria for premenstrual syndrome.
- Discuss the unique characteristics of symptoms that accompany premenstrual syndrome.
- Describe nonpharmacological and pharmacological approaches to care for women who experience premenstrual syndrome.
- Discuss the nurse's role when caring for a patient with a premenstrual disorder.

Introduction

This chapter explores premenstrual syndrome (PMS), a common women's health problem during the childbearing years. In the past, many in the medical profession viewed symptoms of PMS to be wholly attributable to the woman's emotional state and without any physiological basis. PMS-related research was infrequently conducted and consisted mostly of anecdotal experiences. As the women's movement grew in strength and the public's awareness about women's health issues increased, views began to shift. At the same time, a growing body of medical information began to identify various physiological imbalances and theories were proposed to explain the causes of PMS. Today, PMS is viewed as a complex interplay of genetic influences and various hormonal imbalances that can adversely affect a woman's physical, mental, and emotional health (Dickerson, 2007). Various nonpharmacological and pharmacological therapies have been shown to be effective in reducing PMS symptoms. Nurses have traditionally played an important role in promoting women's reproductive health. They can be instrumental in helping women to deal with premenstrual disorders by offering ongoing education and support. These interventions empower women to seek and embrace strategies to help

them gain control over their lives and, ideally, to enjoy life more fully.

Scope of the Problem

Premenstrual disorders affect many women during the reproductive years. *Premenstrual syndrome* (PMS) is defined as the presence of emotional and physical symptoms and behavioral changes that occur during the second half, or luteal phase, of the menstrual cycle and cease at or within a few days after the onset of menses. The timing of the symptoms in relation to the menstrual cycle, rather than the symptoms themselves, constitutes the unique element in this disorder.

A & P Review **Phases of the Uterine (Endometrial) Cycle**

Following menstruation (the "menstrual phase"), follicle-stimulating hormone (FSH) stimulates the growth and development of the ovarian graafian follicle, which secretes estrogen. The first phase of the menstrual cycle is termed the "follicular" or "proliferative" phase; this phase lasts from the end of menses through ovulation (approximately days 7–14). When estrogen production reaches a peak, the pituitary gland releases luteinizing hormone (LH), which triggers ovulation. The "luteal phase" of the ovarian cycle begins at ovulation and ends with the onset of menses. The corpus luteum produces some estrogen but mainly produces progesterone. Eighty percent of all the progesterone secreted during the entire menstrual cycle is secreted during the first 8 days after ovulation. In the absence of fertilization, the life span of the corpus luteum is 14 days. Thus, the luteal phase of the uterine cycle is 14 days in length. As the end of the luteal phase nears, low levels of FSH and LH cause degeneration of the corpus luteum, which is associated with declining levels of estrogen and progesterone. The decreased hormonal levels trigger degeneration of the endometrium and the onset of menses (the "menstrual phase"). ◆

Criteria for Diagnosis

The diagnosis of PMS depends on the determination of the following three criteria:

- The woman's symptoms occur in a cyclic pattern.
- The symptoms are not caused by any underlying physical or mental condition.
- The symptoms greatly disrupt one or more areas of the woman's life.

Since 1987, PMS has been recognized as a mental disorder. More than 150 symptoms, which can affect almost every organ system in various combinations and intensity, have been identified (American College of Obstetricians & Gynecologists [ACOG], 2000, 2007; American Psychiatric Association [APA], 2000; Association of Women's Health, Obstetrical and Neonatal Nurses [AWHONN], 2003; Dickerson, 2007; Polaneczky, 2007).

 Nursing Insight— PMS and PMT

Premenstrual syndrome is sometimes referred to as "premenstrual tension syndrome" (PMT). When first described in 1931, premenstrual tension centered on women's symptoms of tension, self-deprecation, and severe depression during the 7 to 10 days preceding menstruation. By the 1950s, the spectrum of reported symptoms had dramatically increased, and there was a growing realization that the previously described "tension" was just one aspect of the problem. A medical report published in 1953 introduced the term "premenstrual syndrome" to encompass the extensive list of symptoms, and this is the name most often used today.

Prevalence and Economic Impact

Sources vary in estimates of the number of women who experience symptoms of PMS. It has been estimated that over 80% of childbearing-age women experience various emotional and physical changes during the premenstrual period. However, according to experts, most patients who self-diagnose do not actually have PMS (ACOG, 2000, 2007). Of the women with premenstrual symptoms, approximately 20% to 40% regard the emotional and physical changes as difficult, although only 5% to 10%

report a significant degree of impact on their work or lifestyle (ACOG, 2007; Arrowsmith, 2007).

Nevertheless, the disability associated with premenstrual disorders is quite substantial. Women who suffer from PMS reportedly have higher absenteeism from work and make more visits to ambulatory health-care facilities than those who do not experience PMS. On average, women with premenstrual disorders have an increase of $59 in direct annual health-care costs and $4,333 in indirect costs (Borenstein et al., 2003; Whyte & Peraud, 2009).

Symptoms of PMS

Over 100 physical and behavioral symptoms have been experienced by women during the premenstrual period (see Box 2-1). It is important to remember that to meet the criteria for a premenstrual disorder, the symptoms must be confined to the luteal phase of the menstrual cycle and they must resolve after the onset of menstruation.

Clinical criteria from the U.S. National Institute of Mental Health for the diagnosis of PMS include a significant change in the intensity of symptoms between the follicular and late luteal phases. These changes must occur for at least two consecutive cycles (Dickerson, 2007; Whyte & Peraud, 2009). Other definitions, such as symptom intensity, have been developed for research purposes. According to ACOG, at least one of the affective and/or somatic symptoms associated with PMS must be present—and appropriately timed with the menstrual cycle—to meet the diagnostic criteria. Speroff and Fritz (2005) proposed a simple, commonsense definition of PMS: "The cyclic appearance of one or more of a large constellation of symptoms just prior to menses, occurring to such as degree that lifestyle or work is affected,

Box 2-1 Selected Premenstrual Symptoms Reported by Women	
• Irritability	• Joint pain
• Anxiety	• Sore throat
• Mood swings	• Cramps
• Depression	• Nausea
• Hostility	• Insomnia
• Headaches	• Water retention
• Dizziness	• Fatigue
• Fainting	• Increased appetite
• Shakiness	• Cold sweats
• Bloating	• Hot flashes
• Weight gain	• Lack of coordination
• Sugar cravings	• Easy bruising
• Constipation	• Palpitations
• Diarrhea	• Hives
• Backache	• Joint swelling
• Asthma	• Hay fever
• Migraine	• Breast tenderness
• Breast swelling	

followed by a period of time entirely free of symptoms" (p. 247).

It has been noted that PMS symptoms commonly occur in clusters, with some women reporting as many as 10 symptoms at one time. Those who experience severe symptoms may be prone to extremes of behavior, with an increased likelihood of accidents, alcohol abuse, and suicide attempts. For others, PMS symptoms may be described as annoying but mild (Dickerson, 2007).

 Now Can You— **Discuss certain broad aspects of PMS?**

1. Explain why the timing of symptoms is an essential component of premenstrual syndrome?
2. Identify three criteria necessary for a diagnosis of PMS?
3. Identify at least 20 symptoms that may be associated with PMS?

Premenstrual Dysphoric Disorder (PMDD)

Premenstrual dysphoric disorder (PMDD) is a diagnostic term for the most severe form of PMS as defined by the APA's *Diagnostic and Statistical Manual of Mental Disorders* (4th edition, text revision) (*DSM-IV-TR*). It is estimated that nearly 5 million American women have PMDD (Whyte & Peraud, 2009). PMDD pertains to women with PMS who suffer from more severe and disabling emotional symptoms. PMS and PMDD may be viewed as a spectrum of premenstrual disorders that begins with mild emotional and/or physical symptoms that are cyclic but not debilitating and proceeds through PMS to PMDD (Dickerson, 2007; Whyte & Peraud, 2009). Women with PMDD most frequently report the following symptoms: abdominal bloating, anxiety, tension, breast tenderness, crying episodes, depression, fatigue and a lack of energy, irritability, difficulty concentrating, appetite changes, thirst, and swelling of the extremities (Speroff & Fritz, 2005).

 Optimizing Outcomes— **When evaluating a patient for PMS/PMDD symptoms**

When evaluating a patient with PMS/PMDD symptoms, the nurse must always take any report of suicidal thoughts or other indicators of extreme mood change most seriously. The woman will need appropriate medications, close follow-up, and referral to a qualified mental health professional. In the ideal situation, mental examinations are timed to occur during both the luteal and follicular phases of the menstrual cycle. If the patient experiences significant mood symptoms (e.g., suicidal ideation) during both the luteal and follicular phases, referral to a psychiatrist is indicated. Once she is stable, various interventions such as lifestyle changes, dietary alterations, and conventional and complementary care approaches can be initiated that will become an important part of her long-term health promotion and maintenance (Dickerson, 2007; Whyte & Peraud, 2009).

Women who seek care for symptoms associated with premenstrual disorders should be given a complete physical examination and thorough clinical evaluation to rule out illness that may be the source of the symptoms. A detailed health history is the cornerstone in the accurate diagnosis of PMS/PMDD. It is crucial that careful attention be paid to the cyclic timing of symptoms. For most women with PMS, symptoms develop from 2 to 12 days prior to menstruation and resolve within 24 hours following the onset of menses. Women who have symptoms that primarily occur during the menstrual flow or during the first 2 weeks of the menstrual cycle do not have PMS as defined in the literature (Dickerson, 2007; Speroff & Fritz, 2005; Whyte & Peraud, 2009).

 Nursing Insight— *Identifying populations most likely to experience PMS*

Although all age groups are affected, women in their 20s and 30s most frequently report symptoms of premenstrual disorders. It is important to note that premenstrual disorders:

* Occur only in ovulatory women
* Occur only during the luteal phase of the menstrual cycle
* Resolve within 4 days following the onset of menses

The occurrence of premenstrual disorders is not dependent on the presence of monthly menses. Interestingly, women who have had a hysterectomy without bilateral salpingo-oophorectomy (removal of both ovaries) can still have cyclic PMS symptoms (Andolsek & Rapkin, 2006).

Causes of Premenstrual Disorders

Clinical research has not yet determined the exact cause of premenstrual disorders. Variations in the cyclical fluctuation of estrogen and progesterone may well account for symptoms in certain individuals. However, the cause is believed to be multifactorial—that is, a genetic predisposition and multiple biological, psychosocial, and sociocultural factors most likely play a role in the development of premenstrual disorders (Nelson & Baldwin, 2007; Taylor, Schuiling, & Sharp, 2006; Whyte & Peraud, 2009).

Although it was once believed that low levels of progesterone were the primary cause of PMS, research has failed to find a significant difference between PMS sufferers and non-PMS sufferers in levels of various hormones, including progesterone, estradiol, FSH, LH, prolactin, sex hormone binding-globulin (SHBG), and testosterone. It has been proposed, however, that women with PMS may have a greater biological vulnerability to the normal fluctuations in hormone levels than do women without PMS (Nelson & Baldwin, 2008). There appears to be a genetic component to the development of PMS. Women who have a genetic predisposition to the development of PMS are believed to have a heightened sensitivity to various cyclic hormonal changes or a varied response to naturally occurring neurotransmitters (e.g., serotonin). Interestingly, a genetic predisposition to PMS is also known to be associated with a predisposition to other psychiatric disorders (Halbreich, 2003; Whyte & Peraud, 2009).

It has been demonstrated that levels of the gonadal steroids (i.e., androgens, estrogens, progestogens) are the same in patients with and without PMS. However, the responses to fluctuating levels of the hormones are different in women with PMS. Another area of research has explored the role of the neurotransmitters serotonin and gamma-aminobutyric acid (GABA) in the etiology of premenstrual disorders. It has been suggested that a dysregulation in serotonin in particular is linked to many of the psychological symptoms in PMS, such as tension, irritability, and dysphoria (an emotional state characterized by anxiety, depression, or unease) (Clayton, Keller, Leslie, & Evans, 2006; Nelson & Baldwin, 2008; Whyte & Peraud, 2009).

 Optimizing Outcomes— Teaching women about the serotonin–stress relationship

Nurses can empower women with information about the normal workings of their bodies and how certain lifestyle changes may promote an enhanced sense of well-being and diminish PMS symptoms. For example, explaining the relationship between cyclic estrogen fluctuation and changes in serotonin levels may be beneficial in promoting an understanding about serotonin, one of the natural brain chemicals that assists one in coping with life's normal stressors.

Other clinical investigations have focused on the renin–angiotensin–aldosterone system. It has long been noted that many premenstrual symptoms, such as bloating, breast swelling, and weight gain, are caused by fluid retention. Estrogen increases the production of the serum globulin angiotensinogen (a precursor for angiotensin), which leads to increased aldosterone and fluid levels. Under normal circumstances, progesterone competes with aldosterone and prevents excessive fluid retention. However, in the late luteal phase of the menstrual cycle, declining progesterone levels give rise to an increase in the effect of estrogen (Nelson & Baldwin, 2008; Whyte & Peraud, 2009).

 Now Can You— Discuss possible causes of premenstrual disorders?

1. Describe premenstrual dysphoric disorder?
2. List three characteristics common to premenstrual disorders?
3. Describe three possible causes of premenstrual disorders?

Diagnosis

In general, the diagnostic workup for PMS/PMDD consists of four components:

1. A detailed history with a focus on the medical, psychosocial, psychosexual, and substance abuse histories (the gynecological history must include the timing of the symptoms and the regularity of the menstrual cycle)
2. A complete physical examination
3. Laboratory tests (as appropriate to rule out other disorders such as hypothyroidism)
4. A record of the woman's symptoms over a 2- or 3-month period

 Nursing Insight— *Hormonal testing unnecessary in PMS diagnosis*

Laboratory testing of the sex steroid hormonal levels is not necessary for the diagnosis of PMS. Depending on the history and clinical findings, appropriate serum testing may include a chemistry profile, a complete blood cell count, or measurement of the thyroid-stimulating hormone level (Whyte & Peraud, 2009).

 Optimizing Outcomes— Recognizing other conditions that may masquerade as premenstrual disorder

When interviewing patients with premenstrual disorder symptomatology, it is essential to obtain a detailed history. Dysmenorrhea, hypothyroidism, depressive disorders, pain disorders, and generalized anxiety disorders are other conditions that may produce similar symptoms. Hypothyroidism, for example, may be associated with fatigue, bloating, irritability, and depression. Breast disease (breast tenderness) or anemia (fatigue) may be responsible for other common symptoms. Various gynecological disorders such as polycystic ovary syndrome or endometriosis may also cause symptoms that can be confused with PMS (Whyte & Peraud, 2009).

THE SYMPTOM DIARY

The patient must be instructed to record her symptom types, timing, and severity each day. Maintaining a prospective symptom diary for at least two to three consecutive menstrual cycles is an essential element in the diagnostic workup for premenstrual disorders. Because many medical disorders are exacerbated during the luteal phase, the symptom diary is instrumental in determining the severity and the timing of the symptoms (Nelson & Baldwin, 2008; Whyte & Peraud, 2009).

Several symptom inventories are available. The use of a standardized form such as the Daily Record of Severity of Problems (DRSP) was designed to diagnose PMDD. This tool has shown high test/retest reliability and is available on the Internet from the Madison Institute of Medicine at http://www.pmdd.factsforhealth.org (Endicott, Nee, & Harrison, 2006). Other symptom diaries designed to track premenstrual symptoms include the Calendar of Premenstrual Experiences (COPE), the Penn Daily Symptom Report (DSR), and the Premenstrual Symptoms Screening Tool (PSST) (Freeman, DeRubeis, & Rickels, 1996; Steiner, Macdougall, & Brown, 2003).

 Optimizing Outcomes— A daily calendar alternative for tracking PMS symptoms

As an alternative method to using a commercially available symptom inventory form, the nurse may teach the patient how to record her symptoms by taking notes on a regular calendar each day. The woman is taught to write down the symptoms experienced each day, note their severity, and record the dates of her menstrual period. If the number of symptoms is excessive or overwhelming, the patient may record only the three to five symptoms that most profoundly bother her. Under ideal circumstances, the patient's weight, basal body temperature, or home ovulation test results are also documented (Nelson & Baldwin, 2008).

The daily symptom records are useful in that they often heighten the patient's awareness of her symptoms, allow her to gain insights into her problem, and empower her to become more involved in her diagnostic workup and treatment plan. A discussion of cyclic hormonal changes and PMS may be of benefit in heightening an understanding of premenstrual disorders and in promoting a greater sense of control over the situation. If the woman is reluctant to track her daily symptoms, her partner or a family member can be taught to assist with the data collection. It is helpful to ask the patient to continue her charting after therapy has been initiated so that she can identify which interventions improve her symptoms (Nelson & Baldwin, 2008; Whyte & Peraud, 2009).

After the patient has been instructed in the use of a daily symptom diary, she should return in 2 or 3 months for an evaluation of her symptom pattern. Symptoms do not need to recur with equal intensity in each cycle. In fact, the patient may experience different symptoms during different cycles. It is important to recognize, however, that the diagnosis of PMS/PMDD hinges on the timing of symptoms: They must peak in the luteal phase and disappear with the onset of menses (Nelson & Baldwin, 2008).

DIAGNOSTIC CRITERIA FOR PMS AND PMDD

According to ACOG (2000), to meet the diagnostic criteria for premenstrual syndrome, at least one of the following symptoms must be present, occur during the luteal phase of the menstrual cycle, and resolve within 4 days of the onset of menses. Also, the symptoms must not represent an exacerbation of another disorder, and the symptoms should be bothersome but not necessarily debilitating.

PMS Affective Symptoms

- Angry outbursts
- Irritability
- Mild psychological discomfort
- Confusion
- Poor concentration
- Depression
- Sleep disturbances
- Social withdrawal

PMS Somatic Symptoms

- Abdominal bloating
- Headache
- Aches and pains
- Swelling of the extremities
- Breast tenderness
- Weight gain
- Change in appetite

Diagnostic criteria for premenstrual dysphoric disorder defined by the APA include four major symptom categories and seven additional symptoms. To meet the criteria, the woman must report that her symptoms interfere with her usual activities; the symptoms must

not represent an exacerbation of another disorder; at least five symptoms must be present for 1 to 2 weeks premenstrually, with relief by the fourth day of menses; and the criteria must be confirmed by prospective daily ratings for at least two cycles (APA, 2000; Dickerson, 2007; Nelson & Baldwin, 2008).

PMDD Major Symptom Categories (at least one must be present)

- Anger or irritability
- Anxiety, edginess, nervousness
- Depressed mood
- Moodiness

Other, Additional PMDD Symptoms (at least five must be present)

- Appetite changes or cravings
- Decreased interest in usual activities
- Difficulty concentrating
- Fatigue
- Feelings of being overwhelmed or out of control
- Insomnia or hypersomnia
- Physical symptoms (listed in the PMS diagnostic criteria)

 Now Can You— **Discuss aspects of the PMS/PMDD diagnostic workup?**

1. Discuss four components of a diagnostic workup for premenstrual disorders?
2. Teach a patient how to keep a symptom diary?
3. Identify the three components of diagnostic criteria for premenstrual disorders as defined by ACOG?

Patient Care and Management of PMS Symptoms

Women with mild to moderate symptoms of PMS often respond well to reassurance, emotional support, and simple health promotion strategies. Education constitutes a central component in the care of women with PMS. Nurses can teach women about self-help modalities intended to reduce symptoms and enhance coping with various discomforts.

Nonpharmacological therapies are often initiated during the initial visit; patients can then implement them as they complete their daily symptom charting and discuss helpful and non-helpful approaches at the follow-up visit. The first step in treatment centers on validating the woman's experience and acknowledging that the symptoms are real and have a physiological base. For many women, the simple act of validation brings relief and opens the door to healing. Nursing diagnoses, such as Cyclic Pelvic Pain and Related Discomforts (Collins Sharp, Taylor, Thomas, Killeen, & Dawood, 2002) are developed to address the patient's specific symptoms:

- Anxiety related to anticipation of cyclical discomfort
- Depression related to cyclical hormonal changes
- Excess Fluid Volume related to cyclical hormonal changes
- Pain related to cyclical breast changes

" **What to say** " — *Teaching patients about strategies to cope with PMS symptoms*

Nurses can suggest strategies to help women cope with specific PMS symptoms. For example, a fitted support or sports bra may ease the discomfort associated with breast tenderness. Abdominal pain and backache are often relieved with the local application of heat; some women benefit from performing stretching exercises, and NSAIDs are useful in reducing the production of pain-producing prostaglandins. Others may be interested in exploring the possibility of using extended cycle hormonal contraceptives to prevent ovulation. The nurse can also encourage the patient to engage in relaxation techniques and, if available, participate in a PMS support group to help reduce premenstrual tension and anxiety. Support groups provide a forum for the sharing of feelings and concerns and offer an opportunity for learning new strategies for self-care.

PHYSICAL ACTIVITY

Various lifestyle changes have been shown to improve PMS symptoms for many women. These include physical activity, aerobic exercise, stress reduction, and relaxation techniques such as yoga and meditation. Nurses should encourage patients with PMS, as well as all women, to regularly engage in physical activity. Vigorous aerobic exercise may lift the mood, reduce stress, and diminish certain physical symptoms in PMS. The 2008 Physical Activity Guidelines for Americans recommend that adults engage in at least 150 minutes per week of moderate-intensity, or 75 minutes a week of vigorous-intensity, aerobic physical activity or an equivalent combination of moderate- and vigorous-intensity aerobic activity (U.S. Department of Health and Human Services, 2008).

DIETARY ALTERATIONS, VITAMINS, AND MINERALS

Dietary alterations may play a role in reducing certain premenstrual disorder symptoms, although various clinical investigations have not conclusively determined that modification of specific substances, including caffeine, sugar, fat, soy, and complex carbohydrates, ameliorates premenstrual symptoms. Drinking an increased amount of water beginning around 7 to 10 days before menstruation may help to decrease fluid retention.

 Complementary Care: *Enhancing comfort with water and other natural diuretics*

Nurses can encourage women with PMS symptoms related to excessive fluid retention to reduce their sodium intake and consume increased amounts of water during the days preceding the expected menses. The water may serve as a natural diuretic and help reduce edema. Foods that may promote a natural diuresis include peaches, parsley, watermelon, asparagus, and cranberry juice.

Vitamins and minerals have also been prescribed to reduce PMS symptoms. Pyridoxine (vitamin B_6), which plays a role in the biosynthesis of neurotransmitters, may be useful in diminishing premenstrual breast pain and depression. Supplementation with vitamin E (alpha-tocopherol) or magnesium may be beneficial in reducing certain PMS symptoms, although stronger evidence exists for the supplementation of calcium and vitamin D. Calcium may be of benefit in reducing PMS symptoms through its interaction with estrogen and parathyroid hormone (Nelson & Baldwin, 2008; Whyte & Peraud, 2009).

 critical nursing action Counseling About Vitamin Supplements

When counseling about vitamin supplements for premenstrual disorders, the nurse must ensure that women understand the dangers of vitamin overdose. Dosages of vitamin B_6 must remain lower than 100 mg/day, as excessive amounts may lead to peripheral neuropathy. Vitamin E supplements should never exceed 400 IU per day; higher amounts are associated with a number of side effects, including diarrhea, flatulence, bloating, weakness, headache, fatigue, abdominal pain, blurred vision, and an increased risk of bleeding.

HERBAL SUPPLEMENTS AND OTHER COMPLEMENTARY AND ALTERNATIVE MEDICINE MODALITIES

Chasteberry (*Vitex agnus-castus*) has been used throughout the ages to treat a variety of conditions. The fruit of the chaste tree, chasteberry is also known as "monk's pepper." Today this herb is used widely in Europe for a variety of gynecological disorders, including PMS, dysfunctional uterine bleeding, and menstrual cycle irregularities. The German Commission E approved the use of chasteberry for irregularities of the menstrual cycle, cyclical breast discomfort, and PMS (Blumenthal, 2000). Native to western Asia and southwestern Europe, chasteberry is now grown in the southeastern United States. It can be prepared as a medicinal tea and is also available as a tincture and in capsule form. Chasteberry is well tolerated; reported adverse effects are infrequent and include gastrointestinal complaints, dizziness, and dry mouth (Roemheld-Hamm, 2005).

Evening primrose oil (*Oenothera biennis*) has been recommended for relief of PMS-related breast tenderness; but to date, clinical trials of this omega-6 essential fatty acid–rich supplement have failed to demonstrate statistically or clinically significant results.

For many women, various nonpharmacological approaches may diminish PMS symptoms. Trials of cognitive behavioral therapy, group therapy, and relaxation therapy have demonstrated improvement in physical and/or psychological symptoms of PMS, although few studies have randomized patients. For some women, other modalities such as massage, yoga, aromatherapy, biofeedback, acupuncture, hypnosis, reflexology, chiropractic, and light therapy may have a beneficial effect on

PMS symptoms (Andolsek & Rapkin, 2006; Nelson & Baldwin, 2008; Whyte & Peraud, 2009).

Nursing Insight— *Asian medicine and PMS*

Nurses should recognize that the fundamental healing approach offered in Asian medicine may well be of benefit in diminishing symptoms of PMS. With the Asian perspective, premenstrual syndrome is viewed as an energetic imbalance, a blockage and stagnation of vital energy, or "chi," which normally flows through the body and enlivens it. When an individual's vital energy is blocked in the pelvic region, it can be manifest in many of the symptoms associated with PMS. Asian healing approaches are designed to restore and balance the body energies, thereby allowing the hormonal and nervous systems to return to a harmonious equilibrium.

PHARMACOLOGICAL INTERVENTIONS

If the nonpharmacological approaches fail to provide satisfactory symptom relief in 2 to 3 months, medication is often initiated. There are two major pharmacological strategies to treatment. One targets the central nervous system processes that are believed to contribute to premenstrual mood symptoms; the other approach centers on eliminating the hormonal cyclicity by suppressing ovulation. Pharmacological therapy is reserved for women who qualify as having PMDD or severe manifestations of PMS. The U.S. Food and Drug Administration (FDA) has approved two categories of medications for premenstrual disorders: selective serotonin reuptake inhibitors (SSRIs) and an oral contraceptive that contains the progestin drospirenone (Nelson & Baldwin, 2008; Whyte & Peraud, 2009).

The SSRIs that have received FDA approval for the treatment of PMDD are fluoxetine (Prozac, Sarafem), sertraline (Zoloft), and controlled-release paroxetine (Paxil CR). Currently, these medications constitute the mainstay of medical treatment. They have been studied extensively for the treatment of PMS symptoms, and dosing may be administered on a continuous or intermittent schedule. Luteal-phase dosing should be initiated about 14 days before menses and continued until the onset of menstruation. Use of any of the central nervous system agents for treatment of PMS/PMDD does not contraindicate the use of any hormonal or nonhormonal contraceptive method to prevent pregnancy (Nelson & Baldwin, 2008; Whyte & Peraud, 2009).

Be Sure to— Teach about potential adverse effects associated with SSRIs

Although most patients tolerate SSRIs without difficulty, nurses must make certain that the patient is aware of the following side effects associated with these medications: nausea, nervousness, anxiety, headache, drowsiness, dizziness, impaired concentration, decreased libido, and insomnia. The risk of side effects is dose related—lower doses, which often suffice for the symptoms of PMS—are associated with fewer side effects. Also, limiting dosing days to the luteal phase of the cycle has also been shown

to be effective in PMS/PMDD. Teaching women about their specific medications is an important step in helping them to understand their diagnosis and the rationale for the prescribed pharmacological treatment (Deglin & Vallerand, 2009; Nelson & Baldwin, 2008; Whyte & Peraud, 2009).

Spironolactone (Aldactone), a potassium-sparing diuretic, is another nonhormonal medication that has been shown to be beneficial in the treatment of PMS. Administered in a dosage of 25 mg two to four times a day during the luteal phase, this agent reduces bloating and improves mood in many patients. However, it should be noted that use in PMS management is considered to be off-label (Nelson & Baldwin, 2008).

Ovulation suppressants may be beneficial in the treatment of PMS. Although oral contraceptive pills (OCPs) have been used to treat premenstrual symptoms, most clinical trials have not demonstrated any efficacy in this approach. For some women, however, extended-cycle dosing of continuous OCPs or regular administration of Depo-Provera may be useful in providing symptom relief—these agents suppress ovulation and reduce the number of withdrawal bleeding episodes (and associated symptoms) experienced each year (Nelson & Baldwin, 2008).

The FDA has approved one oral contraceptive for the treatment of PMDD in women who desire contraception. Marketed under the trade name Yasmin, this medication contains ethinyl estradiol and drospirenone, a novel progestin. Yasmin is administered for 24 days and followed by a 4-day hormone-free interval. Clinical trials with this medication demonstrated significant improvement in physical, psychological, and behavioral symptoms of PMS/PMDD (Pearlstein, Bachmann, Zacur, & Yonkers, 2005; Yonkers et al., 2005).

case study   Patient with Premenstrual Syndrome

Cassandra Burney is a 29-year-old primigravida who visits the women's health clinic for an evaluation of bothersome premenstrual symptoms. Presently, Cassandra is not sexually active, but she has a diaphragm for birth control and is pleased with her contraceptive method. Her menstrual periods are regular, occur every 28 to 30 days, are moderate in flow, and last 6 to 7 days. Cassandra tells the nurse that each month beginning approximately 1 week before the onset of menstrual flow, she experiences painful, tender, swollen breasts; bloating; weight gain; and feelings of "being down" and irritable.

critical thinking questions

1. What additional information is needed to help confirm the diagnosis of PMS?

2. What can the nurse teach Cassandra about PMS and self-care strategies that may help to minimize her symptoms?

◆ See Suggested Answers to Case Study at the end of this chapter.

Now Can You— **Discuss nursing care for patients with premenstrual disorders?**

1. Describe the nurse's major role when caring for a patient with a premenstrual disorder?
2. Discuss various nonpharmacological therapies for premenstrual disorders?
3. Discuss various pharmacological therapies for premenstrual disorders?

summary points

◆ Premenstrual syndrome may be viewed as a complex constellation of genetic influences and hormonal imbalances that adversely affects a woman's physical, mental, and emotional health.

◆ Women have reported over 100 different physical and behavioral symptoms during the premenstrual period.

◆ The cause of PMS is believed to be multifactorial.

◆ To meet the criteria for PMS, the woman's symptoms must occur cyclically, be unrelated to any physical or mental condition, and greatly disrupt one or more areas of the woman's life

◆ The diagnostic workup for a premenstrual disorder includes the patient history, a physical examination, appropriate laboratory tests, and review of the daily symptom diary.

◆ Management of premenstrual syndrome may include nonpharmacological and pharmacological approaches.

◆ Nurses are instrumental in helping women to deal with premenstrual disorders by offering ongoing education and support.

review questions

Multiple Choice

1. In earlier times, premenstrual syndrome was thought to be related to:
   A. The patient's emotional makeup
   B. Pregnancy
   C. Insanity
   D. Tobacco use

2. One of the criteria for the diagnosis of premenstrual syndrome is that the symptoms:
   A. Occur during the menstrual phase of the uterine cycle
   B. Persist for 25 or more days
   C. Are not caused by any underlying physical or mental condition
   D. Occur during the proliferative phase of the uterine cycle

3. Most women with PMS experience relief of symptoms:
   A. During the luteal phase of the uterine cycle
   B. Within 24 hours following the onset of menstrual flow
   C. Around the time of ovulation
   D. Following removal of the uterus (hysterectomy)

4. An important component in the diagnostic workup for PMS involves:
   A. Obtaining serum levels of iron and prolactin
   B. Evaluating the basal body temperature
   C. Assessing the urine for glucose, protein, and ketones
   D. Evaluating the daily symptom diary

5. The nurse teaches the woman with PMS about self-help strategies to help diminish symptoms. For example, the nurse may suggest:
   A. Decreasing physical activity approximately 1 week before expected menses
   B. Decreasing the intake of water approximately 5 to 7 days before menstruation
   C. Taking evening primrose oil during the menstrual period
   D. Engaging in relaxation techniques and stress-relief therapies such as massage and yoga

REFERENCES

American College of Obstetricians and Gynecologists (ACOG). (2000). *Premenstrual syndrome* (ACOG Practice Bulletin No. 15). Washington, DC: Author

American College of Obstetricians and Gynecologists (ACOG). (2007). *Women's health care: A resource manual* (3rd ed.). Washington, DC: Author.

American Psychiatric Association (APA). (2000). *Diagnostic and statistical manual of mental disorders* (4th ed., text revision). Washington, DC: American Psychiatric Association Press.

Andolsek, K. M., & Rapkin, A. J. (2006). Contraceptive use in women with premenstrual disorders. *Dialogues in Contraception, 10*(4), 4–7.

Arrowsmith, F. M. (2007). Preventing the cycle of migraine: A review of patient issues for NPs. *American Journal for Nurse Practitioners, 11*(8), 42–54.

Association of Women's Health, Obstetrical and Neonatal Nurses. (2003). *Evidence-based practice guideline: Nursing management for cyclic perimenstrual pain and discomfort.* Washington, DC: Author.

Blumenthal, M. (2000). *German Federal Institute for Drugs and Medical Devices. Commission E Herbal Medicine: Expanded commission E monographs.* Newton, MA: Integrative Medicine Communications.

Borenstein, J. E., Dean, B. B., Endicott, J., Wong, J., Brown, C., Dickerson, V., & Yonkers, K. A. (2003). Health and economic impact of the premenstrual syndrome. *Journal of Reproductive Medicine, 48*(7), 515–24.

Clayton, A. H., Keller, A. E., Leslie, C., & Evans, W. (2006). Exploratory study of premenstrual symptoms and serotonin variability. *Archives of Women's Mental Health, 9*(1), 51–57.

Collins Sharp, B. A., Taylor, D. L., Thomas, K. K., Killeen, M. B., & Dawood, M. Y. (2002). Perimenstrual pain and discomfort: The scientific basis for practice. *Journal of Obstetric, Gynecologic, and Neonatal Nursing, 31*(6), 637–649.

Deglin, J. H., & Vallerand, A. H. (2009). *Davis's drug guide for nurses* (11th ed.). Philadelphia: F. A. Davis.

Dickerson, V. M. (2007). Premenstrual syndrome and premenstrual dysphoric disorder: Individualizing therapy. *Female Patient, 32*(1), 38–46.

Endicott, J., Nee, J., & Harrison, W. (2006). Daily record of severity of problems (DRSP): Reliability and validity. *Archives of Women's Mental Health, 9*(1), 41–49.

Freeman, E. W., DeRubeis, R. J., & Rickels, K. (1996). Reliability and validity of a daily diary for premenstrual syndrome. *Psychiatry Research, 65*(2), 97–106.

Halbreich, U. (2003). The etiology, biology, and evolving pathology of premenstrual syndromes. *Psychoneuroendocrinology, 28*(suppl. 3), 55–99.

Nelson, A. L., & Baldwin, S. (2008). Menstrual disorders and related concerns. In R. Hatcher, J. Trussell, A. Nelson, W. Cates Jr., F. Stewart, & D. Kowal (Eds.), *Contraceptive technology* (19th ed., pp. 469–476). New York: Thomson Reuters.

Pearlstein, T. B., Bachmann, G. A., Zacur, H. A., & Yonkers, K.A. (2005). Treatment of premenstrual dysphoric disorder with a new drospirenone-containing oral contraceptive formulation. *Contraception, 72*(5), 414–421.

Polaneczky, M. (2007). Premenstrual syndrome/premenstrual dysphoric disorder. *Female Patient, 32*(9), 40–45.

Roemheld-Hamm, B. (2005). Chasteberry. *American Family Physician, 72*(5), 821–824.

Speroff, L., & Fritz, M. A. (2005). *Clinical gynecologic endocrinology and infertility* (7th ed.). Philadelphia: Lippincott Williams & Wilkins.

Steiner, M., Macdougall, M., & Brown, E. (2003). The premenstrual symptoms screening tool (PSST) for clinicians. *Archives of Women's Mental Health, 6*(3), 203–209.

Taylor, D., Schuiling, K. D., & Sharp, B. A. (2005). Menstrual cycle pain and discomforts. InK. D. Schuiling & F. Liskis (Eds.), *Women's gynecologic health* (pp. 474–500). Sudbury, MA: Jones & Bartlett.

U.S. Department of Health and Human Services. (2008). *Physical activity guidelines for Americans: 2008 activity guidelines for Americans summary*. Retrieved September 1, 2009, from http://www.health.gov/paguidelines/guidelines/summary.aspx

Whyte, J., & Peraud, P. (2009). Premenstrual disorders: A primary care primer. *Consultant, 49*(1), 15–24.

Yonkers, K. A., Brown, C., Pearlstein, T. B., Foegh, M., Sampson-Landers, C., & Rapkin, A. (2005). Efficacy of a new low-dose contraceptive with drospirenone in premenstrual dysphoric disorder. *Obstetrics & Gynecology, 106*(3), 492–501.

suggested answers to case study

1. It is important that the nurse determine the timing and duration of Cassandra's symptoms in order to establish that they are consistent with premenstrual syndrome. To meet the criteria for PMS, the symptoms must occur during the luteal phase of the menstrual cycle and resolve within 4 days after the onset of menstrual flow. Although the patient states that her symptoms occur cyclically, it is important to document this information. The nurse teaches Cassandra how to use a symptom diary to record her premenstrual symptoms each day, note their severity, and record the dates of her menstrual period. Cassandra is asked to bring the diary with her when she returns to the clinic for an evaluation in 3 months.

2. The nurse teaches Cassandra about the relationship between normal cyclic hormonal variations and accompanying physiological changes. This information serves to validate the patient's experience with her monthly discomforts and acknowledges that the symptoms are real and have a physiological base. The information also increases Cassandra's understanding about premenstrual disorders and promotes a greater sense of control over her situation. The nurse counsels Cassandra to wear a supportive bra to minimize breast tenderness. Other self-care strategies are centered on facilitating fluid excretion: limiting the intake of salt- and sodium-containing foods and increasing the consumption of water and other natural diuretic foods such as watermelon, cranberry juice, peaches, asparagus, and parsley approximately 7–10 days before the menstrual period is expected. The nurse can also suggest that Cassandra engage in stress-reduction techniques (e.g., exercise, yoga, meditation, massage therapy) in anticipation of the cyclical hormonal changes each month and participate in a PMS support group, if available.

 For more information, go to http://davisplus.fadavis.com/

Promoting Breast Health
Shelton M. Hisley, PhD, RNC, WHNP-BC

Life begins each morning . . .
Each morning is the open door to a new world—new vistas, new aims, new tryings.

—Leigh Hodges

LEARNING TARGETS *At the completion of this chapter, the student will be able to:*

◆ Describe normal breast anatomy.

◆ Teach a patient how to perform breast self-examination.

◆ Differentiate among various breast abnormalities.

◆ Discuss diagnostic modalities and treatment options for breast cancer.

◆ Describe the nurse's role in promoting breast health.

Introduction

This chapter discusses the promotion of breast health in women. Most concerns about breast care and problems are first voiced in the primary care setting. Nurses who work with women are in an ideal position to educate about the importance of breast health awareness and suggest strategies to promote the early identification of benign and malignant breast disease. As is true with other types of cancers, early detection is key in the successful treatment of breast cancer. Most experts agree that breast cancer is not a singular disease. Instead, it is believed that malignancies of the breast stem from many types of disease, each with distinct histological, biological, and immunological characteristics. A myriad of dietary, socioeconomic, and environmental factors most likely serve as causative or contributing influences in the development of breast cancer. Breast health is an important issue for women; maintaining breast health is an essential strategy for maintaining optimal physical and psychological health.

 Optimizing Outcomes— **A holistic approach to breast care**

Owing to the likelihood that multiple factors play a role in the development of breast cancer, nurses can embrace a holistic approach to women's health care that is centered on health promotion. This strategy focuses on individualized patient education and counseling concerning diet, lifestyle habits, and environmental exposure—all aspects of health over which individuals have control. The general health

benefits of these types of changes have been proven in terms of improved quality of life. Prevention strategies such as these, when combined with early detection, empower women with knowledge and heightened awareness of the normal workings of their bodies and equips them with tools for self-care. The nurse's involvement in patient education and awareness of breast health constitutes an essential action for helping the nation to achieve an extremely important Healthy People 2010 goal: Reduce breast cancer deaths to no more than 20.6 per 100,000 women from a baseline of 23 per 100,000 (USDHHS, 2000).

Benign and Malignant Breast Diseases: The Scope of the Problem

Fibrocystic breast changes, also known as benign breast disease (BBD), are believed to occur in over 50% of women. Benign breast conditions include cysts, tumors, masses, nipple discharge, infection, and inflammation of the ducts. Although not malignant, the discovery of a benign breast mass may evoke feelings of fear, anxiety, and vulnerability and trigger worry about the future. And women have cause for concern, as research has shown that some types of BBD are an important risk factor for the later development of breast cancer (Hartman, Sellers, & Frost et al., 2005; Lee, 2009).

Breast cancer is the most common cancer in women in the United States, except for skin cancer, and it is the second leading cause of cancer deaths in women (American

Cancer Society [ACS], 2009a; Smith, 2007). The American Cancer Society predicts that in 2009, an estimated 192,370 new cases of invasive breast cancer will be diagnosed, and there will be 40,170 deaths from breast cancer. Presently, the chance of a woman developing invasive breast cancer at some time during her life is approximately 1 in 8 (12%). The chance of dying from breast cancer is around 1 in 35 (3%). Women who live in North America have the highest rate of breast cancer in the world. To gain a perspective on the magnitude of the problem, nurses can reflect on the fact that approximately 2.5 million breast cancer survivors are living in the United States today (ACS, 2009a).

 Nursing Insight— *Breast cancer among American women*

Besides skin cancer, breast cancer is the most commonly diagnosed cancer among women in the United States. More than 1 in 4 cancers are breast cancer. From 2001 to 2004, the incidence of breast cancer in this country decreased by 3.5% per year. One theory regarding this decrease centers on the reduced use of hormone therapy by women after the results of the Women's Health Initiative were published in 2002. These results suggest a correlation between hormone therapy and increased breast cancer risk (ACS, 2009a; BreastCancer.org, 2008). Women of different ages have different risks of breast cancer. A woman's risk increases with age until she reaches menopause; breast cancer risk then increases more slowly with the advancing years.

Anatomy of the Breast

To enhance an understanding of the breast, it is helpful to review normal breast anatomy. The female breasts, or mammary glands, are considered to be accessory organs of the reproductive system. The two breasts lie over the pectoral and anterior serratus muscles. Breast tissue, which consists primarily of glandular, fibrous, and adipose tissue suspended within the conical-shaped breasts by Cooper's ligaments, is richly supplied with a dense network of blood vessels and lymph vessels (Fig. 3-1).

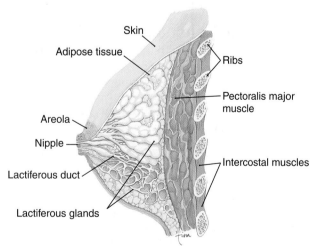

Figure 3-1 Mammary gland shown in a midsagittal section

The glandular tissue contains 15 to 24 lobes that are separated by fibrous and adipose tissue. Each lobe contains several lobules composed of numerous alveoli clustered around tiny ducts that are layered with secretory cuboidal epithelium called alveoli or acini (Fig. 3-2).

The epithelial lining of the ducts secretes various components of milk. The ducts from several lobules come together to form the lactiferous ducts, which are larger ducts that open on the surface of the nipple. The lymphatic vessels carry lymph, an alkaline, clear, colorless tissue fluid, away from the breast. Most of the lymph vessels of the breast lead to the nodes in the axillae. The lymph nodes are small, kidney-shaped organs of lymphoid tissue (Fig. 3-3). An increase in the size of the node (lymphadenopathy) indicates a high level of activity (e.g., infection or cancer).

Outer parts of the breasts include the nipples, areolae, and Montgomery tubercles. The nipples contain several pores that secrete colostrum (breast fluid that precedes breast milk) and breast milk during lactation. The nipples consist primarily of erectile tissue to assist with infant

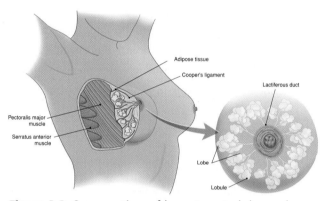

Figure 3-2 Cross section of breast; note lobe and lobule shown in detailed area

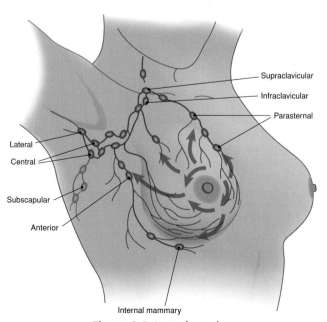

Figure 3-3 Lymph nodes

latch-on during suckling. The areola is a more deeply pigmented area that surrounds the nipple. Its diameter ranges from 1 to 3.9 inches (2.5 to 10 cm). The Montgomery tubercles are papillae located on the surface of the nipple and the areola; they secrete a fatty substance that lubricates and protects the nipple and areola during breastfeeding.

The primary function of the breasts is to provide nutrition to offspring through the process known as lactation. In American culture, the breasts are also closely linked with "womanhood." Many equate large breasts with increased sexiness and eroticism. Because the breasts serve as a source of sensual pleasure for both men and women, injury to or the loss of a breast can trigger major psychological distress for both genders.

The Nurse's Role in Teaching About Breast Health

The promotion of breast health encompasses several areas, including cancer screening, optimal nutrition, and physical activity. It is important for nurses to educate women throughout the life span about strategies for promoting breast health. Personal awareness of the normal appearance and feel of the breasts constitutes an essential first step in promoting and maintaining breast health. Nurses working with women in a variety of settings are perfectly situated to offer information about strategies for promoting breast health and for performing self-examinations. By providing information in a nonthreatening, therapeutic environment, nurses can help to allay women's fears and present self-examination as a positive, empowering experience.

❝ What to say ❞ — *Teaching about breast health*

During a discussion about breast health, the nurse may wish to include the following information:

- As you age, your breasts experience loss of milk glands and shrinkage of collagen. This causes an increase in the fat tissue and loosening of the breast tissue. Instead of getting larger with the increase in fat tissue, however, the breast tissue begins to sag, causing the breasts to drop.
- Breast tissue weighs less than most people think: an A-cup weighs ¼ lb, a B-cup weighs ½ lb, a C-cup weighs ¾ lb, and a D-cup weighs about 1 lb.
- The skin covering the breasts stretches as you grow, causing the skin to become thinner than the skin on other parts of the body.
- It is not uncommon for women to have some degree of hair surrounding their nipples. The darker the skin, the more hair there is likely to be.
- A woman's nipples may be different sizes and may be placed in slightly different locations on each breast. This may cause the nipples to point in different directions, which is considered a normal finding.
- Fluctuating hormone levels during the monthly cycle cause changes in breast tissue. Following menstruation, when hormone levels are at their lowest, the breast tissue is smooth and nontender.

As estrogen levels increase at mid-cycle, the breasts may become more sensitive. Also, just before menstruation, when progesterone is elevated, many women's breasts become swollen and tender, with palpable nodules.

- Ideally, your health-care provider should perform your clinical breast examination 1 week following menstruation, when the breast tissue is nontender and smooth.
- Breast implants still pose health risks, including deflation, leakage, and wrinkling. In addition, capsular contraction can occur, causing the scar tissue surrounding the implant to tighten and the breast to become hard.
- The area between the breasts has several oil and sweat glands, creating an atmosphere conducive to the growth of bacteria.
- Sleeping on your side, with a pillow to support your breasts, provides the best position for maintaining breast shape and contour over time.
- Regular exercise can strengthen the pectoral muscles, reducing sagging over time and creating a natural lift.
- It is not uncommon to have a third nipple, stemming from breast buds that form during early fetal development. These extra nipples, however, rarely contain milk glands.
- Pregnancy darkens the color of the nipple, which is an enhancement for the breastfeeding baby. This darker color does not disappear after pregnancy.
- The left breast is usually larger then the right breast.
- Breasts do not reach their full size until the early 20s.

LIFESTYLE CHOICES AND BREAST HEALTH

Lifestyle choices, including moderate alcohol consumption, weight maintenance, and avoidance of smoking can affect breast health as well. Alcohol consumption is known to be associated with an increased risk of breast cancer. The American Cancer Society (2009b) recommends limiting alcohol intake to one drink per day. The risk of breast cancer is increased 1.5 times in women who consume two to five drinks per day.

Routine exercise, which helps to maintain a healthy weight, is associated with a decreased risk of breast cancer. Maintenance of a healthy weight is recommended for optimum breast health. Obesity is associated with an increased risk of breast cancer, particularly in postmenopausal women. Following menopause, estrogen is produced in the fat cells. In combination with dietary fat, estrogen significantly increases the likelihood of breast cancer development. Smoking is associated with an increased risk of breast cancer, lung cancer and heart disease in women.

🄢 Now Can You— **Discuss breast health promotion?**

1. Describe normal breast anatomy?
2. Discuss the nurse's role in teaching about breast health?
3. Develop an educational program that includes essential information about the breasts?

Breast Awareness and Cancer Screening

Breast self-examination (BSE), clinical breast exams, and mammography (x-ray filming of the breasts) can assist in early detection and early treatment (Fig. 3-4). The initiation and frequency of mammography depends on the woman's age and risk factors. Magnetic resonance imaging (MRI) (a noninvasive nuclear procedure for imaging tissues with high fat and water content) appears to be especially useful in detecting tumors in women with an inherited susceptibility to breast cancer, and recent findings suggest that this diagnostic method can detect cancer in the contralateral breast that was missed by mammography in women with recently diagnosed breast cancer (Lehman, Gastonis, Kuhl, Hendrick, Pisano, Hanna, Peacock, et al., 2007). As a screening tool, MRI may be useful for women with breast implants in whom mammography is difficult or to determine the integrity of the implants. It has been demonstrated that breast MRI is most effective for identifying tissue with increased blood flow, such as neoplastic tumors. However, breast MRI is not a substitute for a mammogram and it should not be used for routine screening of the average-risk woman. Limitations associated with this diagnostic modality include the expense, the limited specificity, and false-positive results (Aliotta & Schaeffer, 2006; Bleicher, Ciocca, Egleston, Sesa, Evers, Sigurdson, & Morrow, 2009; Smith, 2007).

 Optimizing Outcomes— Screening for breast cancer

Best outcome: Monthly breast-self examination, annual clinical breast examinations, and routine mammography allow women and their health-care providers to detect potentially cancerous tumors at the earliest stage possible. This multipronged screening approach facilitates early diagnosis and early treatment, providing the best outcome possible.

 Ethnocultural Considerations . . . Breast Cancer Screening

There are notable differences in breast cancer screening practices among women of different ethnic backgrounds. Although African American women are at a lower risk for developing breast cancer than Caucasian women, they are more likely to die from breast cancer due to late diagnosis. According to Husaini and associates (2001), African American women are more likely to have mammogram screening if they are older, married, have a higher level of education, and believe that early detection could lead to a cure. A positive family history of breast cancer and church affiliation have no influence on the incidence of detection.

Asian American and Pacific Islander women have very low rates of breast cancer screening. Factors responsible for the low screening rates include lack of health insurance, low income, and lack of a primary-care provider (Kagawa-Singer & Pourat, 2000).

Breast cancer causes a significant number of deaths in Filipino women. In a study by Wu and Bancroft (2006), researchers found that women were more likely to follow recommended screenings if there is support from physicians and family members, and if they had insurance. In addition, the presence of physical symptoms, family history of breast cancer, and health literacy promote adherence to recommendations.

BREAST SELF-EXAMINATION

Familiarization with one's breasts facilitates the early detection of problems and allows for prompt evaluation. Breast self-examination is a way for women to learn how their breasts normally feel. Routinely performing BSE is an approach that focuses on the importance of self-awareness and helps women to notice changes in breast tissue (ACS, 2009a). When teaching women about breast self-examination, the nurse can display pictures of breast tissue and discuss the normal irregular contours of breasts. Breast models are also helpful and allow women to feel normal and abnormal masses; these teaching aides may be beneficial in diminishing women's fears about checking their own breasts. Since menstruating women often experience increased discomfort and lumpiness in their breasts during the second half of the menstrual cycle, the ideal time to perform BSE is during the week after menstruation.

Routinely performing BSE helps women to perfect their technique and become familiar with the contours and tissue characteristics unique to their own breasts. Then, if they detect changes that are worrisome to them or that persist, they can schedule an evaluation (Smith, 2007). Nurses can be instrumental in facilitating women's awareness of and comfort with detecting changes in their breasts (Ruhl, 2007).

Breast self-examination is a simple yet powerful self-help behavior that can save lives. Over 75% of breast cancers are discovered by women themselves. The current procedure for performing BSE differs from previous recommendations endorsed by the American Cancer Society. The changes in technique represent an extensive review of the medical literature and input from an expert medical advisory group (ACS, 2008). Despite the advantages of performing BSE, it should be noted that according to the latest (2009) statement from the U.S. Preventive Services Task Force (USPSTF), insufficient evidence was found to recommend for or against teaching or performing routine breast self-examination (http://www.ahrq.gov/clinic/pocketgd09/gcp09s2.htm).

Figure 3-4 Mammogram

Family Teaching Guidelines...
Breast Self-Examination

1. Visually inspect the breasts in front of a mirror. Assess for color, contour, shape, and size. Assess for dimpling or puckering of the skin; change in nipple direction; and redness, rash, or swelling (Fig. 3-5).

2. Repeat first step with the arms slightly raised above the head (Fig. 3-6).

3. Inspect and palpate the nipple. Gently squeeze the nipple between the thumb and forefinger, looking for discharge. Many women, especially those who have had children, are able to express some discharge by squeezing the nipples. Discharge that is of concern is most often spontaneous (ACS, 2008) (Fig. 3-7).

4. Palpate the breast and axillae. Recline on the bed and place a pillow under each shoulder during palpation. Use the left hand to palpate the right breast, and the right hand to palpate the left breast. Using the finger pads of the three middle fingers, palpate the entire surface of the breast. Use overlapping dime-sized

circular motions and apply three different levels of pressure: *light pressure* is best to feel the tissue closest to the skin; *medium pressure* is best to feel a little deeper; and *firm pressure* is used to feel the tissue closest to the chest and ribs (Fig. 3-8).

5. Move around the breast in an up and down pattern, checking the entire breast area until only the ribs are felt; repeat the entire technique on the opposite breast (ACS, 2008)./ftgnl.

The American Cancer Society endorses "breast awareness." Breast awareness, or being aware of how the breasts normally look and feel, may be achieved by feeling the breasts for changes or by using a step-by-step approach (BSE) on a specific schedule (e.g., after menses when the breasts are not tender or swollen) (ACS, 2009a). According to the American College of Obstetricians and Gynecologists (ACOG), despite a lack of definitive data for or against BSE, the technique has the potential to detect palpable breast cancer and can be recommended (ACOG, 2007).

Nursing Insight— *Breast implants and BSE*

If they choose to do so, women with breast implants may perform BSE. Following surgery, it may be helpful for the surgeon to guide BSE teaching by identifying the edges of the implant to enhance the patient's understanding of the new contours of her breasts. For some, the increased prominence of the breast tissue following implant surgery may make it easier to perform the examination. Women who are pregnant or breastfeeding may also choose to examine their breasts regularly (ACS, 2009b).

CLINICAL BREAST EXAMINATIONS

Annual clinical breast examinations (CBE) performed by a trained health-care professional are an important tool in the early detection of breast cancer. Inflammatory breast cancer, a rare and aggressive type that may cause swelling and redness, often does not show up on mammography. Also, the clinical breast examination provides an opportunity for the clinician to reinforce a woman's self-examination technique, discuss concerns, and emphasize the value in becoming intimately familiar with the contour of one's own breasts.

All women should have a clinical breast examination performed at recommended intervals by a skilled healthcare provider. The clinical breast examination should be performed at least every 3 years for women aged 18 to 39, and every year after age 40. According to the American Cancer Society (2009c), the clinical breast examination serves as a complement to mammography, and there may be some benefit in having the CBE performed shortly before the mammogram. It is important for nurses to provide information about the benefits and limitations of the CBE, as well as BSE (ACOG, 2007; ACS, 2009c).

MAMMOGRAPHY

A mammography examination is used to aid in the early diagnosis of breast cancer (Fig. 3-9). The examination, which requires exposure to small doses of ionizing radiation, allows for identification of small breast tissue abnormalities that may require further investigation. In recent times, two enhancements have been made to traditional mammography techniques: digital mammography and computer-aided detection (CAD). Digital mammography, also called full-field digital mammography (FFDM), converts the x-rays to electrical signals, similar to those found in digital cameras. These signals produce images that can be viewed on a computer screen or printed on special film. The images are stored for future comparison. Digital mammography provides improved screening for women determined to be at high risk for developing breast cancer (Pisano et al., 2005). This latest technology is enhanced with the use of computer software that highlights areas of increased density, masses, and calcifications.

 Nursing Insight— *Calcium deposits within breast tissue*

Calcifications (calcium deposits) detected on mammography may be identified as *macrocalcifications* or as *microcalcifications*. Macrocalcifications, degenerative changes resulting from old trauma, inflammation, or aging of the breast arteries, occur in approximately one-half of women in the United States who are over age 50 and are usually not related to malignancy. Microcalcifications are small specks of calcium that may be present as "residue" in areas of rapidly dividing cells (e.g., a neoplasm). A cluster of microcalcifications may be indicative of a small cancer.

Figure 3-9 Mammography showing breast cancer

Screening mammography is beneficial as routine breast surveillance for the asymptomatic woman. Clinical detection through the use of breast self-examination generally does not occur until the tumor approximates the size of a walnut. By the time a palpable mass or lump is detected, the tumor most likely has been growing for some time. Hence, routine screening mammograms provide a much earlier, high-sensitivity study of developing tumors at the lowest possible cost. In addition, a screening mammogram enables the radiologist to identify changes such as calcifications that may point to malignancy (Smith, 2007).

 Nursing Insight— *Differentiating between screening mammography and diagnostic mammography*

Screening mammograms are performed to check for breast cancer in women who have no signs or symptoms of the disease. They usually involve two x-rays of each breast. *Diagnostic* mammograms are performed to check for breast cancer after a lump or other sign or symptom of breast cancer has been detected. They may also be used to evaluate changes discovered during a screening mammogram or to view breast tissue when it is difficult to obtain a screening mammogram because of special circumstances, such as the presence of breast implants. Diagnostic mammography takes longer to perform because more x-rays are taken to obtain views of the breast from several angles (National Cancer Institute [NCI], 2009a).

The value of routine screening mammography for women age 50 and older has been well established. Recommendations for mammography screening in women ages 40 to 49 have been met with some controversy. Analysis of the major studies of women in this age group has shown a marginal benefit in decreasing the death rate from breast cancer. However, it should be noted that:

- Findings from older studies may be flawed because mammography was much cruder 30 years ago.
- Breast cancer in women ages 40 to 49 occurs with less frequency.
- Mammography in premenopausal women historically has not been as accurate owing to the density of breast tissue in women in this age group, as compared with breast tissue in postmenopausal women. Mammography may miss as many as 25% of invasive cancers in women ages 40 to 49 years, as compared with 10% in women age 50 years and older.
- Certain tumors, even when detected early, are not curable. In general, younger women tend to have more rapidly growing tumors than do older women. This finding may be related to the higher levels of estrogen in the blood and tissues of premenopausal women that can stimulate tumor growth or a genetic predisposition that becomes expressed in this age group (Smith, 2007).

In 2002, the U.S. Preventive Services Task Force (USPSTF) issued a recommendation that women undergo screening mammography every 1 to 2 years, beginning at age 40. Guidelines from the American College of

Obstetricians and Gynecologists, the American Medical Association, and the American Academy of Family Physicians are similar, with annual mammography recommended after age 50 (Smith, 2007). Presently, the American Cancer Society recommends that women age 40 and older receive yearly mammograms in addition to clinical breast examinations, and they should continue to perform breast self-examination monthly (ACS, 2009d).

In November 2009, the USPSTF issued new breast cancer screening recommendations for the general population. Based on evidence review, the updated guidelines recommend against routine mammography screening for women before age 50 years, suggest that screening end at age 74 years, and recommend changing the screening interval from 1 year to 2 years. Several professional organizations have voiced their objections to the new recommendations. The American Cancer Society, the American College of Radiology, the American College of Obstetricians and Gynecologists, and several other expert groups recommend that clinicians and patients continue to follow the earlier guidelines (Barclay, 2009; USPSTF, 2009).

Since mammography is considered a less useful screening and diagnostic tool in women younger than age 40, the health-care provider must determine the use of mammography in this patient population on an individual basis. When compared with film mammography, full-field digital mammography has been determined to be more accurate, especially for women younger than age 50, those with dense breast tissue, and those who are premenopausal or perimenopausal (Pisano et al., 2005; Smith, 2007).

 Optimizing Outcomes— **Recognizing mammography barriers to enhance counseling and empower women**

Women may be reluctant to obtain a mammogram for a number of reasons, including a fear of pain associated with the test and a fear of the test findings. Other barriers to breast cancer screening include older age, cultural patterns and health beliefs, lack of knowledge and information, lack of motivation, expense, lack of availability of mammography services, lack of physician referral, lack of health-related social support, cancer fatalism, and the presence of disabilities (Barr, Giannotti, Van Hoof, Mongoven, & Curry, 2008; Farmer, Reddick, D'Agostino, & Jackson, 2007; Kang, Thomas, Kwon, Hyun, & Jun, 2008; Kim & Kim, 2008; Makuc, Breen, Meissner, Vernon, & Cohen, 2007; Wang, Mandelblatt, Liang, Ma, & Schwartz, 2009; Young & Severson, 2005). Nurses can empower women by providing factual information, by addressing specific concerns, and by working with other professionals to help remove barriers to screening. Compliance with mammography guidelines may be improved by strategies such as reminder postcards or telephone calls and direct health-care provider referrals.

❝ What to say ❞ — *Preparing for a mammogram*

Nurses can counsel women about strategies to enhance mammography results and minimize discomfort associated with the procedure. For

example, the nurse can provide the following information:

- Choose a mammography facility that is accredited by the American College of Radiology; ensure that the mammogram is performed by a registered technologist and that the radiologist is trained specifically to interpret mammography.
- Remove powder, deodorant, and perfume prior to the mammogram (these substances may create shadows).
- Schedule the mammogram when the breasts are less tender (e.g., after the menstrual period).
- Ask for the use of a soft pad to cushion the breasts during mammography compression.
- Take acetaminophen, ibuprofen, or aspirin as needed for relief of discomfort.

BREAST TOMOSYNTHESIS: A NEW TOOL FOR BREAST CANCER SCREENING

Mammography, which produces a two-dimensional x-ray image of the breast, is the traditional first-choice modality for the early detection of breast cancer. However, mammography interpretation, especially in women with dense, fibroglandular breasts, has inherent limitations. With a standard mammogram, normal breast structures are superimposed on each other, creating an overlapping image that may mimic or mask a lesion and lead to false-positive or false-negative findings. Tomosynthesis, available in some research settings, is a new advancement in breast imaging. This modality produces breast views in numerous thin slices, providing a three-dimensional image (and better visualization) of breast tissue. Similar to mammography, the breast is compressed with the tomosynthesis technique and the total radiation dose is comparable to the dose of a single-view mammogram. Research is presently underway to determine the clinical utility, guidelines, applications, and cost-effectiveness of this innovative, new diagnostic tool (Buzek, 2009; Diekmann & Bick, 2007; Rafferty, 2004; Rafferty, 2007).

---

where research and practice meet: **Cultural Barriers Toward Mammography Screening**

Kang and associates (2008) explored Korean women's attitudes toward and barriers to mammography screening. The women's beliefs that an absence of symptoms meant there was no need for a breast examination constituted a major finding of the study. Other variables that were identified as barriers to screening included a lack of information and fear about x-rays and test results and fear of discomfort and pain. Other researchers (Wang et al., 2009) investigated the role of knowledge, culture, and attitude as barriers to mammography screening among immigrant Chinese women. Study findings revealed that women who were least likely to obtain mammography were recent immigrants and those with a low income, limited English ability, and lacking regular sources of health care. Findings from both studies underscore the importance of culturally sensitive education and counseling to improve the use of mammography screening services among women of varying ethnic backgrounds.

Now Can You— **Discuss methods of breast awareness and cancer screening?**

1. Explain what is meant by the term "breast awareness" and identify the recommended guidelines for clinical breast examinations and screening mammography?
2. Teach a patient the proper procedure for breast self-examination?
3. Explain how to prepare for a mammogram?

Benign Breast Masses

It has been estimated that at some time during adulthood, 50% of women will experience a breast problem. Fortunately, most breast tumors are benign. Breast cysts are a common finding; they may be fluid-filled or solid. Fluid-filled cysts, also termed "**fibrocystic changes,**" are often tender and fluctuate in size with the menstrual cycle. These changes are the most common benign breast condition and occur most often during the childbearing years. Although the cause is unknown, an imbalance of estrogen and progesterone may play a role in the development of fluid-filled breast masses. It is believed that fibrocystic changes in the breasts are exacerbated by caffeine intake. Therapeutic interventions involve differentiating between fibrocystic changes and breast cancer. Screening methods include clinical breast examinations, mammography, and ultrasonography. The physician may choose to aspirate fluid-filled cysts for evaluation to determine if malignant cells are present. Patients should be advised that although aspiration may eliminate the cysts, they frequently re-form.

Optimizing Outcomes— **Teaching about fibrocystic breast changes**

When teaching women about breast health and BSE, nurses can include information about fibrocystic changes, palpable thickening in the breasts often associated with pain and tenderness that fluctuates with the menstrual cycle. Fibrocystic changes are common, benign, and tend to appear during the second and third decades of life. Treatment for the condition centers on relief of symptoms and may include analgesics, nonsteroidal anti-inflammatory drugs (e.g., ibuprofen), diuretics, use of a supportive bra, avoidance of caffeine and other stimulants (called methylxanthines), tobacco, and alcohol, and the application of heat to the breasts.

Fibroadenomas are solid cysts composed of stromal (connective) and glandular tissue. They are usually moveable and nontender. Fibroadenomas are the second most common benign breast condition (fibrocystic changes are the most common) and are usually located in the upper outer quadrant of the breast. This tumor occurs most often in women who are in their 20s and 30s. The use of oral contraceptives before age 20 has been linked to the risk of fibroadenomas (ACS, 2009b).

Lipomas are mobile, nontender fat tumors that are soft with discrete borders. Lipomas may develop anywhere in the body, including the breasts. **Intraductal papillomas** are small, wartlike growths in the lining of the milk ducts near the nipple. These rare, benign tumors usually produce a clear or bloody nipple discharge. They may be felt as a small lump behind or next to the nipple.

Mammary duct ectasia is an inflammation of the ducts located behind the nipple. Occurring most often in peri- and postmenopausal women, this condition produces a thick, sticky nipple discharge that may be purple, brown, or white in color. Upon inspection, the nipple and adjacent breast tissue may be tender and red and the nipple may be pulled inward. Duct ectasia may resolve spontaneously, or it may require treatment with warm compresses and antibiotics. In some situations, surgical removal of the abnormal duct is necessary. This lesion does not increase the risk of breast cancer.

Nursing Insight— Nonproliferative and proliferative breast lesions

The presence of cysts in the breasts does not necessarily increase a woman's risk for breast cancer. It has been estimated that approximately 70% of fibrocystic changes are *nonproliferative lesions*; 26% of changes are *proliferative lesions* without atypical or unusual growing cells (termed "atypia"), and *proliferative lesions with atypical hyperplasia* represent the remainder of fluid-filled breast lesions. Nonproliferative (multiplying) lesions do not affect breast cancer risk. Proliferative lesions without atypia may slightly increase cancer risk, and proliferative lesions with atypical hyperplasia raise the risk of cancer (ACS, 2009c).

Mastitis is an infection of the breast that occurs when bacteria enter the mammary ducts through a nipple. Most often, bacteria are introduced during breastfeeding. Localized pockets of infection produce tender, warm lumps and the adjacent axillary lymph nodes are frequently enlarged and painful. Mastitis is usually treated with antibiotics and warm compresses. If there is no improvement in symptoms following antibiotic therapy, further screening is indicated to rule out inflammatory carcinoma, a rare form of breast cancer that may cause redness, warmth, swelling, and skin texture changes in the affected breast.

Breast trauma or injury may produce an accumulation of blood at the site (hematoma) or destruction of the mammary fatty tissue ("fat necrosis"), which can appear as a lump. A biopsy may be performed to rule out malignancy. There is no evidence that breast injury causes cancer.

Evaluating Breast Abnormalities

Over the past decade, breast cancer screening methods, especially mammography, have become more precise, allowing for earlier diagnosis. Improved screening and increased public awareness have accounted for the dramatic increase in the detection of breast cancer. Earlier diagnosis has resulted in a decrease in mortality rates.

If an area of abnormal breast tissue is detected during the clinical breast examination, unless there is a high index of suspicion, the woman is usually asked to return for a second evaluation after her next menstrual period. In many situations, she is also referred for a mammography. A limitation of mammography is the inability of this modality to differentiate between solid and cystic masses. An ultrasound examination (ultrasonography; sonography) may be performed at the time of the mammography to determine whether the lump is solid or fluid-filled.

Further testing is indicated if the breast mass persists after the next menstrual period, or if any abnormality is identified on mammography or sonography. If the ultrasound examination reveals that the lump is solid, the suspicious tissue is biopsied for further analysis. If the mass is fluid-filled, a needle aspiration is performed, and the woman is monitored for the development of additional cysts. Ultrasound may be used to guide the needle aspiration. If a distinct, palpable lump persists despite normal findings on mammography, immediate follow-up and evaluation are indicated.

A biopsy of any suspicious area is needed to provide a tissue sample for analysis so that a definitive diagnosis can be made. Although mammography is considered to be the best detection method for early breast cancer, it is often unable to distinguish between benign and malignant tumors. The American Cancer Society estimates that four out of every five biopsy results are not cancer (ACS, 2009c).

Breast MRI is used with increasing frequency to evaluate abnormal breast findings and to screen women at high risk for breast cancer. This screening modality is especially beneficial for breast masses that are not visualized mammographically, for lobular cancers, and for patients at risk for bilateral disease. MRI of the breast has shown an overall sensitivity to breast cancer of 95% (Esserman, Lane, Ewing, & Hwang, 2005; Knutson & Steiner, 2007; Smith, 2007). Recent evidence suggests that this diagnostic method can detect cancer in the contralateral breast that was missed by mammography in women with recently diagnosed breast cancer (Lehman et al., 2007; Pomeranz, 2007).

The American Cancer Society recommends both MRI scans and mammograms once per year for women considered as high risk—those whose chance of developing breast cancer during their lifetime is greater than 20%—beginning at age 30. Younger women frequently develop more aggressive cancers and they tend to have more dense breasts, a factor that makes it more difficult to detect cancerous changes via mammography alone (ACS, 2009c; Pomeranz, 2007).

BIOPSY

Most often, the diagnosis and treatment of breast abnormalities is a two-step process: A biopsy is obtained and evaluated and then based on this information, decisions are made regarding the treatment. Palpation alone cannot determine whether or not a suspicious mass or lump is cancer. Likewise, neither the clinical breast examination nor available technology can provide definitive proof that a suspicious lesion is cancerous. All that can be concluded from these modalities is that "no evidence of cancer is found." Confirmation of cancer can be made only by examining the suspicious tissue (Smith, 2007). A number of different biopsy procedures may be used to obtain a sample of breast tissue or fluid within the breast tissue for evaluation. These include fine needle aspiration, core needle aspiration, and surgical or open biopsy.

Fine Needle Aspiration (FNA)

The FNA technique involves the use of a fine needle that is carefully guided into the suspicious area while the practitioner palpates the lump. It is usually conducted in the office setting. If the abnormality is too small to feel, ultrasound or a stereotactic biopsy can be used to help locate and ensure an adequate sampling of the suspicious tissue. In the latter technique, the biopsy is conducted with the aid of mammography. The needle is guided to the area by computer-assisted x-ray, which can help the examiner precisely control the needle placement. Then suction is applied to the needle. FNA is used to determine whether the lump is a fluid-filled cyst or a solid tumor (Smith, 2007) (Fig. 3-10).

 clinical alert

Indications for breast biopsy

A biopsy obtained by FNA with a stereotactic core needle or by surgical excision is usually recommended for any breast mass that does not resolve spontaneously within one or two menstrual cycles and for all postmenopausal women. It is important to note that negative results from mammography and ultrasonography are not always accurate enough to rule out cancer (Venes, 2009).

If fluid is aspirated, the FNA procedure may eliminate the lump altogether and provide a preliminary diagnosis. In some situations it is necessary to perform further testing. Additional evaluation may be indicated if the fluid is dark in color, or if the fluid-filled cyst has recurred several times, or if the sample has been obtained from a postmenopausal woman, who would not be expected to have breast cysts because of low estrogen levels. Clear fluid is usually indicative of a benign cyst; cloudy or bloody fluid may be present in benign or malignant tumors (Smith, 2007).

If no fluid is aspirated or if a residual thickened area remains after aspiration of the fluid, a core needle biopsy is performed. The false-positive rate for needle aspiration is almost zero. False-negative results occur more frequently because the needle may have missed the abnormal tissue. If no abnormalities are found with aspiration, follow-up mammography or sonography is recommended in

Figure 3-10 Fine needle breast biopsy

approximately 2 to 4 months to assess for recurrence of the cyst (Smith, 2007).

Core Needle Biopsy

In this technique a large-bore needle is used to remove a small cylinder of tissue. The needle placement is often guided as with the fine needle aspiration procedure. Core needle biopsy may be performed with the use of a local anesthetic in the office setting. The procedure may be painful, but there is usually little or no scarring. Core biopsy samples can identify invasive cancer and they can also provide prognostic biomarkers to help direct the course of treatment (Smith, 2007).

 Optimizing Outcomes— **With stereotactic biopsy**

The Mammotome and the Advanced Breast Biopsy Instrument (ABBI) are stereotactic biopsy methods that remove more tissue than a core needle biopsy. The Mammotome is a type of vacuum-assisted biopsy that uses a hollow probe instrument to remove about twice as much tissue as a core biopsy. Performed in the outpatient setting under local anesthesia, this procedure requires no stitches and leaves minimal scarring. The ABBI method uses a rotating circular knife equipped with a thin heated electrical wire to remove a large cylinder of abnormal tissue. This procedure requires sutures and is more likely to leave a minimal scar. In some centers, the biopsy is guided by an MRI, which locates the tumor, plots its coordinates, and precisely aims the stereotactic biopsy instrument into the tumor. Automated Tissue Excision and Collection (ATEC) is a biopsy technique that combines vacuum-assisted breast biopsy with MRI-assisted guidance. This method, which allows many samples to be taken through one small cut in the skin, requires only a local anesthetic. It is being studied in women who have had a personal or family history of breast cancer, in those who have had previous breast surgery, and in women with dense breast tissue who cannot be accurately screened with tests such as mammography or sonography (ACS, 2009d).

Surgical or Open Biopsy

In many instances, removal of all or a portion of the tissue for microscopic analysis may be indicated. When this is the case, a number of decisions must be made concerning the amount of tissue needed, since the goal is to obtain surgical margins that are free of possible malignant tissue. If possible, the incision is made near the areola of the nipple to minimize scarring and disfigurement. The surgical or open biopsy is considered the most accurate biopsy technique for large masses or for large areas of suspicion and may involve removal of the entire tumor (excisional biopsy) or a small part of a large tumor (incisional biopsy) (ACS, 2009d; Smith, 2007). Depending on the situation, the procedure may be performed using local anesthesia or regional anesthesia; if the tumor is deep inside the chest, general anesthesia may be required.

Skin ("Punch") Biopsy

A punch biopsy may be used to confirm a diagnosis of inflammatory breast cancer or Paget's disease (carcinoma of the mammary ducts) of the nipple.

Testing for Estrogen and Progesterone Receptors

Normal breast tissue contains hormone receptors that respond to the stimulatory effects of estrogen and progesterone. An estrogen receptor is a cellular protein that binds the female sex steroid hormones. When circulating estrogens attach to it, they stimulate the cells to transcribe DNA and manufacture proteins. This process typically leads to cellular growth and proliferation. Many types of breast cancers retain estrogen receptors, and for these particular tumors, estrogen enhances proliferation of the malignant cells. The same situation occurs with tumors having progesterone receptors.

An important component in the evaluation of a woman with early breast cancer is to test for the presence of hormone receptors. The estrogen and progesterone receptor proteins are present in the cell cytoplasm and may be located on the surface of some of the breast cancer cells. When present, the receptors bind to the estrogen or progesterone, and the binding promotes growth of the malignant cells. A malignant breast tumor may have estrogen receptors, progesterone receptors, or both types. Determining the patient's hormone receptor status through biologic testing of the tumor type provides valuable information concerning the predicted response to hormone manipulation therapy. Tumors that lack hormone receptors will not respond to hormone therapy. In general, postmenopausal women tend to be estrogen receptor positive; premenopausal women tend to be estrogen receptor negative (Venes, 2009).

Evaluating Breast Symptoms

Breast symptoms may occur in benign and malignant conditions. For example, the woman may experience nipple discharge, skin changes, or breast pain. It is important that each symptom be evaluated to determine its significance and the need for further testing or treatment.

NIPPLE DISCHARGE

Any spontaneous nipple discharge should be promptly evaluated. In most cases, nipple discharge results from a physiological event (e.g., infection) or hormonal imbalance. However, a small percentage of women who experience this symptom are diagnosed with a serious pituitary disorder or malignancy.

 Optimizing Outcomes— **Use of the ductogram to evaluate nipple discharge**

A ductogram is sometimes performed to determine the cause of nipple discharge. Also called a "galactogram," this test involves the placement of radiopaque dye (instilled via a tiny plastic tube) into the nipple. An x-ray is then taken to determine the presence of a ductal mass.

Galactorrhea (the continuation of milk secretion after breastfeeding has ceased) is characterized by a spontaneous bilateral, milky, sticky discharge. Galactorrhea normally occurs during pregnancy due to increased circulating levels of prolactin. Elevated prolactin levels may also be associated with a thyroid disorder, a pituitary tumor, chest wall surgery, or trauma. Some women develop galactorrhea during therapy with certain neuroleptic drugs or oral contraceptives. In addition to evaluation of serum prolactin levels, diagnostic testing may also include a ductogram, microscopic analysis of the nipple discharge, a thyroid profile, pregnancy testing, and mammography.

Serous or bloody nipple discharge may be caused by an intraductal papilloma, a rare, benign condition of unknown etiology that develops in the terminal nipple ducts. Purulent nipple discharge is typically associated with breast infection. Occasionally, breast cancer produces a spontaneous unilateral discharge that may be bloody, serous, or watery. The bloody discharge associated with breast cancer ranges from bright red to black and the serous discharge is thin, sticky, and yellow to light orange in color (Smith, 2007).

False discharge is a term that refers to fluid that appears on the nipple or areola but is not secreted by breast tissue. False discharge may be bloody, clear, colored, purulent, serous, or viscous. Various conditions such as eczema, dermatitis, nipple trauma, and Paget's disease may be associated with false nipple discharge.

 Nursing Insight— *Recognizing symptoms that may point to Paget's disease*

Paget's disease is an inflammatory, malignant neoplasm that originates in the nipple. This rare tumor accounts for only 1% of all cases of breast cancer. It usually occurs with invasive ductal carcinoma and can cause scaling, bleeding, oozing, and crusting of the nipple. The woman may complain of burning or itching in the affected area. Nurses should remind women that an important component of breast awareness and self-examination involves visualization and inspection of the nipples and that any changes should be promptly reported.

SKIN CHANGES

Erythema, or reddening of the skin, may be related to benign or malignant conditions. Infection, the most common cause of breast erythema in young women, is usually accompanied by increased tenderness and localized warmth. Infection is treated with a course of antibiotic therapy. Reddening that occurs at the end of the nipple may be associated with Paget's disease, and a biopsy is required for diagnosis. Changes in the breast skin color and texture that resemble orange peel (*peau d'orange*) may result from inflammatory breast cancer and require immediate evaluation. Other skin changes associated with inflammatory breast cancer include the presence of pink, purplish, or bruised skin; a pitting or ridging of the skin; and a nipple newly turning inward (Ruhl, 2007). **Mondor disease** of the breast is a rare, self-limiting condition characterized by thrombophlebitis of the superficial veins. Symptoms include skin redness, edema, and pain in the affected area. The condition may occur after trauma or appear without apparent cause. Although Mondor disease is usually benign, it may be associated with breast cancer and hypercoagulability (Marcovici, 2007; Venes, 2009).

BREAST PAIN

The most common type of breast pain occurs cyclically and is associated with the period of time that immediately precedes the onset of menses. While the exact etiology is unknown, cyclical breast pain has been linked to hormonal imbalances. The pain may be experienced in one or both breasts. An association between methylxanthines (a group of chemicals present in tea, colas, coffee, and chocolate) and premenstrual breast pain has been established. In general, breast pain is not associated with breast cancer, although women with breast cancer may complain of a localized tightening or pulling sensation or a localized burning or itching.

 Now Can You— **Discuss breast abnormalities?**

1. Describe the following types of breast masses: fibrocystic changes, fibroadenomas, intraductal papillomas, mammary duct ectasia?
2. Identify and describe four methods for evaluating breast abnormalities?
3. Explain the significance of testing for estrogen and progesterone receptors?

Breast Cancer

RISK FACTORS

Risk factors for breast cancer may be related to demographics, personal health history, lifestyle choices, and defects in certain genes. As is the case with many other diseases, the greater the number of risk factors that are present, the greater the likelihood of developing breast cancer. A listing of specific risk factors is presented in Box 3-1. It is important to note, however, that approximately 70% to 80% of women who develop breast cancer have none of the known risk factors (ACS, 2009b; Smith, 2007). Nurses may assist women in assessing their personal risk for breast cancer with the Breast Cancer Risk Assessment Tool.

 Optimizing Outcomes— **The Breast Cancer Risk Assessment Tool**

The National Cancer Institute (NCI) and the National Surgical Adjuvant Breast and Bowel Project (NSABP) have developed an interactive computer tool to estimate a woman's risk of developing invasive breast cancer. The tool, designed for use by health professionals, has recently been updated for African American women. The tool predicts a woman's risk of breast cancer in 5 years and over the lifetime (to age 90 years). Various risk factors, including present age, number of first-degree relatives affected, age at menarche, age at first live birth, the number of breast biopsies, and a history of abnormal hyperplasia in breast biopsy specimens, are assessed. The tool is available at the Web site http://www.cancer.gov/bcrisktool/ (NCI, 2009b).

Demographics and Personal Health History

Advancing age constitutes the single most important risk factor for breast cancer. A woman's risk increases as her age increases. According to the American Cancer Society,

Box 3-1 Risk Factors Associated with Breast Cancer

- Defects in breast cancer gene 1 (*BRCA1*) or breast cancer gene 2 (*BRCA2*)
- Gender: 100 times more likely to occur in females than in males
- Age: Increasing age—2 out of 3 invasive breast cancers occur in women age 55 and older
- Personal history of breast cancer in at least one breast
- Family history of breast cancer
- Exposure to chest radiation
- Excess weight
- Exposure to estrogen: early onset of menarche, late menopause, or use of hormonal therapy
- Race: Caucasians more likely to develop breast cancer than Hispanics or African Americans
- Smoking
- Exposure to carcinogens
- Excessive use of alcohol
- Diagnosis of precancerous breast changes
- Increased breast density revealed on mammography
- Exposure to diethylstilbestrol (DES)—mothers and female offspring

Source: American Cancer Society (2009b).

Lifestyle-Related Factors

Women who have had no children or who had their first child after age 30 have a slightly increased risk of breast cancer, owing to increased exposure to estrogen. Also, women who use oral contraceptives (OC) have a slightly greater risk of breast cancer than women who never used them. However, after discontinuation of OC use, the risk decreases; approximately 10 years after discontinuing the OC, there is no increased risk of breast cancer. Postmenopausal combined hormone therapy (i.e., estrogen + progestin) is associated with an increased risk of breast cancer; the use of estrogen alone for less than 10 years does not appear to increase the risk. Breastfeeding, especially for 1 to 2 years, appears to slightly reduce the risk for breast cancer (ACS, 2009b).

Being overweight or obese increases breast cancer risk, especially for postmenopausal women, and especially if the extra weight has been gained in adulthood and is accumulated at the waist. Following menopause, adipose tissue becomes the primary source of estrogen. Postmenopausal weight loss lowers circulating estrogen levels, and since estrogens are directly related to the risk of breast cancer, it is believed that weight loss may decrease the risk. Regular exercise also appears to reduce breast cancer risk; the American Cancer Society recommends 45 to 60 minutes of intentional physical activity 5 or more days a week (ACS, 2009b; Eliassen, Colditz, Rosner, et al., 2006; Hellwig, 2007; Theroux, 2007).

Alcohol use increases breast cancer risk, especially for women who drink more than 1 alcoholic beverage per day. Women who consume 2 to 5 alcoholic drinks daily have about 1½ times the risk of women who consume no alcohol. According to the American Cancer Society (2009b), women should limit their alcohol consumption to no more than 1 drink a day. Smoking or secondhand

approximately 1 out of 8 invasive breast cancer diagnoses are among women younger than age 45; approximately 2 out of 3 women with invasive breast cancer are age 55 or older when they are diagnosed (ACS, 2009b). Breast cancer is more prevalent in women than in men. In males, breast cancer accounts for only 0.7% of all breast cancer diagnoses (ACS, 2009b; Smith, 2007).

Caucasian women are more likely to develop breast cancer than are African American women. Statistically, however, African American women are more likely to die from their disease than are Caucasian women, and they are also more likely to be diagnosed with higher-grade tumors associated with a poorer prognosis. Reasons for this finding may include an inability to obtain health care or screening mammography, not following up after receiving abnormal test results, distrust of the healthcare system, and the belief that mammograms are not needed (U.S. Department of Health and Human Services [USDHHS], 2008). Also, higher-grade tumors may occur more frequently in African American women, even those who receive regular screening (Smith-Bindman, Miglioretti, Lurie, Abraham, Barbash, Strzelczyk, et al., 2006). Asian, Hispanic, and Native American women have an overall lower risk of developing and dying from breast cancer (ACS, 2009b; Centers for Disease Control and Prevention [CDC], 2009).

Women who currently have or have been previously diagnosed with cancer in one breast have three to four times the risk of developing new cancer in the same or other breast than do their counterparts who have never had breast cancer (ACS, 2009b). A history of a family member, especially a mother or sister, who received a diagnosis of breast cancer also increases the risk, especially if the cancer occurred prior to menopause. Interestingly, however, approximately 70% to 80% of women who develop breast cancer do not have a family history of this disease.

Family Teaching Guidelines...
Tips for Reducing Breast Cancer Risk

Nurses can teach families about simple at-home strategies that may reduce breast cancer risk:

Diet and exercise: Reducing calories and engaging in regular exercise may slow tumor growth and lower the amount of circulating leptin, a fat-released protein that has been linked to breast cancer.

Extra-virgin olive oil: Contains polyphenol compounds that suppress a breast cancer-promoting gene.

Apples: Phenols found in apples may combat malignant tumors.

Vitamin D: Prevents the division of cancer cells and activates a tumor-suppressing protein.

Folate: Consuming foods that contain the B-vitamin folate (e.g., leafy green vegetables, beans, and fortified cereals) may help to mitigate the increased breast cancer risk associated with drinking alcohol.

Soy supplements: Soy contains isoflavones, substances that act like estrogen and may stimulate the growth of certain types of breast cancer. Supplements that contain concentrated amounts of isoflavones should be avoided. However, healthy soy foods such as edamame, soy milk, and tofu are not considered harmful.

exposure to tobacco smoke as a risk factor for breast cancer is controversial; all women should be counseled to stop smoking and avoid secondhand smoke as a health-promoting strategy (ACS, 2009b).

 Nursing Insight— *Controversial breast cancer risk factors*

It has been suggested that various factors, including dietary fat, antiperspirants, bras, breast implants, environmental chemicals, abortions, and night work, increase the risk for breast cancer. It is important for nurses to know about these claims so that they can address their patients' concerns and provide appropriate counseling. The dietary intake of fat has not been clearly linked with an increased risk for breast cancer. However, high-fat diets can lead to obesity, which is a breast cancer risk factor. Although one postulate is that the absorption of chemicals in underarm antiperspirants may lead to cancer, there is no evidence to support this theory. Bras, purported to obstruct lymph flow, have also been implicated in the development of breast cancer. However, there is no scientific evidence to support this claim. Although breast implants do not increase breast cancer risk, scar tissue associated with the silicone implants may make mammography interpretation more difficult. Presently, there are no data supporting a definite link between breast cancer and environmental chemicals (e.g., DDE [a pesticide]; polychlorinated biphenyls [PCBs]). Neither induced nor spontaneous abortions are related to an increased risk for breast cancer. Some researchers have proposed that, owing to a disruption in the hormone melatonin, there is a link between working at night and breast cancer; this theory is currently undergoing investigation (ACS, 2009b).

Gene Defects

Approximately 5% to 10% of breast cancer cases are hereditary, resulting from gene defects, or mutations, passed on from a parent. The identification of the *BRCA1* and *BRCA2* genes was a pivotal discovery that clearly demonstrated the role of heredity and genetic mutations in the development of breast and ovarian cancer. It is estimated that approximately 10% of ovarian cancer cases and 3% to 5% of breast cancer cases are due to genetic mutations in *BRCA1* and *BRCA2*. Hereditary breast and ovarian cancer syndrome is an inherited cancer-susceptibility syndrome (ACOG, 2009; ACS, 2009b; Lessick, 2007).

 Clinical Alert

Recognizing Hallmarks of Hereditary Breast and Ovarian Cancer Syndrome

When taking the patient history, nurses must be aware of the following indicators of hereditary breast and ovarian cancer syndrome: multiple family members with breast cancer or ovarian cancer or both; the presence of both breast cancer and ovarian cancer in a single individual; and early age of breast cancer onset. Women with these risk factors can be referred for clinical genetic testing for gene mutations. Information gained from the testing allows for the identification of individuals who are at substantial risk of breast cancer and ovarian cancer and the timely institution of screening and prevention strategies to reduce the woman's personal risk (ACOG, 2009).

Approximately 1 in 300 to 1 in 800 individuals in the general population are estimated to carry a mutation in *BRCA1* or *BRCA2*. Normally, *BRCA1,* located on chromosome 17, and *BRCA2,* located on chromosome 13, help to prevent cancer by manufacturing proteins that halt the abnormal growth of cells. However, individuals who inherited a mutated copy of either gene from a parent have an increased risk of developing breast and/or ovarian cancer. For a woman with a *BRCA1* mutation, the risk of ovarian cancer is 39% to 46%. For a woman with a *BRCA2* mutation, the risk of ovarian cancer is 12% to 20%. The estimated lifetime risk of breast cancer with a *BRCA1* or *BRCA2* mutation is 65% to 74%. For women with breast cancer, the 10-year actuarial risk of developing subsequent ovarian cancer is 12.7% for *BRCA1* mutation carriers and 6.8% for *BRCA2* mutation carriers. In the United States, *BRCA* mutations occur most often in Jewish women of Ashkenazi (Eastern European) origin. In fact, an estimated 1 in 40 Ashkenazi Jews carries a specific "founder mutation" in *BRCA1* or *BRCA2*. Other rare gene mutations, such as ATM, p53, CHEK2, PTEN and CDH1, are less common causes of inherited breast cancer. Genetic testing to identify mutations in the *BRCA* and other genes is available; women who seek this testing should be offered counseling to help them make an informed decision (ACOG, 2009; ACS, 2009b; Hughes & Ravnikar, 2009).

TUMOR TYPES

There are several types of breast cancer. The majority of breast cancers represent a type of adenocarcinoma, which arises from the glandular tissue (i.e., ducts and lobules of the breast). Four subtypes account for most breast cancers. Occasionally, a single breast tumor can have a combination of these types or a mixture of invasive and in situ cancer. The term *in situ* indicates that the cancer cells remain confined to the ducts (ductal carcinoma in situ) or lobules (lobular carcinoma in situ); they have not penetrated into deeper breast tissues or spread to other organs in the body. Invasive carcinomas have grown beyond the layer of cells where the cancer originated. Most breast cancers are invasive carcinomas—either invasive ductal carcinoma or invasive lobular carcinoma (ACS, 2009e).

Ductal Carcinoma In Situ (DCIS) and Lobular Carcinoma In Situ (LCIS)

The most common type of noninvasive breast cancer, ductal carcinoma in situ, is confined within the ducts and has not spread into the surrounding breast tissue. DCIS accounts for approximately 1 in 5 new breast cancer cases. It is most often detected by mammography and has an excellent cure rate (ACS, 2009e).

Lobular carcinoma in situ (LCIS) (sometimes termed "lobular neoplasia") begins in the milk-producing glands and does not penetrate the wall of the lobules. LCIS is not considered a true cancer, although this neoplasm is sometimes classified as a type of noninvasive breast cancer. LCIS is rarely an invasive cancer, but women with this type have a higher risk of developing an invasive breast cancer in the same breast or in the opposite breast (ACS, 2009e).

Figure 3-11 Invasive ductal carcinoma

Invasive (Infiltrating) Ductal Carcinoma (IDC)

The most common type of breast cancer, invasive ductal carcinoma (IDC), originates in a mammary duct, penetrates through the ductal wall, and grows into the fatty tissue of the breast. (Fig. 3-11) Metastasis (spread) to other parts of the body may occur through the lymphatic system and bloodstream. Approximately 8 out of 10 invasive breast cancers are infiltrating ductal carcinomas. Women with this type of tumor usually present with a discrete, solitary breast mass (ACS, 2009e; Smith, 2007).

Invasive (Infiltrating) Lobular Carcinoma (ILC)

Invasive (infiltrating) lobular carcinoma (ILC) originates in the lobules (milk-producing glands). Like invasive ductal carcinoma, this neoplasm has spread into the fatty tissue and can metastasize to other parts of the body. Approximately 1 out of 10 invasive breast cancers is an ILC, and women with this type are more likely than those with other cancers to have bilateral disease. ILC may be harder to detect by mammography; breast MRI is often helpful in the diagnosis (ACS, 2009e; Capobianco, Spaliviero, Dessole, Rocca, Cherchi, Ambrosini et al., 2007; Smith, 2007).

Inflammatory Breast Cancer (IBC)

Inflammatory breast cancer (IBC) is a rare neoplasm that tends to grow more quickly and aggressively than the more common types of breast cancer. There is usually no lump or tumor, and the skin often exhibits changes similar to an infectious process such as mastitis. The affected breast may appear inflamed: red, thickened, tender, itchy, or larger than the unaffected breast. Because metastasis has usually occurred by the time of diagnosis, the cure rate is lower with IBC than with other types of breast cancer (Smith, 2007).

 Optimizing Outcomes— **Teaching about inflammatory breast cancer**

Although inflammatory breast cancer is rare, nurses should educate women about the signs and symptoms (ACS, 2009f):

* Breast swelling, which is usually sudden with one breast much larger than the other
* Itching
* A pink, red, or dark-colored area, sometimes with a texture like the skin of an orange (*peau d'orange*)
* Ridges and thickened areas of the skin

* Breast feeling warm to the touch
* Nipple retraction
* Breast pain

In the early stages, IBC may be mistaken for infection, resulting in a delay in diagnosis. Also, because there is no defined lump, this neoplasm may not be detected by mammography. MRI, which allows for precise measurement of the associated skin changes, is the most sensitive imaging test for IBC. Positron emission tomography (PET) scanning combined with computed tomography (CT) may be used to detect areas of metastasis (lymph nodes and organs) (ACS, 2009f).

 Ethnocultural Considerations… African American Women and Inflammatory Breast Cancer

Inflammatory breast cancer accounts for approximately 1% to 3% of all breast cancers diagnosed in the United States. Symptoms (e.g., redness, increased warmth, changes in the skin texture termed *peau d'orange* ["orange peel"]) that occur with this rare type of breast cancer are related to interference with lymph drainage by the malignant cells. Inflammatory breast cancer tends to occur more often in younger women; African American women appear to be at a higher risk than Caucasian women (ACS, 2009f).

INDICATORS OF DISEASE PROGNOSIS

A number of variables, such as the cancer stage, type, and tumor size, the presence of lymph node involvement (Fig. 3-12), and the presence of hormone receptor levels and HER2/neu (human epidermal growth factor receptor 2) in the tumor tissue, are associated with the likelihood of breast cancer recurrence.

 Nursing Insight— *Understanding about human epidermal growth factor receptor 2 (HER2/neu)*

Human epidermal growth factor receptor 2, a protein involved in normal cell growth, is found on some types of cancer cells, including breast and ovarian. Approximately 20% of breast cancers have an amplification (or overexpression) of the *HER2/neu* gene. Overexpression of this receptor in breast cancer is associated with increased disease recurrence and a worse prognosis. All newly diagnosed breast cancers should be tested for HER2/neu because HER2-positive cancers are more likely to benefit from treatment with medications that specifically target the HER2/neu protein, such as trastuzumab (Herceptin) and lapatinib (Tykerb) (ACS, 2009e; NCI, 2009c).

Identification of these factors allows for development of an individualized plan of treatment. The majority of women with negative lymph nodes (approximately 60% of women diagnosed with breast cancer today) will be cured by surgery alone. Approximately 30% of women with breast cancer will develop recurrent disease within 10 years of the initial treatment. In addition to identifying hormone receptor status and the histological tumor type,

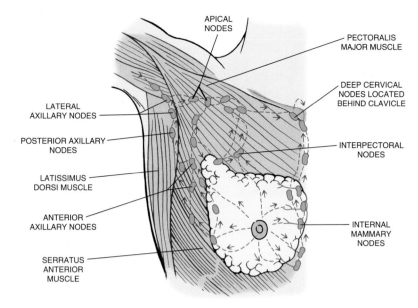

APICAL NODES

PECTORALIS MAJOR MUSCLE

DEEP CERVICAL NODES LOCATED BEHIND CLAVICLE

LATERAL AXILLARY NODES

POSTERIOR AXILLARY NODES

INTERPECTORAL NODES

LATISSIMUS DORSI MUSCLE

ANTERIOR AXILLARY NODES

INTERNAL MAMMARY NODES

SERRATUS ANTERIOR MUSCLE

Figure 3-12 Breast cancer: possible paths of lymphatic spread

information concerning the status of the axillary lymph nodes and the overall tumor size is useful in determining the disease prognosis (ACS, 2009e).

Axillary Nodes

It has long been recognized that tumor involvement of the axillary nodes is an important indicator for breast cancer prognosis. Clinical assessment of the axillary nodes is associated with a 30% false-positive and false-negative rate. Thus, pathological staging of the patient's lymph nodes is an essential step in the development of the treatment plan. Seventy percent of women with negative nodes survive 10 years following their breast cancer treatment. The disease prognosis worsens as the number of positive lymph nodes increases. Recurrence of breast cancer occurs in approximately 75% of women who have multiple positive nodes (Smith, 2007).

Sentinel node biopsy is a technique that targets selected lymph nodes during biopsy. A radioactive tracer (dye) injected into the region of the tumor travels through the lymphatic system to a lymph node. This node, termed the "sentinel node," is the first node that receives lymphatic drainage from the tumor. If no cancer is detected in this node, the patient is able to avoid more extensive lymph node surgery with its accompanying side effects, such as lymphedema (swelling of the arm) (ACS, 2009e).

Tumor Size

There is a direct relationship between the size of the tumor and the risk of recurrence. Prior to the widespread use of mammography, fewer than 8% of women with node-negative breast cancer had tumors that were less than 1 cm in diameter. Tumors of this size are associated with a relative 5-year survival that approaches 99%. Women with tumors that measure 1–3 cm have a relative 5-year survival rate of approximately 91%, and those with tumors that measure greater than 3 cm have a 5-year survival of approximately 85%. Women whose tumors are

greater than 3 cm have a breast cancer recurrence rate that exceeds 50% (Smith, 2007).

CANCER STAGING SYSTEM

The stage of cancer is based on the size of the tumor, the number of lymph nodes involved, and whether the cancer has spread. The American Joint Committee on Cancer TNM system is the most commonly used system to describe the stages of breast cancer. The *clinical stage* is based on findings from the physical examination, biopsy, and imaging tests; the *pathologic* stage combines these three diagnostic modalities with the results of surgery. Pathologic staging, which includes detailed information about the breast mass and adjacent lymph nodes, provides a more accurate description of the tumor.

 Optimizing Outcomes— Staging cancer to guide development of a treatment plan

The TNM staging system classifies cancers based on their T, N, and M stages:

- **T** = Tumor: size and spread within the breast and to nearby organs
- **N** = Nodes: spread to the lymph nodes
- **M** = Metastasis: spread to distant organs

Additional letters or numbers are added after the T, N, and M to provide further details about the tumor, lymph nodes, and metastasis to distant organs, such as the bones, lungs, brain, and liver. Breast cancer stage grouping is a process that combines the T, N, M information to allow for the identification of cancers with similar stages, which are usually treated in a similar way. Stage is delineated in Roman numerals and progresses from Stage I (least advanced) to Stage IV (most advanced); Stage 0 identifies noninvasive cancer (ACS, 2009g) (Box 3-2).

Box 3-2 The Breast Cancer Staging System

Stage 0: Ductal carcinoma in situ (DCIS), the earliest form of breast cancer.

Stage I: The tumor measures 2 cm in diameter or less and there is no involvement of the lymph nodes and no distant metastasis.

Stage II: The tumor measures 2.0 cm in diameter (or less) to 5.0 cm. Depending on the specific findings, the cancer may have spread to the axillary or internal mammary lymph nodes but has not spread to distant sites.

Stage IIIA: One of the following applies:

1. The tumor is not more than 5 cm across and has spread to 4–9 axillary lymph nodes, or it has enlarged the internal mammary lymph nodes; no distant metastasis.

2. The tumor is larger than 5 cm across and does not grow into the chest wall or skin. It has spread to 1–9 axillary nodes or to internal mammary nodes; no distant metastasis.

Stage IIIB: The tumor has grown into the chest wall or skin and one of the following applies:

1. No spread to the lymph nodes; no distant metastasis.

2. Spread to 1–3 axillary lymph nodes and/or small amounts of cancer are found in the internal mammary lymph nodes (per sentinel lymph node biopsy); no distant metastasis.

3. Spread to 4–9 axillary lymph nodes, or enlargement of the internal mammary lymph nodes; no distant metastasis.

Stage IIIC: The tumor is any size, and one of the following applies:

1. Cancer has spread to 10 or more axillary lymph nodes; no distant metastasis.

2. Cancer has spread to the lymph nodes beneath the clavicle; no distant metastasis.

3. Cancer has spread to the lymph nodes above the clavicle; no distant metastasis.

4. Cancer involves the axillary lymph nodes and there is enlargement of the internal mammary lymph nodes; no distant metastasis.

5. Cancer has spread to 4 or more axillary lymph nodes, small amounts of cancer are present in the internal mammary lymph nodes (per sentinel lymph node biopsy); no distant metastasis.

Stage IV: The cancer can be any size (any "T"), may or may not have spread to nearby lymph nodes (any "N"). It has metastasized ("M") to distant organs or to distant lymph nodes.

Source: ACS (2009g).

 Now Can You— **Discuss aspects of breast cancer diagnosis and staging?**

1. Identify and describe at least 12 risk factors associated with breast cancer?

2. Describe at least 6 signs and symptoms associated with inflammatory breast cancer?

3. Explain why the hormone receptor status, tumor type and size, and presence of positive axillary lymph nodes are important indicators for the overall breast cancer prognosis?

4. Explain what is meant by the TNM cancer staging system and why this information is useful?

BREAST CANCER TREATMENT

Medical management of breast cancer is complicated and may require a multitreatment approach, including surgery and adjunctive treatment, such as radiation, chemotherapy,

and hormone therapy. The simplest surgical treatment option is a lumpectomy: The lump and an area of surrounding normal tissue are removed. The lumpectomy is usually followed by radiation treatment to remove any remaining cancerous cells. A partial or segmental mastectomy involves removal of the tumor, the surrounding breast tissue, a portion of the lining of the chest wall, and some of the axillary lymph nodes. This procedure is usually followed with radiation therapy as well. A simple mastectomy involves the removal of all the breast tissue along with the area surrounding the nipple and areola. Radiation, chemotherapy, or hormone therapy may follow this surgical procedure. In a modified radical mastectomy, the entire breast and several axillary lymph nodes are removed, leaving the chest wall intact. While this procedure makes breast reconstruction easier for the patient, complications including lymphadenopathy and paresthesia are more likely to occur (ACS, 2009c).

 Optimizing Outcomes— **Counseling women about chemotherapy side effects**

When counseling patients about expected side effects from chemotherapy, nurses can reassure them that there are medications available now that are highly effective in reducing nausea and vomiting, the major symptoms traditionally associated with chemotherapy. Other side effects include a change in appetite, loss of hair, mouth or vaginal sores, suppression of the immune system that leads to an increased chance of infection, anemia, fatigue, menstrual cycle changes, and infertility. With the exception of infertility, most of the side effects are temporary (Smith, 2007).

Many women choose to undergo breast reconstruction after a mastectomy. This surgical option, performed by a plastic surgeon, is a personal decision that requires considerable individualized counseling and education. Since the reconstruction can be performed at the same time as the mastectomy, it is important to consider the options early. Breast reconstruction methods include use of a synthetic breast implant or reconstruction using one's own tissue. Synthetic implants typically are composed of a silicone shell filled with a saline solution. A tissue expander may be needed to cover the implant. To accomplish tissue expansion, an empty implant shell is placed under the skin and muscles and is gradually filled with the saline solution over several months. Once the skin is stretched sufficiently, the expander is removed and replaced with a permanent implant. Recovery usually takes several weeks.

Women who choose to undergo breast reconstruction using their own tissue may have a transverse rectus abdominis myocutaneous (TRAM) flap procedure. The breast is reconstructed using fat and muscle tissue taken from the abdomen, back, and buttocks. Recovery following the procedure usually takes 6 to 8 weeks, and there is an increased risk of infection and tissue necrosis. Deep inferior epigastric perforator (DIEP) reconstruction is a slightly less complicated surgical procedure. This method is similar to the TRAM flap procedure, but the abdominal muscles are left intact. The DIEP procedure is associated with fewer complications and less postoperative pain. Following reconstruction of the breast tissue, the surgeon can reconstruct the nipple and areola using tissue from other areas of the body. A small mound is constructed to resemble a nipple, and tattooing may be used to create an areola. In this situation, the surgeon applies a skin graft to the areolar region, slightly raises the skin, and then tattoos the skin graft.

Adjuvant therapies may include radiation therapy, chemotherapy, or hormone therapy. Radiation is usually begun 3 to 4 weeks after surgery, and treatments are given 5 days per week for 5 to 6 weeks. Chemotherapy that includes a combination two or more drugs may also be prescribed. Chemotherapeutics may be administered orally or intravenously and usually require four to eight treatments over 3 to 6 months. Hormone therapy is most commonly used to treat advanced metastatic cancer or as an adjuvant treatment to prevent recurrence of cancer. Normally, estrogen and progesterone bind to receptor sites in the breast tissue and encourage growth of cancerous cells. Prescribed hormone medications bind to the sites instead and prevent estrogen from reaching them. Medications used in hormone treatment include tamoxifen (Nolvadex), a selective estrogen receptor modulator (SERM), and aromatase inhibitors, which block the conversion of androgens into estrogen.

Nursing Insight— *Anti-angiogenesis therapy for cancer treatment*

Angiogenesis, which comes from the Greek words *angio* ("making new blood vessels") and *genesis* ("beginning"), is the process of making new blood vessels. Anti-angiogenesis is a targeted therapy that uses drugs or other substances to halt the tumor's production of new blood vessels. New anti-angiogenesis drugs that may prove useful in the treatment of breast cancer are currently under development and investigation (ACS, 2009h).

Optimizing Outcomes— **Using genomics to guide breast cancer care**

Genomic medicine encompasses the disciplines of gene mapping and sequencing and the study of the functions and interactions of all genes in the genome (a complete copy of the genetic material in an organism). Genomics focuses on developing tests that are both prognostic (i.e., based on factors such as tumor size, lymph node involvement, hormone receptor status) and predictive. *Prognostic* testing identifies the likelihood of cancer recurrence; *predictive* testing identifies the relative resistance of a cancer to specific treatments. Breast cancer specialists use information from genomics-driven specialized tests (e.g., Mammoprint; Oncotype DX; HOXB13/IL17BR) to develop an individualized treatment approach based on recurrence risk and predicted benefits of specific therapies (Moeller, 2008).

NURSING CARE FOR WOMEN DEALING WITH BREAST CANCER

Nurses must be sensitive to the fact that once a woman has received a diagnosis of breast cancer, her life is forever changed. Compassionate care during this difficult time

where research and practice meet:
Enhancing patient follow-up after breast cancer surgery

After surgery, women diagnosed with early stage breast cancer often benefit from treatment with chemotherapy, radiation, or hormonal therapy. For this reason, surgeons typically refer these patients to oncologists and assume that the cancer specialist is following up on them appropriately. Unfortunately, some women, especially African Americans and Hispanics, never see an oncologist. To keep these patients from being lost to follow-up, researchers developed a tracking system to determine if patients visited an oncologist and alert the surgeon to those who did not so that they could provide timely follow-up.

Bickell and colleagues (2008) compared the treatment of 639 women with early stage breast cancer who were seen at six city hospitals between January 1999 and December 2000 to 300 women who were seen between September 2004 and March 2006, the time period in which the tracking system was used. The rates of oncology consultations, chemotherapy, and hormonal therapy were higher for all women after the tracking system was in place. According to the investigators, the tracking system eliminated the racial disparity for African American and Hispanic women regarding the underuse of radiation, chemotherapy, and hormonal therapy. For example, after the tracking system was implemented, underuse of radiotherapy declined from 23% to 10%, underuse of chemotherapy decreased from 26% to 6%, and underuse of hormonal therapy diminished from 27% to 11% for African American and Hispanic women.

The researchers suggest two strategies to ensure that patients receive proper care for early stage breast cancer: Ensure that the tumor registry personnel follow up with patients to determine if they have visited an oncologist; and mandate that insurers require an oncology consultation for all patients diagnosed with invasive breast cancer to ensure that the women receive appropriate treatment. Nurses can be instrumental in ensuring proper oncology follow-up by counseling women about the importance of continued specialized cancer care after surgery and by participating in tracking efforts to prevent loss of patient contact after surgical intervention.

includes providing emotional support; empowering the patient and her family with current, evidence-based information; assisting them with immediate needs; and directing them to available resources. Personal and professional resources are essential as the woman works her way through the diagnostic process, the necessary decision-making concerning treatment and possible breast reconstruction, the surgery and adjuvant therapies, and the future with its uncertainties. Women who are confronted with breast cancer frequently discover an inner strength that they did not know existed. Examples of appropriate nursing diagnoses for women who have received a diagnosis of breast cancer are listed in Box 3-3.

Nurses can be a tremendous source of support and advocacy for women who are diagnosed with breast cancer. It is important to encourage patients to carefully consider all options and seek other opinions or other providers if they do not feel comfortable with recommendations. Nurses can direct women to the wealth of reliable information about breast cancer treatment and recovery available in books and on Internet sites and to the opportunities for personal sharing through local and national support groups.

Box 3-3 Examples of Nursing Diagnoses for Women Diagnosed With Breast Cancer

- Anticipatory grieving
- Anxiety
- Body image disturbance
- Denial
- Dysfunctional grieving
- Fear
- Grief
- Hopelessness
- Impaired skin integrity
- Ineffective individual or family coping
- Knowledge deficit
- Low self-esteem
- Pain
- Powerlessness
- Spiritual distress

 Collaboration in Caring— *Resources for women with cancer*

An important nursing role in the care of women with cancer centers on sharing information about the various resources that are available to them. These include:

- National Breast and Cervical Cancer Early Detection Program, NCCDPHP, CDC
- National Cancer Institute, NIH, HHS
- Office of Minority Health, OPHS, OS, HHS
- American Cancer Society
- Cancer.net
- BreastCancerTrials.org
- Celebrating Life Foundation
- Sisters Network® Inc.
- Susan G. Komen Breast Cancer Foundation
- Lance Armstrong Foundation and University of Pennsylvania
- NCI Community Cancer Centers Program
- National Coalition for Cancer Survivorship

For many, holistic medicine offers an additional healing approach to assist the body, mind, and spirit through the rigors of cancer diagnosis and treatment and to foster healing throughout the recovery process. The woman's immune system can be supported and enhanced naturally through dietary and safe herbal remedies, along with practices that reduce stress and help restore physical and emotional harmony and balance. For example, patients may benefit from imagery, aromatherapy, meditation, music therapy, dance therapy, journal writing, humor, art therapy, and hypnosis. Other modalities such as acupuncture, Ayurveda, Qigong, yoga, and tai chi may provide relief from unpleasant symptoms and be instrumental in lifting the body and spirit during the journey to recovery.

 Optimizing Outcomes— **Complementary and alternative therapies for cancer patients**

Many women find that various complementary and alternative therapies help to relieve cancer side effects and discomforts and enhance and enrich their lives during treatment and into recovery. Nurses can empower women with specific information and direct them to available resources. The American Cancer Society provides an up-to-date Internet source for complementary and alternative therapies. It is available at http://www.cancer.org/docroot/ETO/ETO_5.asp?sitearea5ETO.

Today there are an estimated 11 million cancer survivors living in the United States. Nurses who care for women across the life span are likely to see patients who are dealing with the psychosocial and physical effects of cancer treatments, which may occur for months or years after the treatment has ended. Development of a cancer survivorship care plan can help to ensure coordination of care and appropriate follow-up and empower the woman to understand and participate in her continuing care (Ruhl, 2009). Cancer survivorship care plans have been recommended by a variety of groups, including the Institute of Medicine (IOM), which, along with the National Research Council, produced a major report on cancer survivorship in 2005 (Greenwood & Stovall, 2005).

 Optimizing Outcomes— **With a cancer survivorship care plan**

First introduced for survivors of childhood cancers, cancer survivorship care plans have recently been recommended for adult survivors. Components of the survivorship plan, which should be provided to the patient's primary care physician, include a summary of treatment, the possible short- and long-term effects of treatment, late toxicity monitoring, monitoring for primary cancer recurrence or a second cancer, identification of the provider responsible for survivor care, psychological and vocational needs, community support resources, and recommendations for preventive care and practices. For women, additional information should include genetic issues, the effects of treatment on future pregnancy and fertility, and menopausal issues (Cox, 2009; Ganz & Hahn, 2008; Ruhl, 2009; Ruhl & Moran, 2008).

Nurses are perfectly situated to provide cancer survivor care. With a holistic and family-centered approach that emphasizes patient education, health promotion, and preventive care practices, nursing can fully embrace the cancer survivorship movement to empower women and their providers with a comprehensive, holistic plan for continuing care in the aftermath of cancer. Owing to the dynamic nature of the survivorship plan, evolving scientific evidence about the specific cancer type, management of short- and long-term treatment sequelae, and the need for screening for recurrence and other cancers can be readily incorporated into the plan. This information can help to inform the woman's decision-making and allow her and her care provider to be proactive in both the planning and management of her health after cancer (Ruhl, 2009).

case study: Midlife Woman Treated for Breast Cancer

Dorothy is a 56-year-old postmenopausal Caucasian woman who received a diagnosis of early stage breast cancer approximately 6 months ago. Dorothy's treatment, which included a lumpectomy followed by radiation therapy, was uncomplicated and her physician has told her that her chance for a cure is "excellent."

Today, during an interview at the woman's health clinic, Dorothy confides in the nurse that she is concerned about herself because she feels "down and out." She admits that physically, she feels just fine and is very relieved to have the treatment behind her. Lately, however, she has been concerned about "the way my body looks." As a result of the surgery and radiation therapy, Dorothy has experienced a decrease in breast size in the affected breast. Although she acknowledges that "in the grand scheme of things, this change is a minor thing," the alteration in breast appearance is concerning to her.

critical thinking questions

1. What is a priority nursing intervention for Dorothy?
2. What information should the nurse provide to Dorothy?
3. What other actions should the nurse take?

♦ See suggested answers to case studies on DavisPlus.

 Now Can You— Discuss aspects of breast cancer treatment?

1. Identify four treatment modalities for breast cancer?
2. Describe the nurse's role in breast cancer treatment care?
3. Identify the components of a cancer survivorship care plan and explain why this information is useful?

summary points

♦ Maintaining breast health is an essential strategy for maintaining optimal physical and psychological health.

♦ Nurses are in an ideal position to educate women about breast health and strategies for the identification of benign and malignant breast disease.

♦ Breast cancer is the most common cancer in women in the United States, except for skin cancer, and it is the second leading cause of cancer deaths in women.

♦ Dietary, socioeconomic, and environmental factors most likely contribute to the development of breast cancer.

♦ A number of screening and diagnostic methods, including mammography, ultrasonography, magnetic resonance imaging, and biopsy, may be used in the clinical evaluation of the breasts.

• Risk factors for breast cancer may be related to demographics, personal health history, lifestyle choices, and defects in certain genes.

• The cancer staging system, based on the size of the tumor, the number of lymph nodes involved, and the presence of metastasis, is used to guide the development of a treatment plan for breast cancer.

• Breast cancer treatment may include surgery, radiation, chemotherapy, hormone therapy, and complementary and alternative therapies.

• The nursing role in caring for women with breast cancer includes providing emotional support, empowering the patient and her family with current information, assisting them with immediate needs, and directing them to available resources.

review questions

Multiple Choice

1. When teaching women how to perform proper breast self-examination (BSE), the nurse advises:
   a. Avoid the axillary area
   b. Refrain from squeezing the nipples
   c. Place the arm adjacent to the breast being examined in a relaxed position alongside the thigh
   d. Use the finger pads to apply light, medium, and firm pressure

2. Breast magnetic resonance imaging (MRI) is useful in screening:
   a. Women with recently diagnosed breast cancer
   b. Postmenopausal women
   c. All women
   d. Women whose screening mammograms are satisfactory

3. Ultrasound can reveal whether a breast mass is:
   a. Malignant
   b. Benign
   c. Fluid-filled or solid
   d. Potentially malignant

4. Known risk factors for breast cancer include:
   a. Slender body type
   b. Pregnancy before the age of 20
   c. Age greater than 50
   d. Menopause before the age of 50

5. Treatment for breast cancer may include:
   a. Estrogen therapy
   b. Anti-angiogenesis drugs
   c. Lactation suppressants
   d. Oral contraceptives

REFERENCES

Aliotta, H.M., & Schaeffer, N.J. (2006). Breast conditions. In K.D. Schuiling & F. E. Likis (Eds.), *Women's gynecologic health*. Sudbury, MA: Jones & Bartlett Publishers.

American Cancer Society (ACS). (2008). *How to perform a breast self-exam*. Retrieved from http://www.cancer.org/docroot/CRI/content/CRI_2_6x_How_to_perform_a_breast_self_exam_5.asp (Accessed October 1, 2009).

American Cancer Society (ACS). (2009a). *How many women get breast cancer?* May 6, 2009. Retrieved from http://www.cancer.org/docroot/CRI/content/CRI_2_2_1X_How_many_people_get_breast_cancer_5.asp (Accessed September 13, 2009).

American Cancer Society (ACS). (2009b). *What are the risk factors for breast cancer?* Retrieved from http://www.cancer.org/docroot/CRI/content/CRI_2_4_2X_What_are_the_risk_factors_for_breast_cancer_5.asp?sitearea= (Accessed October 29, 2009).

American Cancer Society (ACS). (2009c). *Cancer reference information*. Retrieved from http://www.cancer.org/docroot/CRI/content/CRI_2_4_6x_For_Women_Facing_a_Breast_Biopsy.asp (Accessed October 5, 2009).

American Cancer Society (ACS). (2009d). *Mammograms and other breast imaging procedures*. Retrieved from http://www.cancer.org/docroot/CRI/content/CRI_2_6X_Mammography_and_other_Breast_Imaging_Procedures_5.asp?sitearea= (Accessed October 6, 2009).

American Cancer Society (ACS). (2009e). *What is breast cancer?* Retrieved from http://www.cancer.org/docroot/CRI/content/CRI_2_4_1X_What_is_breast_cancer_5.asp?sitearea= (Accessed October 15, 2009).

American Cancer Society (ACS). (2009f). *Inflammatory breast cancer*. Retrieved from http://www.cancer.org/docroot/CRI/content/CRI_2_6X_Inflammatory_Breast_Cancer.asp (Accessed October 16, 2009).

American Cancer Society (ACS). (2009g). *How is breast cancer staged?* Retrieved from http://www.cancer.org/docroot/CRI/content/CRI_2_4_3X_How_is_breast_cancer_staged_5.asp?rnav=cri (Accessed October 16, 2009).

American Cancer Society (ACS). (2009h). *Anti-angiogenesis treatment*. Retrieved from http://www.cancer.org/docroot/ETO/eto_1_3_Antiangiogenesis_Therapy.asp (Accessed October 17, 2009).

American College of Obstetricians and Gynecologists (ACOG). (2007). *Guidelines for women's health care: A resource manual*. (3rd ed.). Washington, DC: Author.

American College of Obstetricians and Gynecologists (ACOG). (2009). *Hereditary breast and ovarian cancer syndrome* (Practice Bulletin No. 103). *Obstetrics and Gynecology, 113*(4), 957–966.

Barclay, L. (2009). *New breast cancer screening guidelines opposed*. Retrieved from http://www.medscape.com/viewarticle/712720?src (Accessed January 5, 2010).

Barr, J.K., Giannotti, T.E., Van Hoof, T.J., Mongoven, J., & Curry, M. (2008). Understanding barriers to participation in mammography by women with disabilities. *American Journal of Health Promotion, 22*(6), 381–385.

Bickell, N.A., Shastri, K., Fei, K., Oluwole, S., Godfrey, H., Hiotis, K., Srinivasan, A., & Guth, A.A. (2008). A tracking and feedback registry to reduce racial disparities in breast cancer care. *Journal of the National Cancer Institute, 100*(23), 1717–1723.

Bleicher, R.J., Ciocca, R.M., Egleston, B.L., Sesa, L., Evers, K., Sigudson, E.R., & Morrow, M. (2009). Association of routine pretreatment magnetic resonance imaging with time to surgery, mastectomy rate and margin status. *Journal of the American College of Surgeons, 209*(2), 180–187.

BreastCancer.org. (2008). *Breast cancer statistics*. Retrieved from http://www.breastcancer.org/symptoms/understand_bc/statistics.jsp (Accessed October 11, 2009).

Buzek, N. (2009). Breast tomosynthesis: The future of breast imaging? *Advance for Nurse Practitioners, 17*(10), 25–28.

Capobianco, G., Spaliviero, B., Dessole, S., Rocca, P.C., Cherchi, P.L., Ambrosini, G., Meloni F., & Meloni, G.B. (2007). Lymph node axillary metastasis from occult contralateral infiltrating lobular carcinoma arising in accessory breast: MRI diagnosis. *Breast Journal, 13*(3), 305–307.

Centers for Disease Control and Prevention (CDC). (2009). *Breast cancer rates by race and ethnicity*. Retrieved from http://www.cdc.gov/cancer/breast/statistics/race.htm (Accessed October 12, 2009).

Cox, T. (2009). *Breast cancer survivorship*. Oncology Nursing Society Special Interest Group Newsletter, 7:1. Retrieved from http://onsop-content.ons.org/Publications/SIGNewsletters/sur/sur7.1.html (Accessed October 29, 2009).

Diekmann, F., & Bick, U. (2007). Tomosynthesis and contrast-enhanced digital mammography: Recent advances in digital mammography. *European Journal of Radiology, 17*(12), 3086–3092.

Eliassen, A.H., Colditz, G.A., Rosner, B., Willet, W.C., & Hankinson, S. C. (2006). Adult weight change and risk of postmenopausal breast cancer. *Journal of the American Medical Association, 296*(2), 193–201.

Farmer, D., Reddick, B., D'Agostino Jr., R., & Jackson, S.A. (2007). Correlates of mammography screening in older African American women. *Oncology Nursing Forum, 34*(1), 117–123.

Ganz, P.A., & Hahn, E.E. (2008). Implementing a survivorship care plan for patients with breast cancer. *Journal of Clinical Oncology, 26*(8), 659–767.

Hartman, L.C., Sellers, T.A., Frost, M.H, Lingle, W.L., Degnim, A.C., Ghosh, K., Vierkant, R.A., Maloney, S.D., Pankratz, S., Hillman, D. W., Suman, V.J., Johnson, J., Blake, C., Tlsty, T., Vachon, C.M., Melton, L.J., & Visscher, D.W. (2005). Benign breast disease and the risk of breast cancer. *New England Journal of Medicine, 353*(3), 229–237.

Hellwig, J.P. (2007). Breast cancer: Lower fat intake may reduce recurrence. *Nursing for Women's Health, 11*(2), 121–122; 124–128.

Hughes, K.S., & Ravnikar, V. (2009 Suppl). Risk assessment and management of women with BRCA mutations. *The Female Patient, 34*(11), 1–4.

Kang, H.S., Thomas, E., Kwon, B.E., Hyun, M.S., & Jun, E.M. (2008). Stages of change: Korean women's attitudes and barriers toward mammography screening. *Health Care for Women International, 29*(2), 151–164.

Kim, J.H., & Kim, O. (2008). Predictors of perceived barriers to mammography in Korean women. *Asian Nursing Research, 2*(2), 74–81.

Knutson, D., & Steiner, E. (2007). Screening for breast cancer. Current recommendations and future directions. *American Family Physician, 75*(11), 1660–1666.

Lee, E. (2009). Evidence-based management of benign breast diseases. *The American Journal for Nurse Practitioners, 13*(7/8), 22–31.

Lehman, C.D., Gastonis, C., Kuhl, C., Hendrick, R.E., Pisano, E.D., Hanna, L., Peacock, S., et al. (2007). MRI Evaluation of the contralateral breast in women with recently diagnosed breast cancer. *The New England Journal of Medicine, 356*(13), 1295–1303.

Lessick, M. (2007). Genetic testing for breast and ovarian cancer: Ethical, legal, and psychosocial considerations. *Nursing for Women's Health, 11*(4), 390–401.

Makuc, D.M., Breen, N., Meissner, H.I., Vernon, S.W., & Cohen, A. (2007). Financial barriers to mammography: Who pays out-of-pocket? *Journal of Women's Health, 16*(3), 349–360.

Marcovici, I. (2007). Mondor disease of the breast. *Female Patient, 32*(10), 53–58.

Moeller, M. (2008). Genomics in breast cancer care. *Women's Health Care: A Practical Journal for Nurse Practitioners, 7*(9), 19–24.

National Cancer Institute (2009a). *Fact sheet: Mammograms*. Retrieved from http://www.nci.nih.gov/cancertopics/factsheet/Detection/screening-mammograms (Accessed October 11, 2009).

National Cancer Institute (2009b). *Breast Cancer Risk Assessment Tool*. Retrieved from http://www.cancer.gov/bcrisktool/Default.aspx (Accessed October 15, 2009).

National Cancer Institute. (2009c). *General information about breast cancer*. Retrieved from http://www.cancer.gov/cancertopics/pdq/treatment/breast/HealthProfessional/page2 (Accessed October 16, 2009).

Pisano, E., Gastonis, C., Hendrick, E., Yaffe, M., Braum, J., Acharyya, S., et al. (2005). Diagnostic performance of digital versus film mammography for breast cancer screening: The results of the American College of Radiology Imaging Network (ACRIN) digital mammographic imaging screening trial (DMIST). *The New England Journal of Medicine, 353*(17), 1773–1783.

Pomeranz, S.J. (2007). Breast MRI scans: What women need to know. *Radiology Today, 8*(10), 8–10.

Rafferty, E.A. (2004). Tomosynthesis: New weapon in breast cancer fight. *Imaging Economics*. Retrieved from http://www.imagingeconomics.com/issues/articles/2004-04_12.asp (Accessed October 11, 2009).

Rafferty, E.A. (2007). Digital mammography: Novel applications. *Radiologic Clinics of North America, 45*(1), 831–843.

Ruhl, C. (2007). Breast health screening: What all women should know. *Nursing for Women's Health, 11*(3), 326–330.

Ruhl, C. (2009). Cancer survivor care planning: A dynamic approach to cancer survivors' futures. *Nursing for Women's Health, 13*(5), 427–431.

Ruhl, C., & Moran, B. (2008). The clinical content of preconception care; preconception care for special populations. *American Journal of Obstetrics and Gynecology, 199*(6), (Suppl. B), S384–S388.

Smith, E.C. (2007). Breast cancer fundamentals. *Clinician Reviews, 17*(10), 32–40.

Smith-Bindman, R., Miglioretti, D.L., Lurie, N., Abraham, L., Barbash, R.B., Strzelczyk, J., et al. (2006). Does utilization of screening mammography explain racial and ethnic differences in breast cancer? *Annals of Internal Medicine, 144*(8), 541–553.

Theroux, R. (2007). Breast cancer after menopause: Do weight and exercise affect risk? *Nursing for Women's Health, 11*(3), 319–321.

U.S. Department of Health & Human Services (USDHHS). (2000). *Healthy People 2010.* Washington, DC: Author.

U.S. Department of Health & Human Services (USDHHS). (2008). *Minority women's health: Breast cancer.* Retrieved from http://64.94.16.210/minority/africanamerican/bc.cfm (Accessed October 12, 2009).

U.S. Preventive Services Task Force. (2009a). *Screening for breast cancer. Guide to preventive services, 2009, Section 2. Recommendations for adults.* Retrieved from http://www.ahrq.gov/clinic/pocketgd09/gcp09s2.htm (Accessed October 1, 2009).

U.S. Preventive Services Task Force. (2009b). Screening for breast cancer: U.S. Preventive Services Task Force recommendation statement. *Annals of Internal Medicine, 151*(10), 716–726.

Venes, D (Ed.). (2009). *Taber's cyclopedic medical dictionary* (21st ed.). Philadelphia: F.A. Davis.

Wang, J.H., Mandelblatt, J.S., Liang, W., Yi, B., Ma, I-Jung, & Schwartz, M.D. (2009). Knowledge, cultural, and attitudinal barriers to mammography screening among nonadherent immigrant Chinese women. *Cancer, 15*(20), 4828–4838.

Young, R.F., & Severson, R.K. (2005). Breast cancer screening barriers and mammography completion in older minority women. *Breast Cancer Research and Treatment, 89*(2), 1573–1577.

 For more information, go to http://davisplus.fadavis.com/

Promoting Reproductive Health Through an Understanding of Various Gynecological Disorders

Shelton Hisley, PhD, RNC, WHNP-BC

Both within the family and without,
our sisters hold up our mirrors,
our images of who we are and of
who we can dare to become.

—Elizabeth Fishel

LEARNING TARGETS *At the completion of this chapter, the student will be able to:*

◆ Describe various gynecological disorders and discuss implications for patient counseling and teaching.

◆ Describe various causes of abnormal uterine bleeding.

◆ Develop a nursing plan of care for a patient with a diagnosis of endometriosis.

◆ Develop a nursing plan of care for a patient with a diagnosis of polycystic ovary syndrome.

◆ Identify signs and symptoms that may be associated with vaginal, ovarian, endometrial, and vulvar carcinoma.

◆ Describe a strategy for increasing women's awareness of potential ovarian cancer symptoms.

◆ Teach a woman how to perform vulvar self-examination.

Introduction

This chapter explores several gynecological disorders in women. To deliver safe, effective care, nurses who care for women should be familiar with the special aspects of various gynecological conditions. It is important to remember that the human body functions as a whole system. Although a gynecological problem may initially appear to be confined to the pelvis, it could actually result from a host of other influences, activities, and imbalances. For example, amenorrhea, or absence of menses, may be related to excessive exercise, eating disorders, obesity, weight loss, stress, chronic illness, or endocrine disorders that adversely affect the normal functioning of the menstrual cycle (American College of Obstetricians and Gynecologists [ACOG], 2007).

Mutual trust and respect in the nurse–patient relationship help to facilitate appropriate discussion of questions and concerns about various health issues. Women's emotional responses to certain gynecological disorders may profoundly affect their quality of life and ability to function. The nurse must always remain sensitive to women's unique problems related to the functioning of their reproductive systems and offer holistic, individualized care that empowers them to seek and embrace strategies to restore balance and control over their lives.

Menstrual Disorders

Menstrual disorders, specifically amenorrhea, irregular bleeding, and dysmenorrhea, constitute some of the most common reproductive problems in women. Premenstrual syndrome, another problem frequently encountered in the clinical setting, is discussed in Chapter 2. Potential nursing diagnoses for women with various menstrual disorders are presented in Box 4-1.

AMENORRHEA

Under normal circumstances, the menstrual cycle is dependent on the integrated functioning of the hypothalamus, pituitary gland, ovaries, uterus, cervix, and vagina. Amenorrhea, or a lack of menstruation, may result from abnormalities of the structure or function of any of these organs.

The term *amenorrhea* is rooted from the Greek "a" = no + "men" = month + "rhoia" = flow = "no monthly flow." Amenorrhea may be classified as "primary" or "secondary." With primary amenorrhea, menstruation never takes place. With secondary amenorrhea, menstruation starts but then stops. The nurse should refer the patient for an evaluation for amenorrhea when the following circumstances are present.

Primary

- Lack of secondary sex characteristics by age 14–15
- Lack of menarche (the initial menstrual period) by age 15
- Lack of menses within 3 years after breast development (thelarche) or the appearance of pubic or axillary hair (pubarche or adrenarche) (ACOG, 2007)

Primary amenorrhea may be caused by a number of conditions, including pregnancy, lactation, missed abortion, eating disorders (e.g., anorexia nervosa, bulimia), obesity, hyperthyroidism, hypoglycemia, cystic fibrosis, Crohn's disease, genetic abnormalities, congenital absence of the cervix and/or vagina, and polycystic ovary syndrome.

Secondary

Secondary amenorrhea is defined as an absence of menses for at least 3 months in a woman who has previously had regular monthly menses, or a lack of menses for at least 6 to 12 months in a woman who normally experiences irregular menses. The term *delayed menses* is used in situations where the amenorrhea is for a shorter period of time (ACOG, 2007; Hatcher et al., 2008). Pregnancy, lactation, premature ovarian failure (menopause before age 40), weight loss, eating disorders, and obesity are conditions that may cause secondary amenorrhea. Other causes include hormonal contraceptive effects and post–oral contraceptive pill amenorrhea, pituitary gland dysfunction (e.g., hyperprolactinemia), polycystic ovary syndrome,

emotional or physical stress, frequent strenuous exercise, chronic illness (e.g., colitis, kidney failure, cystic fibrosis), cancer chemotherapy, ovarian cysts or tumors, and certain endocrine disorders such as Cushing's syndrome and thyroid dysfunction (ACOG, 2007).

When evaluating a patient for amenorrhea, the first step is to test for pregnancy. Once pregnancy has been ruled out, the patient undergoes a thorough physical examination and, depending on the findings, additional testing that may include laboratory and diagnostic testing (e.g., ultrasonography). In many situations, a careful review of the woman's health history can provide clues as to the cause(s) of the amenorrhea (ACOG, 2007; Hatcher et al., 2008).

 Nursing Insight*— *Perspectives on amenorrhea

Amenorrhea is a symptom, not a condition. In the United States, approximately 2% to 5% of all women of childbearing age are affected by amenorrhea. Although the cause is generally not a life-threatening condition, amenorrhea can be associated with significant potential morbidity. In most situations, amenorrhea is reversible with treatment for the underlying condition (ACOG, 2007).

ABNORMAL GENITAL BLEEDING

Any bleeding other than what is expected in a normal ovulatory cycle is considered abnormal genital bleeding. This condition constitutes one of the most frequent reasons for patient visits to the clinic or private office and accounts for approximately 19% of all gynecological complaints. The source of the bleeding may be the rectum, urinary tract, vulva, vagina, cervix, or uterus. Conditions that may cause abnormal bleeding include pregnancy and pregnancy-related complications, trauma, infection, endocrine abnormalities, lesions, or tumors (ACOG, 2007; Nelson & Baldwin, 2008).

 Nursing Insight*— *Understanding correct terminology for abnormal genital bleeding

Nurses who care for women should be familiar with terminology for abnormal genital bleeding, which is classified by the timing of the bleeding and the duration of the flow. The use of accurate terminology helps to promote effective communication and justifies appropriate work-ups and therapies. Patient-recorded menstrual calendars are beneficial in facilitating the accurate documentation of bleeding patterns.

- *Metrorrhagia* is bleeding that occurs at abnormal times during an ovulatory cycle—that is, the woman experiences bleeding more frequently than every 21 days.
- *Menorrhagia* is excess bleeding (80 mL or more, or bleeding that lasts longer than 7 days) during the expected time of menstrual flow.
- *Menometrorrhagia* is a combination of the above two bleeding abnormalities—the woman experiences excessive bleeding and frequent bleeding at abnormal times during the cycle.
- *Polymenorrhea* is bleeding that occurs at short intervals (less than 21 days).

Intermenstrual bleeding is bleeding of variable amounts that occur between regular menses.

Postcoital bleeding is bleeding that occurs after sexual intercourse (ACOG, 2007; Nelson & Baldwin, 2008; Stern, 2009).

A number of possible diagnoses are associated with bleeding disorders. Although many factors influence a woman's menstrual patterns, one of the first considerations is the patient's age. In an adolescent female, approximately 20 hormonal cycles occur before ovulation takes place on a regular basis. Bleeding that is irregular in both timing and amount tends to be the rule rather than the exception during early adolescence. Similarly, perimenopausal women commonly experience an increased variation in their menstrual intervals and in the quantity of flow during the 5 years that precede menopause. The cause of abnormal genital bleeding can range from simple to complex. Evaluation requires a careful and thorough history and work-up, including a physical examination, laboratory tests, and appropriate diagnostic tests such as ultrasonography (Nelson & Baldwin, 2008; Speroff & Fritz, 2005).

 Optimizing Outcomes— Using patient age to guide the work-up for abnormal genital bleeding

The patient's age is an important consideration in the evaluation of abnormal genital bleeding. For example, during *adolescence*, a common cause is persistent anovulation, or failure to ovulate, which may be related to contraception, pregnancy, polycystic ovary syndrome, or coagulopathies.

During *mid-life* (30s–40s), women most often develop abnormal genital bleeding from pregnancy, structural lesions (e.g., leiomyomata [fibroid tumors], polyps), and anovulation, including that caused by polycystic ovary syndrome, hormone therapy, and endometrial hyperplasia.

During *menopause*, bleeding most often results from hormone therapy, endometrial atrophy, leiomyomata, endometrial hyperplasia, and malignancy (ACOG, 2007; Nelson & Baldwin, 2008).

DYSMENORRHEA

Dysmenorrhea, defined as painful menstruation, is one of the most common gynecological problems occurring in women of all ages. For most, the pain develops during or shortly before the onset of menstruation and is most intense in the suprapubic region or in the lower abdomen. Symptoms including nausea, vomiting, diarrhea, headaches, and lightheadedness may accompany the pain. Dysmenorrhea can cause significant disruption with daily activities each month, resulting in absence from school and missed time from work. Dysmenorrhea may be classified as primary (intrinsic and usually early onset) or secondary (results from some other physical cause and usually has a later onset) (Nelson & Baldwin, 2008).

Primary dysmenorrhea usually begins within 1 to 3 years following menarche and results from physiological causes—no pathology is present. In general, women with primary dysmenorrhea are ovulatory and thus produce progesterone in the luteal phase. Progesterone stimulates the production of prostaglandins in the base of the endometrium. Found in various tissues throughout the body, prostaglandins are substances that control local functions such as vasodilation and vasoconstriction. Women with primary dysmenorrhea produce excessive amounts of prostaglandin F2-alpha, which increases the force of the uterine contractions. Uterine contractions reduce blood flow to the uterus, causing ischemia and pain. The pain usually begins at the onset of menstrual flow and persists for 8 to 48 hours. During menstruation, the highest levels of prostaglandins are released during the first 48 hours. When the prostaglandins are introduced into the general circulation by uterine contractions, they can produce symptoms of headache, nausea, vomiting, and diarrhea (ACOG, 2007; Nelson & Baldwin, 2008).

Secondary dysmenorrhea is due to some other physical cause and usually is of a later onset. Women with secondary dysmenorrhea also complain of painful uterine cramping with menstruation but frequently have other accompanying complaints, such as dyspareunia or nonmenstrual pelvic pain. By definition, pain that occurs with secondary dysmenorrhea is related to uterine or pelvic pathology. The treatment for secondary dysmenorrhea should be targeted to the underlying cause and should be reflective of the patient's desire for fertility. When surgical intervention is not required, the treatments helpful for primary dysmenorrhea are often successful in reducing the symptoms of secondary dysmenorrhea (ACOG, 2007; Nelson & Baldwin, 2008).

The most common causes of secondary dysmenorrhea are adenomyosis, endometriosis, pelvic adhesions, and neoplasia. Adenomyosis is a condition characterized by the presence of endometrial glands and stoma that are embedded in the myometrium (the deep muscle layer of the uterus). Adenomyosis most commonly occurs in parous women. Each month, normal ovarian hormonal changes cause stimulation of the ectopic (abnormally located) endometrial tissue and produce sloughing within the myometrium. In addition to dysmenorrhea, women with adenomyosis may also experience heavy menses and perimenstrual pain. The uterus is enlarged, boggy, and tender immediately before and during menses (ACOG, 2007; Nelson & Baldwin, 2008).

Endometriosis is a condition characterized by implantation of endometrial tissue outside the uterus. Women with endometriosis experience painful menses due to the cyclic shedding of the ectopic endometriotic implants and the local inflammatory response triggered by the shedding. The pain associated with endometriosis often occurs just prior to the onset of menses. (See later discussion of endometriosis.) Pelvic adhesions may also cause secondary dysmenorrhea. Pelvic adhesions are fibrous bands that may result from previous pelvic inflammatory disease, appendicitis, and pelvic or abdominal surgery. *Neoplasia* is a term that refers to the abnormal proliferation of benign or malignant cells (ACOG, 2007; Bloski & Pierson, 2008; Nelson & Baldwin, 2008). (See later discussion about various neoplastic processes.)

Health-care teaching for women experiencing dysmenorrhea should be holistic in nature and include relaxation and breathing techniques, the use of heat to reduce uterine contractions and increase blood flow to the uterine tissues, exercise or rest, and the use of NSAIDs to inhibit the synthesis of prostaglandin. These drugs not only improve the cramping pain but also reduce backache, headaches, and gastrointestinal symptoms. When taken at the onset of menses, NSAIDs reduce the release of prostaglandins and considerably decrease menstrual blood loss. Other therapeutic interventions for dysmenorrhea include hormonal contraceptives (e.g., combined oral contraceptive pills, depo medroxyprogesterone acetate [Depo-Provera], the levonorgestrel-releasing intrauterine system [LNG-IUS]), which reduce menstrual blood loss and decrease the production of prostaglandins (Nelson & Baldwin, 2008).

 Complementary Care: *Measures for Relief From Dysmenorrhea*

Throughout the ages, women have resorted to the use of various herbal remedies such as cramp bark, wild yam, black haw, ginger, and raspberry leaf to ease the pain of menstrual cramps. The nurse should counsel patients that because herbal preparations may be toxic and also interact with other medications, only preparations obtained from reputable companies should be used. Other strategies for relief from menstrual pain include the application of heat or cold, massage, meditation, and progressive relaxation. Exercise is beneficial for some women. Physical activity enhances blood flow to the pelvis and reduces pelvic congestion. Dietary strategies include the use of natural diuretics such as peaches, parsley, and cranberry juice to reduce edema and limiting the intake of meat.

 Now Can You— **Discuss abnormal genital bleeding, dysmenorrhea, and vaginal infections?**

1. Define the terms *metrorrhagia, menorrhagia, menometrorrhagia, and polymenorrhea*?
2. Differentiate primary dysmenorrhea from secondary dysmenorrhea and identify three possible causes of secondary dysmenorrhea?
3. Develop a holistic teaching plan for women who experience dysmenorrhea?

Common Vaginal Infections

Under normal circumstances, the vaginal environment functions as an ecosystem that maintains a steady state as it interacts with the environment outside the vagina. Many organisms, including certain bacteria and yeast, normally reside in the vagina. In fact, at any given time, from 5 to 10 different types of microorganisms are normally present in the vaginal flora. *Lactobacillus* is the dominant bacterial genus. It plays an essential role in helping to maintain the vaginal balance by producing byproducts such as lactic acid and hydrogen peroxide. These byproducts allow the vagina to maintain a healthy acidic pH of less than 4.5, which prevents the overgrowth of less desirable vaginal microorganisms. If the delicate balance of microorganisms is upset, the potentially pathogenic minor bacteria can proliferate to a concentration that causes symptoms (ACOG, 2007; Hatcher et al., 2008; Nyirjesy & Sobel, 2005).

 Nursing Insight— Understanding vaginal infections

During the reproductive years, the normal vaginal pH range is between 3.8 and 4.2, which falls within the acidic spectrum of the pH scale. Anaerobic bacteria are unable to colonize and thrive in the normally acidic vaginal environment, and lactobacilli become the predominant bacteria. When anaerobic bacteria are able to colonize, they eradicate the lactobacilli, creating an alkaline environment that allows continued colonization. Vaginal infections primarily occur in two ways: An imbalance and overgrowth of organisms that normally inhabit the vagina proliferate and cause symptoms, or organisms are introduced into the vagina, usually from intimate sexual contact. Factors that may cause an alteration in the normal vaginal environment include stress, douching, feminine hygiene products, harsh soaps, dietary changes (e.g., sugar, caffeine), sexual intercourse, barrier contraceptive methods (e.g., condoms, diaphragms), spermicides, synthetic underwear or tight-fitting pants, illness, chronic metabolic conditions (e.g., diabetes), immunosuppression, certain medications, and pregnancy (Coughlin & Secor, 2010; Hatcher et al., 2008).

 Optimizing Outcomes— **Teaching women strategies for promoting vaginal health**

Nurses can be instrumental in promoting vaginal health by teaching women about the normal functioning of their bodies. Women can be taught that leukorrhea is a normal vaginal discharge that undergoes hormonally mediated changes throughout the menstrual cycle. In the early (proliferative) phase, estrogen promotes a clear, thin, stretchy vaginal discharge. Later, the discharge becomes thick and tacky in response to the effects of progesterone, the dominant hormone during the second half of the cycle. The normal vaginal discharge varies in quantity from woman to woman, and often from cycle to cycle. Nurses can help patients explore ways to promote a balanced vaginal environment through alterations in lifestyle and choice of birth control method. Women should be taught that douching is discouraged, as it has a drying effect on the vagina and disrupts the normal vaginal flora. Douching can also cause an increase in the amount of vaginal discharge normally present and has been shown to contribute to serious infection of the upper reproductive tract (ACOG, 2007; Hatcher et al., 2008; Vermund & Allen, 2009).

A number of infections and conditions that involve the vaginal environment are commonly seen in women with gynecological disorders. These include bacterial vaginosis, candidiasis, sexually transmitted diseases (STDs), cervicitis, and pelvic inflammatory disease (PID). Cervicitis may be accompanied by a purulent discharge, which may be a symptom of infection with gonorrhea or chlamydia. Less commonly encountered conditions include vaginal carcinoma (primary, which is rare, or secondary, which results from the spread of cancer to the vagina from another site), cancer associated with in utero exposure to diethylstilbestrol (DES), and toxic shock syndrome (TSS). STDs and PID are discussed in a separate chapter.

BACTERIAL VAGINOSIS

Bacterial vaginosis (BV) was previously called "nonspecific vaginitis," *Haemophilus vaginitis*, or *Gardnerella*. BV is the most common vaginal infection in women, and although it is a sexually associated condition, it is not usually considered to be a specific STD. This vaginal infection is related to a lack of hydrogen peroxide–producing lactobacilli (microorganisms that normally maintain a low vaginal pH) and a dramatic overgrowth of the vaginal resident bacterium *Gardnerella vaginalis* and anaerobic bacteria (e.g., *Mycoplasma hominis*, *Mobiluncus*, *Bacteroides*, *Prevotella*, *Peptostreptococcus*, *Eubacterium*, *Escherichia coli*, and group B streptococci). Anaerobic bacteria thrive in a low-oxygen environment (ACOG, 2007; Coughlin & Secor, 2010; Hatcher et al., 2008).

Ethnocultural Considerations— Prevalence of bacterial vaginosis

Bacterial vaginosis affects approximately 30% of reproductive-age women. In the United States, African American women are infected with BV at three times the rate of Caucasian women. The prevalence rate of BV is highest in African American women without Hispanic heritage (50.3%) and Mexican American women (28.8%) when compared with non-Hispanic Caucasian women (22.4%) (Coughlin & Secor, 2010; Koumans et al., 2007).

Women with BV may be asymptomatic. When present, symptoms include a thin white or gray adherent vaginal discharge with a "fishy" amine odor, and women often report that the odor is worse after intercourse and following menses. The diagnosis is made on the basis of a positive finding on the "whiff" test—the characteristic amine odor is produced when a sample of the discharge is combined with a 10% solution of potassium hydroxide (KOH). Microscopic examination of the vaginal fluid (i.e., a wet mount) reveals the presence of clue cells, which are sloughed vaginal epithelial cells coated with bacteria that cling to the edges of the cells. Clue cells have a granular appearance with indistinct, blurry borders (Fig. 4-1).

Nursing Insight— The vaginal wet mount

A wet mount, also known as a "wet-prep" or "wet smear," is frequently used in the clinical setting to diagnose three of the most common vaginal infections: bacterial vaginosis, trichomoniasis, and yeast (candidiasis). To perform this test, the clinician inserts a speculum and uses a moist cotton swab to take a sample of the discharge from the posterior vaginal fornix. The discharge is then placed on a glass slide and viewed under a microscope. Alternately, a dry swab may be used: The sample is placed in 1 mL of saline, mixed, and placed on a slide or a drop of saline is placed on a slide and the sample is added to it. A cover slip is then applied and the slide is promptly viewed.

Typically, when BV is present, the vaginal pH is above the normal value of 4.5. Because BV may occur concurrently with other STDs (e.g., chlamydia, gonorrhea, genital herpes), it is important to screen for STDs as well (ACOG, 2007; Coughlin & Secor, 2010; Elkins & Mayeaux, 2010; Hatcher et al., 2008).

Optimizing Outcomes— With vaginal pH testing kits for home and clinical use

Self-diagnosis of vaginal infections based on symptoms alone is inaccurate approximately 50% of the time. Over-the-counter vaginal pH screening tests (e.g., Vagisil Screening Kit for vaginal infections, VI-SENSE) can help distinguish vaginal symptoms that require attention from a health-care provider. The Vagisil Screening Kit contains plastic wands with attached pH paper; the woman touches the wand to the vaginal wall to moisten the pH paper and withdraws the device. The vaginal pH level is then compared to the color on the pH guide. A pH value of 4.5 suggests that the vaginal symptoms are due to candidiasis (yeast); a pH reading of 5.0 or higher indicates that the vaginal symptoms are likely due to BV, trichomoniasis, or a mixed infection, and office follow-up is necessary (Dunican, 2008; Scolaro, Lloyd, & Helms, 2008; Wysocki, 2009).

The VS-SENSE is a swab-based test to detect vaginitis in the clinical setting. The VS-SENSE indicates by color change the elevated vaginal acidity levels associated with bacterial vaginosis and trichomonas. This new screening test offers immediate results and assists in detecting BV and trichomonas even when *Candida* (yeast) symptoms mask the more serious infections.

When BV is detected in an asymptomatic woman, it is usually not treated unless the patient will be undergoing an invasive surgical procedure, such as abortion, hysterectomy, or insertion of an intrauterine device. These procedures increase the risk of pelvic infection in the presence of BV. Bacterial vaginosis has also been shown to be associated with various pregnancy complications, such as spontaneous abortion, preterm birth, and infection following cesarean birth (ACOG, 2007; Coughlin & Secor, 2010; Hatcher et al., 2008).

Symptomatic women are typically treated with metronidazole (Flagyl), which is given either orally (500 mg twice a day for 7 days) or vaginally (metronidazole gel, 0.75% [Metro-Gel], 5 grams intravaginally for 5 days). Flagyl should not be used in women with a history of seizures. No alcohol should be ingested 24 hours before or after taking this medication, since the combination of metronidazole and alcohol causes abdominal discomfort, nausea, vomiting, and headache. Since nausea is the most common side effect, nurses should advise women to always take the medication with food. Metronidazole

Figure 4-1 Clue cell (Venes, D. (Ed.). (2009). *Taber's cyclopedic medical dictionary* (p. 397, 21st ed.). Philadelphia: F. A. Davis)

readily crosses the placenta and should not be taken during the first trimester of pregnancy; it is also contraindicated in breastfeeding women. Clindamycin (Cleocin) given orally (300 mg twice a day for 7 days) or in a 2% vaginal cream (5 grams intravaginally for 7 days) or in a vaginal ovule (100 mg at bedtime for 3 days) is also used to treat bacterial vaginosis. This medication is especially useful in individuals with an allergy or intolerance to metronidazole. Tinidazole (Tindamax), an oral medication, may also be used to treat BV in non-pregnant, adult women. The recommended dose is 2 grams once daily for 2 days, or 1 gram once daily for 5 days, and this medication should be taken with food. The half-life of this medication is twice as long as that of metronidazole, and it has fewer side effects. Alcohol should be avoided during the 3 days after taking tinidazole because of its longer half-life. Because treatment of male sexual partners has no effect on the recurrence rate in female partners, male treatment is not indicated (ACOG, 2007; Centers for Disease Control and Prevention [CDC] 2006a; Coughlin & Secor, 2010; Elkins & Mayeaux, 2010; Hatcher et al., 2008). Health professionals should consult the CDC Web site (http://www.cdc.gov/std/treatment/2006/vaginal-discharge.htm#vagdis2) for the most current guidelines on BV treatment.

✗ CANDIDIASIS

Commonly known as a yeast infection, candidiasis is generally caused by *Candida albicans* (Fig. 4-2). Other related yeast species (e.g., *C. tropicalis, C. glabrata, C. parapsilosis, C. krusei, C. lusitaniae*), however, can also be causative agents as well. Infection with candidiasis is usually characterized by intense vulvar pruritus (itching) and irritation and a thick, white, cottage cheese–like vaginal discharge that may have a sour odor. The discharge may be observed on the vaginal walls, cervix, and labia, and the vulva and labial folds are red and edematous. The patient may complain of dyspareunia and dysuria, although symptoms are subtler in some women. The diagnosis of candidiasis is made on the basis of microscopic examination of the vaginal discharge. A saline and KOH wet smear reveals budding yeast or pseudohyphae. The vaginal pH is usually unaltered, although it may be slightly more acidic than normal. During the examination, it is important to rule out STDs (Watson & Ng, 2008).

Figure 4-2 Gram's stain of *Candida albicans* (purple) in blood (× 640) (Venes, D. (Ed.). (2009). *Taber's cyclopedic medical dictionary* (p. 354, 21st ed.). Philadelphia: F. A. Davis)

 Optimizing Outcomes— **Recognizing factors that are associated with vulvovaginal candidiasis**

Certain factors are associated with vulvovaginal candidiasis, such as the use of broad-spectrum antibiotics and systemic corticosteroids, which can cause a reduction in the normal protective vaginal flora (Pirotta & Garland, 2006; Sheary & Dayan, 2005); high-dose oral contraceptives; and uncontrolled diabetes and allergies, especially allergic rhinitis (White, Vanthuyne, Wood, & Ayres, 2004). Spermicidal creams have also been associated with vaginal yeast infections. Nurses can advise women who use these medications or products about strategies to enhance the normal vaginal environment and reduce the likelihood of vulvovaginal candidiasis (Watson & Ng, 2008).

Candidiasis is treated with antifungal medications, and many over-the-counter agents such as miconazole (Monistat) and clotrimazole (Gyne-Lotrimin) are available. Most of the commercial products are fungistats that inhibit the organisms from reproducing, so the woman's immune system can suppress the yeast. Patients can apply a topical antifungal cream to the vulva as well as the intravaginal cream or suppositories. It is important to remind women that creams and vaginal suppositories are oil based and may weaken latex condoms or diaphragms (CDC, 2006a). Although these medications are available without prescription, the nurse should advise patients to avoid self-treatment without first undergoing a clinical evaluation to confirm the diagnosis of vulvovaginal candidiasis. Treatment of asymptomatic sexual partners is not generally necessary (ACOG, 2007; Watson & Ng, 2008).

 Complementary Care: *Measures for Vaginal Candidiasis*

Nurses can educate women about strategies to relieve symptoms of candidiasis and help prevent recurrent yeast infections. For example, women can be advised to take sitz baths for comfort and add Aveeno powder to the bath. Boric acid, 600 mg in size 0 gelatin capsules inserted in the vagina each night for 14 days, has been reported to be effective against resistant infections. Vaginal suppositories containing acidophilic bacteria, as well as long-term (6 months) daily ingestion of dairy products or powders, capsules, or tablets that contain *Lactobacillus acidophilus* are other strategies that anecdotally have been associated with prevention and relief of symptoms, although the evidence supporting this intervention is conflicting (Falagas, Betsil, & Athansion, 2006; Goodman, Herman, Murdaugh, Moneyham, & Phillips, 2007). Nurses can also teach women to wear cotton underwear to enhance ventilation of the genital area, avoid wearing tight-fitting pants or wet clothing (e.g., bathing suits) for prolonged periods of time, and avoid potential irritants such as perfumed soaps; bubble baths; hot tubs; and the application of perfumes, sprays, or powder near the vaginal area.

Stronger antifungal prescription medications are available in creams or suppositories, along with oral preparations, including fluconazole (Diflucan), itraconazole (Sporanox), and ketoconazole (Nizoral). Although the oral medications are associated with various side effects (e.g., nausea, vomiting, diarrhea, abdominal pain, headache), they tend to be well tolerated by most women. Ketoconazole is associated with hepatotoxicity, and baseline and ongoing liver function monitoring is recommended. Oral antifungals and boric acid suppositories should not be used during pregnancy. Topical antifungals have limited systemic absorption and are considered safe for maternal use. Women who have recurrent yeast infections should be evaluated for diabetes and infection with HIV (CDC, 2006a; Hatcher et al., 2008; Watson & Ng, 2008).

 Now Can You— **Discuss various aspects of vaginitis?**

1. Develop an educational tool for teaching women about promoting healthy vaginal environment.
2. Compare and contrast bacterial vaginosis and vaginal candidiasis.
3. Describe strategies intended to relieve symptoms and help prevent recurrence of vaginal candidiasis.

Vaginal Carcinoma

Vaginal carcinoma is any type of cancer that forms in the tissues of the vagina. Vaginal carcinomas can be primary or secondary or related to in utero diethylstilbestrol (DES) exposure. Vaginal cancer is extremely rare, occurs primarily in women over age 50, and accounts for only 1% to 2% of gynecological malignancies. It is frequently asymptomatic and first detected during a routine gynecological examination. Abnormal vaginal bleeding constitutes the most common symptom of this type of cancer, and the bleeding may be postcoital, intermenstrual, prepubertal, or postmenopausal. Other symptoms include foul-smelling vaginal discharge, dysuria, dyspareunia, and pelvic pain.

There are two primary types of vaginal cancer: squamous cell carcinoma and adenocarcinoma. Most lesions (85% of cases) are squamous cell carcinomas that arise from the thin, flat, squamous cells that line the vagina. These kinds of cancers develop over a period of many years and are usually found in women between the ages of 60 and 80. Vaginal squamous cell carcinoma occurs most often in women with a history of infection with human papillomavirus (HPV) (genital warts) or cervical or vulvar cancer. The time from HPV infection to the development of invasive cancer is believed to be from 5 to 10 years. In most cases, the cancer initially spreads superficially within the vaginal wall and later invades the paravaginal tissues and the parametria (the connective tissue and fat adjacent to the uterus). Distant metastases occur most commonly in the lungs and liver (National Cancer Institute [NCI], 2009).

Vaginal adenocarcinoma (occurring in approximately 15% of cases) arises from the glandular or secretory cells that line the vagina and produce some vaginal fluids. Adenocarcinoma is more likely than squamous cell cancer to spread to the lungs and lymph nodes. The most common type of vaginal adenocarcinoma usually develops in women over the age of 50. Clear cell adenocarcinoma is another type of vaginal cancer that usually occurs in women who were exposed to diethylstilbestrol (DES) in utero.

 Nursing Insight— *Understanding diethylstilbestrol (DES)*

Diethylstilbestrol (DES) is a nonsteroidal, synthetic estrogen that is several times more potent than natural estrogens. In the United States, DES was prescribed to approximately 5 to 10 million mothers during the late 1930s until the early 1970s as a preventative treatment to reduce the likelihood of spontaneous abortion or preterm birth (Smith, 1948). It was taken off the market when study results revealed that DES was linked to abnormalities in both male and female offspring of women who received this drug during pregnancy. Structural alterations, changes in the tissue of the vagina and cervix, and infertility have been linked to in utero DES exposure. The incidence of DES-related clear cell adenocarcinoma is highest for those women who were exposed during the first 3 months of their mother's pregnancy. The highest incidence of occurrence is between ages 17 and 21. The incidence of vaginal clear cell adenocarcinoma peaked in the early 1970s and is now rare, since DES use during pregnancy diminished during the early 1960s and was banned in the early 1970s (Helming, 2009; Stern, 2007).

Other less common forms of vaginal cancer include germ cell tumors (e.g., teratoma, endodermal sinus tumors), which are rare and found most often in infants and children; malignant melanoma; and sarcoma botryoides, a rhabdomyosarcoma that is also found most often in infants and children. Screening for malignancies of the vagina is similar to screening for cervical cancer. In addition to a history and physical examination, diagnostic testing for vaginal carcinoma includes a pelvic exam, Pap smear, biopsy, and colposcopy (an examination of the cervix, using a lighted instrument that magnifies the tissues). Other diagnostic modalities may include laboratory testing and imaging studies (ACOG, 2007; NCI, 2009; Stern, 2007).

The prognosis for vaginal carcinoma depends primarily on the type and stage of the condition at the time of diagnosis, but survival is reduced in women who are older than 60 years of age, are symptomatic at the time of diagnosis, have lesions of the middle and lower third of the vagina, or have poorly differentiated tumors. Treatment modalities depend on the stage of the condition; surgery or radiation therapy is highly effective in the early stages, while radiation therapy is the primary treatment for the more advanced stages. Chemotherapy has not been shown to be curative for advanced vaginal cancer (ACOG, 2007; NCI, 2009; Stern, 2007).

Toxic Shock Syndrome

Toxic shock syndrome (TSS) is a rare, sometimes fatal condition that affects many body systems. Although this disorder is not well understood, TSS is believed to be associated with tampon use during menses. However, TSS can also occur in children, men, and non-menstruating women. Non-menstrual TSS risk is increased for women who use vaginal barrier contraceptives. The incidence of TSS peaked during the late 1970s and 1980s, most likely because of the widespread availability of superabsorbent tampons. A few specific tampon designs and high-absorbency tampon materials were found to have some association with an increased risk of TSS; these products are no longer sold in the United States. Today, the overall rate of TSS is 1 to 3 cases per 100,000 people per year, and only 55% of current cases are associated with menstruation (Hatcher et al., 2008).

 Be sure to— Teach about toxic shock syndrome

Women who use a diaphragm, cervical cap, or contraceptive sponge should be aware of the possible association between these devices and toxic shock syndrome. Common signs of TSS include fever of sudden onset greater than 102.2°F (38.9°C), diffuse rash, vomiting, diarrhea, malaise, muscle aches, and hypotension with a systolic blood pressure less than 90 mm Hg. Patients who experience these symptoms should seek medical care immediately; left untreated, TSS can be fatal within hours (CDC, 2005).

Toxic shock syndrome is caused almost exclusively by toxins produced by some strains of the colonized bacterium *Staphylococcus aureus*. Toxins produced from the bacterium *Streptococcus pyogenes* may also cause TSS (sometimes referred to as "Toxic Shock–Like Syndrome" [TSLS] or "Streptococcal Toxic Shock Syndrome" [STSS]). Although the exact mechanism of cause is unknown, several conditions are believed to contribute to the development of menstrual TSS. These include alterations in the normal vaginal flora, a neutral vaginal pH, mechanical blockage of menstrual flow, contamination of tampons by the bacteria *S. aureus*, absorption of bacteria-resistant cervical fluids, the superabsorbent or synthetic materials found in some tampons, and damaged cervical or vaginal tissue. The toxin implicated in menstrual TSS is capable of entering the bloodstream by crossing the vaginal wall in the absence of ulcerations (Hatcher et al., 2008).

 Optimizing Outcomes— Strategies to reduce risk for menstrual TSS

Nurses can teach women about strategies to minimize the risk of contracting menstrual TSS. For example, menstruating women may use sanitary pads or choose a tampon with the minimum absorbency needed to manage the menstrual flow and use the tampons only during active menstruation. Women can be taught to change tampons frequently (at least every 6 hours) and alternate sanitary pads with tampons, especially during the night. Nurses should emphasize that if symptoms suggestive of TSS occur, the tampon should be removed and medical attention sought immediately.

The diagnosis of TSS is made on the basis of physical examination findings and symptoms, along with results of a complete blood count, which often shows an elevated white blood cell count indicative of an acute infectious process. Treatment of this potentially life-threatening condition involves immediate hospitalization with fluid replacement and aggressive antibiotic therapy. Antibiotics should cover both *S. aureus* and *S. pyogenes* and may

include a combination of cephalosporins, penicillins, and vancomycin, along with clindamycin or gentamicin. With appropriate care and prompt treatment, patients usually recover within 2 to 3 weeks (Hatcher et al., 2008).

 Nursing Insight— Formulating appropriate nursing diagnoses for patients with TSS

Nursing diagnoses for patients with TSS may focus on Hyperthermia (related to the inflammatory process/hypermetabolic state and dehydration), Deficient Fluid Volume (related to increased gastric losses, fever, and decreased intake), Acute Pain (related to the inflammatory process, effects of circulating toxins, and skin disruptions), and Impaired Skin/Tissue Integrity (related to the effects of circulating toxins and dehydration).

Urinary Tract Infections

Because of the widespread prevalence of urinary tract infections in women, a brief description of the problem is included in this discussion of gynecological disorders. Urinary tract infection (UTI) is defined as significant bacteriuria in the presence of symptoms. UTIs occur more frequently in women than in men because of the shorter route from the external environment to the bladder in women, along with the close proximity of the urethra to the vaginal and anal areas. UTIs account for a significant number (>6 million) of physician/health clinic visits each year, and it is estimated that 20% of women will be affected by a UTI at some time during their lifetime (ACOG, 2008a).

Under normal circumstances, the flow of urine keeps bacteria flushed from the urinary tract, and the entire urinary system remains sterile. The bladder wall possesses antibacterial properties, and the urine is usually acidic, which inhibits growth of bacteria.

A & P review **The Female Urinary Tract and Bacterial Exposure**

The female and male urinary tracts are relatively the same except for the length of the urethra. Owing to this difference, women are 30 times more likely to develop UTIs than are men. The female urethra is approximately 1.5 inches long; the male urethra is approximately 8 inches long. In women, bacteria from fecal matter can be easily transferred to the vagina or the urethra (Figs. 4-3 and 4-4). Most UTIs arise from one type of bacteria, *Escherichia coli*, which normally lives in the colon. Other common culprits include *Enterococcus faecalis*, *Staphylococcus saprophyticus*, *Klebsiella pneumoniae*, and *Proteus mirabilis*. Chlamydia and mycoplasma may also cause UTIs in both women and men, but these infections tend to remain limited to the urethra and reproductive system. Unlike *E. coli*, chlamydia and mycoplasma may be sexually transmitted (Sadovsky, 2007). ◆

Risk factors for UTIs include extremes of age, altered immunity, diabetes, urinary tract obstructions, pregnancy, sexual activity, and diaphragm use. Irritation of the urethra during sexual activity can cause bacteria to migrate upward

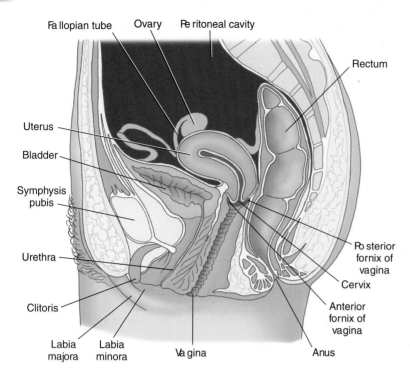

Figure 4-3 Internal female genitalia (Dillon, P. M. (2007). *Nursing health assessment: A critical thinking approach* (2nd ed., p. 612). Philadelphia, F. A. Davis)

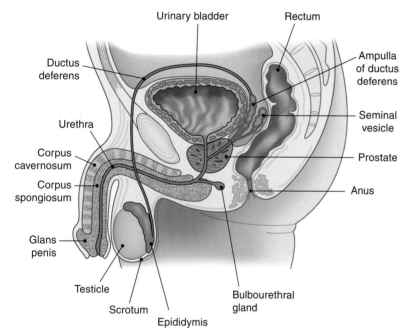

Figure 4-4 Male genitourinary system (Dillon, P. M. (2007). *Nursing health assessment: A critical thinking approach* (2nd ed., p. 651). Philadelphia, F. A. Davis)

into the urinary tract. Spermicides may alter the vaginal pH and decrease levels of normal protective bacteria, allowing harmful bacteria to grow in the vagina, which can then migrate to the bladder. Allergy to certain ingredients in soaps, vaginal creams, bubble baths, or other chemicals used in the genital area may cause tissue injury that can allow for the introduction of bacteria.

> ### ✿ *Nursing Insight— Recognizing signs and symptoms of a UTI*
>
> Nurses should be alert to certain patient symptoms that may be indicative of a UTI. Dysuria (pain with urination),

urinary frequency, urgency, a sensation of bladder fullness, suprapubic tenderness, and cloudy, foul-smelling urine are classic symptoms associated with a UTI. If the infection has ascended to the kidneys, the woman may experience pain in the lower back region where the vertebrae and ribs meet (costovertebral angle tenderness), and fever may be present.

Diagnosis for a UTI varies according to the location and extent of the infection. For uncomplicated infection of the lower urinary tract, the diagnosis is made on the basis of symptoms and urinalysis, including the microscopic examination of a clean-catch urine sample (Procedure 1) for the presence of white or red blood cells and

Procedure 1 Obtaining a Midstream Urine Sample

Preparation

1. Complete the information requested on the container label. Include the patient's full name and the date and time of collection of the specimen. If a requisition is needed, note the date and time on the requisition.

2. Explain the procedure to the woman to ensure she understands why a urine sample is requested, the purpose of any tests to be performed, and directions on how to obtain a midstream urine sample.

Equipment

Approved empty sterile container for collection
Towelette for cleaning in between the labia
Tissue

Procedural Steps

Instruct the patient to do the following:

1. Wash and dry your hands thoroughly or use an alcohol-based hand rub

   RATIONALE: *To reduce the risk of specimen contamination. Alcohol-based hand rubs are fast acting, reduce the number of microorganisms on the skin, and may cause less skin irritation or dryness.*

2. Remove the container cap and set it on a clean, even surface with the inner surface pointing up. Do not touch the inner surface of the lid or the container.

   RATIONALE: *To reduce the risk of specimen contamination.*

3. Sit on the toilet seat and separate the labia (vaginal lips) using your nondominant hand. Clean the urogenital area from the front to back with the towelette provided. Wipe for only one stroke and then discard the towelette.

   RATIONALE: *To reduce the risk of specimen contamination and to reduce the number of microorganisms on the skin. Cleansing from front to back prevents bringing rectal contamination forward.*

4. Holding the labia apart, begin to pass urine. Allow the beginning urine go directly into the toilet.

   RATIONALE: *The initial stream of urine washes urethral microorganisms and other debris away from the urethral meatus. The midstream collection ensures that a sterile specimen is obtained.*

5. Continue to urinate and hold the container under the urine stream. Avoid touching the inside of the container. Remove the container when it is approximately half full.

6. Carefully replace the cap and secure tightly.

   RATIONALE: *Placing the cap on the container prevents inadvertent spilling and possible contamination of the urine specimen.*

7. Wash your hands again after the specimen collection.

Clinical Alert Pregnant women are at an increased risk for developing urinary tract infections, especially if they are diabetic or have gestational diabetes. Urinary tract infections may also predispose to the onset of preterm labor.

bacteria. Complicated cases require a urine culture and sensitivity. In some practice settings, a leukocyte esterase or nitrite urine dipstick screening test to detect bacteriuria in women with suspected uncomplicated urinary tract infections is used (ACOG, 2008a).

Teach the patient to recognize common signs of a UTI:

- Dysuria—pain (burning sensation) on urination
- Urinary frequency associated with small amounts of urine
- Hematuria—blood or red blood cells in the urine

Treatment for uncomplicated lower urinary tract infections may be initiated in non-pregnant women with antibiotic therapy given over a 3-day course. Medications commonly used include co-trimoxazole (e.g., Bactrim, Septra), nitrofurantoin macrocrystals (e.g., Macrodantin), and amoxicillin/clavulanate (e.g., Augmentin). If the woman complains of intense dysuria, a bladder analgesic such as phenazopyridine (Pyridium), given for 1 to 2 days, is beneficial in alleviating the bladder discomfort (ACOG, 2008a).

 Optimizing Outcomes— **Strategies to promote bladder health and decrease the incidence of UTI**

Nurses can teach women about strategies to promote bladder health and decrease the likelihood of developing a UTI. For example, the nurse may advise the patient to:

- Void frequently (every 2–4 hours); avoid postponing urination (allowing urine to remain in the bladder allows bacteria to multiply).
- Empty the bladder before and after intercourse; drink liquids before and after intercourse.
- Remain hydrated to keep bacteria flushed out of the urinary tract system.
- Drink fruit juices to acidify the urine; take vitamin C regularly to inhibit bacterial growth.
- Wipe the urethral meatus and perineum from front to back after voiding.
- Avoid harsh soaps, powders, sprays; avoid bubble baths and bath oils.
- Wear cotton underwear; avoid tight-fitting underwear and pants.

Now Can You— **Discuss various aspects of vaginal carcinoma, toxic shock syndrome, and urinary tract infections?**

1. Identify risk factors for vaginal carcinoma?
2. Develop an educational program to teach women about toxic shock syndrome?
3. Discuss urinary tract infections and describe five strategies to reduce risk for a UTI?

✗ Endometriosis

First described by Dr. John Sampson in the 1920s, endometriosis is defined as the growth, adhesion, and progression of endometrial glands and tissue outside of the uterine cavity with cellular activity evident in lesions, nodules, and cysts. Women ages 30 to 40 are most likely to develop endometriosis, and the condition is found in 20% to 40% of infertile women and in up to 33% of women with chronic pelvic pain. Endometrial lesions have been discovered on the ovaries, fallopian tubes, lining of the inside of the pelvic cavity, cervix, bladder, bowel, brain, nostrils, liver, and lungs (Fig. 4-5) (Audebert et al., 1992; Bloski & Pierson, 2008; Sampson, 1940).

Each month, the misplaced endometrial tissue responds to cyclic hormonal stimulation during the secretory and proliferative stages of the menstrual cycle, growing and thickening in a similar fashion to the endometrial tissue normally lining the uterus. During the ischemic and menstrual phases of the cycle, however, the misplaced endometrial tissue breaks down and bleeds into the surrounding tissue, causing inflammation. The released blood becomes trapped in the surrounding tissues, causing the development of blood-containing cysts. The recurrence of inflammation in the areas outside of the uterus eventually results in scarring, fibrosis, and the development of adhesions, scar tissue that binds the organs together, causing increased abdominal pain and a risk of infertility (Guo & Wang, 2006; Bloski & Pierson, 2008; Speroff & Fritz, 2005; Woodson, 2007).

 Nursing Insight— Understanding terms associated with endometriosis

Endometriosis is the presence of endometrial glands and tissue outside the uterus. An *endometrioma* is a solitary, non-neoplastic mass that contains endometrial tissue. An endometrioma is also referred to as an *endometrioid cyst*. Endometrioid cysts, often filled with dark, reddish-brown blood, may range in size from 0.75 to 8 inches (19.05 mm–20.32 cm). An endometrioid cyst is sometimes called a "chocolate cyst" because it is filled with old blood.

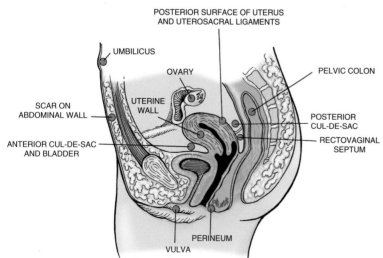

Figure 4-5 Possible sites of occurrence of endometriosis (Venes, D. (Ed.). (2009). *Taber's cyclopedic medical dictionary* (p. 768, 21st ed.). Philadelphia: F. A. Davis)

ETIOLOGY AND PATHOGENESIS

The exact cause and pathogenesis of endometriosis is not known. One of the most widely accepted theories is Sampson's theory, or "retrograde menstruation." This theory postulates that during menstruation, endometrial tissue is transported through the fallopian tubes into the peritoneal cavity, where it implants on the ovaries and other structures. Although retrograde menstruation occurs in most women, it is not clear why some develop endometriosis and others do not. The level of functioning of the immune system is thought to be a factor in the development of endometriosis, although the exact mechanism is unknown. Interestingly, women with endometriosis tend to develop additional symptoms such as allergies, fibromyalgia, asthma, eczema, autoimmune inflammatory disease, chronic fatigue syndrome, and hypothyroidism. Also, there is a higher risk of breast cancer in women diagnosed with endometriosis after age 40 because of their prolonged exposure to elevated endogenous estrogen (Bertelsen et al., 2007; Bloski & Pierson, 2008; Sinaii, Cleary, Ballweg, Nieman, & Stratton, 2002).

SIGNS AND SYMPTOMS

The signs and symptoms of endometriosis vary from woman to woman, and the severity of symptoms may increase over time. However, the most common symptom is pelvic pain. The pain, which usually begins 1 or 2 days before the expected menses, may be unilateral or bilateral and frequently lasts until the end of menstruation. Some patients experience a constant, debilitating pain that interferes with their normal daily activities. Bowel symptoms such as diarrhea, pain with defecation, constipation, and rectal bleeding with significant bowel involvement may also occur. Other symptoms include dyspareunia, dysuria, various gastrointestinal symptoms, low back pain, infertility, and menstrual dysfunction. Interestingly, the severity of pain does not correlate well with the extent of the condition. Thus, severe disease may go undetected (Bloski & Pierson, 2008; Chopin et al., 2006; Denny & Mann, 2007; Ninia, 2007).

DIAGNOSIS

The diagnosis of endometriosis can be difficult to confirm owing to the wide variation in symptoms. Diagnostic laparoscopy to allow for visualization and biopsy of the lesions remains the gold standard for diagnosis, after other causes of pelvic pain (e.g., upper genital tract infection, pelvic inflammatory disease) have been ruled out. A vaginal ultrasound may also be performed to provide imaging of the displaced endometrial tissue or cyst(s), although it may be difficult to differentiate between other pathological entities such as tubal cysts, abscesses, and ectopic pregnancy (Bazot et al., 2003; Bloski & Pierson, 2008).

Optimizing Outcomes— Endometriosis staging to guide care

The American Society for Reproductive Medicine (ASRM) has developed classification and staging guidelines to assist with endometriosis diagnosis, prognosis, treatment, and progress and communication among health professionals.

Staging is based on the extent of the spread of the lesions, the density of pelvic adhesions, involvement of pelvic organs, and the degree of fallopian tube occlusion. In the standardized schema, endometriosis is classified into four stages: Stage 1—minimal, Stage 2—mild, Stage 3—moderate, and Stage 4—severe. Interestingly, women with minimal or mild endometriosis have been shown to have high degrees of pain and infertility while women with Stage 4 disease have been asymptomatic and diagnosed during laparoscopy for various procedures such as tubal ligation (ASRM, 2006; Bloski & Pierson, 2008).

TREATMENT OPTIONS

Because endometriosis can persist during a woman's entire reproductive life, her treatment plan should be individualized and holistic. When determining the best approach for therapy, many factors must be taken into account, such as the woman's desire for future pregnancy, the size of her current family, and general lifestyle patterns. Although there are no ideal treatments for endometriosis, the planned course of therapy is based on the severity of symptoms and the woman's or couple's goals. Treatment plans generally begin with the least invasive approach and progress to more invasive therapies. Regardless of the treatment, however, approximately 10% to 20% of women with endometriosis experience a recurrence of the condition.

Medical Therapy

The goal of medical treatment is to reduce the amount of estrogen in the body so that menstruation and the subsequent growth of endometrial tissue are suppressed. To accomplish the suppression of endogenous estrogen, two main classes of drugs are used: GnRH-agonists and gonadotropin inhibitors. GnRH-agonists such as leuprolide (Lupron), goserelin (Zoladex), and nafarelin (Synarel) suppress the secretion of pituitary gonadotropins. This action causes anovulation and amenorrhea, which result in shrinkage of the endometrial tissue. The patient experiences significant pain relief and an interruption in the further development of endometrial lesions. Common side effects are similar to those associated with natural menopause and include hot flashes; vaginal dryness; loss of libido; emotional lability; and mild, reversible bone loss. Treatment is limited to 5 months due to the decrease in bone mineral density associated with these medications (Bloski & Pierson, 2008; Crosignani, Olive, Bergqvist, & Luciano, 2006; Deglin & Vallerand, 2009).

Danazol (Danocrine, Cyclomen) is a synthetic androgen that acts as a pituitary gonadotropin inhibitor. This medication causes anovulation by suppressing the secretion of follicle-stimulating hormone (FSH) and luteinizing hormone (LH). Pain relief results from the hypoestrogenic environment, endometrial atrophy, and regression of the endometrial lesions. Because this medication is an androgenic synthetic steroid, masculinizing side effects such as acne, hirsutism, deepening of the voice, weight gain, decreased breast size, and oily skin are common. Other side effects include headaches, flushing, sweating, atrophic vaginitis, and edema. The duration of treatment is approximately 6 months, due to the multitude of adverse side effects (Blosky & Pierson, 2008; Deglin & Vallerand, 2009).

Contraceptive medications are also used to treat endometriosis. Combination oral contraceptives contain progestins and estrogen—hormones that suppress gonadotropins, prevent ovulation, and cause endometrial atrophy. Pain relief, related to a thinning of the endometrial lining and regression of the endometriotic implants, is achieved in approximately 75% of patients. Side effects include irregular bleeding, weight gain, headache, thrombophlebitis, benign liver tumors, and gallbladder disease. Medroxyprogesterone (Depo-Provera) is an injectable progesterone that also suppresses gonadotropins and thins endometrial tissue. Potential adverse side effects associated with this medication include weight gain, headache, abdominal discomfort, and irregular bleeding. Treatment outcomes are similar to those achieved with oral contraceptives (ASRM, 2006; Bloski & Pierson, 2008; Brankin & Cackovic, 2010; Deglin & Vallerand, 2009).

Anastrozole (Arimidex) and letrozole (Femara) are aromatase inhibitors that decrease levels of circulating estrogen by inhibiting the peripheral conversion of androgens. Potential adverse effects include headache, nausea, diarrhea, hot flashes, and an increased risk of osteoporosis with long-term use. Treatment is limited to 6 months due to the decrease in bone mineral density. Up to 90% of patients experience alleviation of symptoms during and up to 15 months post-treatment (Ailawadi, Jobanpufra, Kataria, Gurates, & Bulun, 2004; Bloski & Pierson, 2008; Deglin & Vallerand, 2009; Shippen & West, 2004).

Surgical Treatment

Laparoscopy with biopsy of the lesions is the only accurate method to diagnose and determine the severity of endometriosis. During the laparoscopy, surgical removal of the lesions, adhesions, and cysts may be conducted via excision, electrocautery, or laser vaporization. The recurrence rate of endometriotic lesions after 5 years is 19% with laparoscopic removal of the lesions and 10% with hysterectomy (removal of the uterus) and bilateral oophorectomy (removal of the ovaries). Women who undergo a bilateral oophorectomy are usually treated with hormone therapy, as the benefits outweigh the risk of endometriosis recurrence (ASRM, 2006; Bloski & Pierson, 2008).

IMPLICATIONS FOR NURSES

Counseling and support constitute the cornerstone of nursing care for women diagnosed with endometriosis. It is incumbent upon nurses who care for women with this chronic condition to remain knowledgeable about endometriosis so that they can provide factual information about treatment options, including the risks and benefits of each. Therapeutic listening reflects respect and encourages patients to share intimate details about sensitive issues, such as dyspareunia. Teaching patients about endometriosis empowers them to participate in their treatment plan and explore approaches such as alternative methods of pain control and lifestyle and diet modifications that may enhance well-being and improve functionality (Bloski & Pierson, 2008; Huntington & Gilmour, 2005). Potential nursing diagnoses for women with endometriosis are presented in Box 4-2.

Box 4-2 Potential Nursing Diagnoses for Women with Endometriosis

- Knowledge Deficit related to endometriosis diagnostic workup and treatment
- Acute Pain related to menstruation secondary to endometriosis
- Situational Low Self-Esteem related to infertility secondary to endometriosis
- Anxiety related to possible invasive surgical interventions secondary to endometriosis
- Risk for Tissue Injury related to progression of endometriosis

Collaboration in Caring— *Assisting women with endometriosis*

Women with endometriosis can benefit from a multidisciplinary approach to treatment. The health-care team, composed of professionals with skills to address the many difficulties associated with this chronic condition, may include dietitians, physiotherapists, psychologists, and chronic pain specialists. Also, nurses may suggest referral to local support groups and national organizations such as Resolve (http://www.resolve.org), an organization for infertile couples, or the Endometriosis Association (http://www.endometriosisassn.org). Nurses can remain up-to-date on evidence-based guidelines for the treatment of endometriosis through the European Society for Human Reproduction & Embryology (SHRE) Web site (http://www.guidelines.endometriosis.org) or the National Guideline Clearinghouse Web site (http://www.guideline.gov) (Bloski & Pierson, 2008).

Now Can You— Discuss various aspects of endometriosis?

1. Describe the chronic condition of endometriosis, and define the term *endometrioma*?
2. Discuss the modalities and goals of medical and surgical treatment for endometriosis?
3. Develop a nursing plan of care for a patient with endometriosis?

Leiomyomas (Fibroids)

Uterine leiomyomas (also called fibroids) are the most common solid pelvic tumors in women and the leading indication for hysterectomy. Fibroids arise from a singular neoplastic smooth muscle cell in the uterus and grow slowly. Although the exact cause is unknown, the growth of leiomyomas is dependent on estrogen. They are almost always benign (ACOG, 2008b).

Nursing Insight— *Understanding terminology for uterine fibroid tumors*

A leiomyoma, or fibroid, is a benign tumor composed of nonstriated muscular tissue. The plural form of leiomyoma is either *leiomyomas* or *leiomyomata*.

Leiomyomas may be located in various places in and around the uterus. The most common fibroids form within the uterine wall. They can vary greatly in size and may protrude into the uterine cavity, bulge outward through the uterine wall and into the pelvic cavity, or grow on a stalk called a "pedicle" that can become twisted and cause pain. Leiomyomas are more common in African American women, and some studies report the presence of fibroids in 70% of Caucasian women and more than 80% of African American women by age 50 years. Stimulated by estrogen and progesterone, the tumors occur more frequently with increasing age and regress after menopause (ACOG, 2008b; Day Baird, Dunson, Hill, Cousins, & Schectman, 2003).

SIGNS, SYMPTOMS, AND DIAGNOSIS

The two most common symptoms of uterine leiomyomas for which women seek medical treatment are abnormal uterine bleeding and pelvic pressure. Frequently, however, fibroids cause no symptoms and are first discovered during a routine bimanual pelvic examination. When abnormal bleeding is present, it is usually reported as heavy or prolonged menstrual bleeding, which may result in iron-deficiency anemia. In some situations, the bleeding significantly disrupts the woman's normal daily activities. The pelvic and abdominal discomfort is often described as "pressure." Depending on the location of the leiomyoma, pressure may be experienced in the bladder or rectal regions, leading to difficulty with urination or defecation or dyspareunia. Also, depending on their size and location, leiomyomas can interfere with fertility (ACOG, 2008b; Fraser, Critchley, Munro, & Broder, 2007).

On examination, the uterus is nontender and may feel enlarged, irregularly shaped, or both. Pregnancy must always be ruled out. An ultrasound examination can confirm the presence of the leiomyoma and provide baseline measurements. Sometimes a hysteroscopy, an office procedure that uses an instrument to view the uterine cavity, or a laparoscopy, an outpatient hospital procedure that uses an instrument to view the uterus and surrounding structures, is performed to aid the diagnosis (ACOG, 2008b).

TREATMENT

In general, patients with leiomyomas are seen in the office every 3 to 6 months as long as they are experiencing mild symptoms. If heavy and prolonged bleeding or severe pain occurs, however, referral to a specialist for further evaluation is indicated. Interventions may include drug therapy, uterine artery embolization, myomectomy, hysterectomy, and laser surgery, electrocauterization, or magnetic resonance imaging (MRI)–guided focused ultrasound surgery.

Drug Therapy

Contraceptive steroids (estrogen and progestin combination and progestin alone) may be prescribed to control heavy periods and dysmenorrhea. Gonadotropin-releasing hormone (GnRH) agonists including leuprolide acetate (Lupron, Synarel) suppress the production of estrogen and progesterone and shrink the tumors, although the effects of these agents is temporary, with gradual recurrent growth of leiomyomas within several months following the cessation of treatment. Also, the significant menopausal symptoms such as vaginal dryness, hot flashes, and mood changes along with decreased bone mineral density limit use of these medications to no more than 6 months. Antiprogesterone agents such as mifepristone (Mifeprex) may also be useful in controlling leiomyoma symptoms. Recurrence of tumor growth following cessation of treatment tends to be slower than with other medications; however, further study is needed. Potential side effects include endometrial hyperplasia and alterations in liver functioning (ACOG, 2008b).

Uterine Artery Embolization (UAE)

Performed by interventional radiologists, this treatment involves the injection of polyvinyl alcohol pellets into selected blood vessels to block the blood supply to the fibroid and cause shrinkage and resolution of symptoms. UAE is performed under local anesthesia and conscious sedation. An incision is made into the groin, a catheter is threaded from the femoral artery into the uterine artery, and an arteriogram identifies the major blood vessels that supply the leiomyoma. Most tumors shrink in size by 50% within 3 months following treatment. Women who wish to undergo this procedure should be advised that data are lacking about the long-term effects on fertility and future pregnancies (ACOG, 2008b; Society of Obstetricians and Gynaecologists of Canada, 2005; Spies et al., 2005).

Myomectomy and Hysterectomy

For women who desire uterine preservation, myomectomy (removal of the leiomyoma) may be an option. Depending on the size and number of tumors, this surgical procedure may be accomplished during a laparotomy, a laparoscopy, or a hysteroscopy. Myomectomy can be performed through a laparoscopic or abdominal incision approach or a vaginal (hysteroscopic) approach. The uterus (and therefore childbearing potential) is preserved, although most myomectomy patients will require a cesarean birth. Hysterectomy (removal of the uterus) may be the treatment of choice if heavy, persistent bleeding cannot be controlled by any other means (ACOG, 2008b).

Laser Surgery, Electrocauterization, and MRI-Guided Focused Ultrasound Surgery

Laser surgery and electrocauterization may be used to destroy small leiomyomas with a vaginal (hysteroscopic) or abdominal (laparoscopic) approach. Laser coagulation vaporizes the fibroids and produces necrosis. However, although the uterus remains intact, endometrial scarring may diminish future fertility (ACOG, 2008b).

In 2004, the U.S. Federal and Drug Administration (FDA) granted approval for the use of an MRI-guided system for the localization and treatment of uterine leiomyomas with focused ultrasound therapy. This treatment is a noninvasive approach that uses high-intensity ultrasound waves directed into the leiomyoma. The ultrasound energy penetrates soft tissue and causes necrosis. Adverse effects include heavy menses and persistent pain; further studies regarding the long-term efficacy of this treatment modality are indicated (ACOG, 2008b).

Optimizing Outcomes— **Following surgical intervention for leiomyomas**

Nurses can educate women undergoing surgical interventions for leiomyomas about strategies to enhance comfort and promote healing. Nurses can teach women to:

- Take all prescribed medications.
- Contact the physician for symptoms including bleeding, cramping, fever of 39°C (102.2°F) or greater, gastrointestinal changes, signs of wound infection (redness, swelling, heat, or pain at the incision site), urinary retention, abnormal vaginal discharge.
- Consume foods high in protein, iron, and vitamin C to facilitate tissue healing; drink plenty of fluids.
- Avoid straining during bowel movements.
- Follow the physician's recommendations regarding physical activity and driving.
- Follow the physician's orders regarding tub baths and the resumption of intercourse.

Abnormal Uterine Bleeding

Abnormal uterine bleeding, a common problem for women, may be associated with major disruptions in daily functioning. Typically, the abnormal uterine bleeding is categorized as either *structural* or *dysfunctional*. Dysfunctional uterine bleeding is a diagnosis that is made only after all pathological causes of bleeding, such as leiomyomata, polyps, endometrial hyperplasia, and cancer, have been excluded. An accurate diagnosis for the cause of the bleeding should be established. Based on age alone, endometrial assessment to exclude cancer should be performed on any woman older than 35 years. In addition to a physical examination, diagnostic tests used to evaluate women with abnormal uterine bleeding may include a pregnancy test to rule out ectopic pregnancy, Pap smear, complete blood count, evaluation for endocrine dysfunction, endometrial biopsy, transvaginal ultrasound, hysteroscopy, and dilatation and curettage (D & C) (ACOG, 2007).

ABNORMAL BLEEDING RELATED TO STRUCTURAL CAUSES

Structural causes of uterine bleeding include leiomyomata, polyps, and infection. Uterine fibroid tumors are often asymptomatic and first detected during a bimanual pelvic examination. Precancerous or cancerous conditions of the uterus or cervix can also cause abnormal bleeding (ACOG, 2007).

ABNORMAL BLEEDING RELATED TO DYSFUNCTIONAL CAUSES

Dysfunctional uterine bleeding is defined as noncyclic menstrual blood flow that is derived from the endometrium. The bleeding may range from spotty to excessive and may be prolonged. It is most commonly caused by hormonal imbalances, which account for approximately 75% of cases of irregular bleeding. Heavy bleeding is a common problem for women during the perimenopausal period between the ages of 40 and 50. As ovulation becomes more erratic, levels of progesterone decrease. An important function of progesterone is to stabilize the uterine endometrial lining. In the absence of progesterone, the bleeding may become unpredictable, excessive, or prolonged. Abnormal uterine bleeding may also occur during adolescence, before a pattern of regular ovulatory cycles has been established. Other conditions that may cause abnormal bleeding include thyroid or adrenal gland disorders, polycystic ovary syndrome, clotting disorders, liver or kidney disease, leukemia, herbal preparations such as ginseng, or medications such as anticoagulants (ACOG, 2000, 2007; Keehbauch & Nystrom, 2007; Speroff & Mishell, 2007; Wolfe, 2006).

 Nursing Insight— *Clotting disorders may cause abnormal uterine bleeding*

Nurses should be aware that abnormal uterine bleeding may be related to an undiagnosed coagulopathy such as defects in primary hemostasis, platelet deficiency (e.g., leukemia, idiopathic thrombocytopenia), platelet dysfunction (e.g., von Willebrand disease), and abnormalities of secondary homeostasis (congenital factor deficiencies). von Willebrand disease is a genetic bleeding disorder caused by a defect or deficiency of a blood-clotting factor (von Willebrand factor). This condition occurs in approximately 1% of all women and is the most common medical disorder associated with menarche (ACOG, 2007).

TREATMENT

Depending on the cause, treatment for abnormal uterine bleeding may include drug therapy and/or surgery. Medical management is the preferred method of therapy for anovulatory uterine bleeding. The goals of medical treatment are to alleviate the acute bleeding, prevent future episodes of noncyclic bleeding, decrease the woman's risk of long-term complications from anovulation, and improve her overall quality of life. It is important for nurses to counsel patients that the treatment may initially cause heavy menstrual bleeding related to buildup of the endometrium. However, the bleeding should diminish over the course of 3 to 4 months.

Depending on the patient's age and physical findings, medications used include conjugated equine estrogens, low-dose combination oral contraceptives, cyclic progestogens, iron supplementation, prostaglandin synthetase inhibitors (e.g., indomethacin [Indocin]), and NSAIDs (e.g., aspirin, ibuprofen, naproxen). The FDA recently approved an oral nonhormonal product to treat heavy menstrual bleeding. Tranexamic acid (Lysteda) works by stabilizing a protein that helps blood to clot. Because the use of this medication while taking hormonal contraceptives may increase the risk of blood clots, stroke, or heart attack, women using hormonal contraception should take tranexamic acid only if there is a strong medical need and the benefits outweigh the potential risks (ACOG, 2007; FDA, 2009).

Surgical procedures to treat abnormal uterine bleeding include dilation and curettage (D & C), hysteroscopic-assisted endometrial ablation, thermal balloon ablation, and hysterectomy. These interventions are indicated for patients who fail to improve with medical therapy and who desire no future fertility. Women with significant acute bleeding may need a D & C for the immediate control of bleeding as well as for diagnosis. However, the beneficial effects associated with this surgical intervention are only temporary, and the D & C procedure is no longer the mainstay of treatment (ACOG, 2007; Nelson & Baldwin, 2008).

A surgical alternative to hysterectomy is endometrial ablation, a procedure that uses a lighted viewing instrument (hysteroscope) and other instruments to destroy (ablate) the uterine lining. Endometrial ablation is generally performed in an outpatient facility or hospital. The procedure may be done using a local or spinal anesthesia, although general anesthesia is sometimes used. Recovery following endometrial ablation generally ranges from a few days to a couple of weeks.

 Nursing Insight— *Understanding endometrial ablation*

Endometrial ablation is used to control heavy, prolonged vaginal bleeding for the following circumstances: The bleeding has not responded to other treatments; childbearing is completed; the patient prefers not to have a hysterectomy to control the bleeding; or other medical problems prevent a hysterectomy. The five FDA-approved methods use a variety of energy sources to achieve endometrial destruction, and each is designed to ablate down to the basal layer to prevent regeneration and subsequent menstrual flow. Endometrial ablation may be accomplished by laser beam (laser thermal ablation), electricity, freezing, microwave, or heat (thermal ablation, using radiofrequency or a balloon filled with heated saline solution). With thermal balloon ablation, a flexible balloon attached to a thin probe is inserted through the cervix and inflated in the uterus with sterile saline. The saline, heated to approximately 85°C, destroys the uterine lining. With all ablation techniques, the endometrium heals by scarring, which usually reduces or prevents uterine bleeding. Fertility is not preserved, although there is a remote possibility of pregnancy if a portion of the endometrium is left intact. Contraception is recommended for women who have not completed menopause (ACOG, 2000; Fothergill & Sulak, 2010; Song, 2007).

Hysterectomy

A hysterectomy is a surgery to remove the uterus. After cesarean section, hysterectomy is the second most frequently performed major surgical procedure for women of reproductive age in the United States. Each year in this country, approximately 600,000 hysterectomies are performed, and an estimated 20 million women have had a hysterectomy. The three conditions most commonly associated with hysterectomy are uterine leiomyomata, endometriosis, and uterine prolapse. Other indications include cancer (i.e., uterine, ovarian, cervical, endometrial), adenomyosis (a condition in which endometrial tissue grows into the myometrium), chronic pelvic pain, and abnormal vaginal bleeding (ACOG, 2007, 2009a; CDC, 2006b).

During the surgery, the whole uterus or a part of it may be removed. A *partial*, *subtotal*, or *supracervical* hysterectomy involves removal of the upper part of the uterus, leaving the cervix in place. A *total* hysterectomy removes the whole uterus and cervix, and a *radical* hysterectomy removes the whole uterus, along with the tissue on both sides of the cervix and the upper part of the vagina. This particular surgery is done mostly when there is cancer present.

❝ **What to say** ❞ — *"What to say" — When explaining surgical approaches for hysterectomy*

Several different surgical approaches are used to perform removal of the uterus. To determine the most appropriate method, the physician assesses a number of factors, including the patient's health history, reason for the surgery, and personal preference. The nurse can explain the various procedures:

Abdominal hysterectomy: A 5- to 7-inch incision is made in the low abdomen, just above the pubic hairline. The incision may be in a vertical or horizontal direction. The uterus is removed through the incision. Recovery time varies from 4 to 6 weeks.

Vaginal hysterectomy: An incision is made in the vagina, and the uterus is removed through the vagina.

Laparoscopic hysterectomy: An instrument with a thin, lighted tube and small camera (laparoscope) is inserted into the abdomen to allow for visualization of the pelvic organs. Three or four small cuts are made in the abdomen for insertion of the laparoscope and other instruments. The uterus is divided into small segments and removed through the incisions.

Laparoscopically assisted vaginal hysterectomy (LAVH): The uterus is removed through the vagina, and the laparoscope is used to guide the procedure.

Robotic surgery: The doctor uses a special machine to perform the surgery like laparoscopic surgery. This method is most often used when a patient has cancer or is very obese and vaginal surgery is considered unsafe.

Recovery from vaginal or laparoscopic surgery generally takes from 3 to 4 weeks.

Prior to the surgery, a psychological assessment is an essential component of care. The nurse should ensure that the woman has an opportunity to consider the personal significance of the loss of her uterus, discuss misconceptions about the effects of the surgery, and ensure that she has an adequate support system for postoperative care and concerns. Recovery from a hysterectomy is a very personal experience that is shaped by a myriad of factors, such as the woman's age, her physical and emotional health, reason for the surgery, and type of surgery performed. The nurse can help to empower women facing uterine surgery by creating a therapeutic environment where the patient feels safe in sharing feelings and expressing concerns. Other nursing actions to help prepare the woman for the surgery and promote a healthy recovery include providing information, engaging the assistance of other health professionals, and making referrals when appropriate.

Now Can You— **Discuss leiomyomas, abnormal uterine bleeding, and hysterectomy?**

1. Identify common treatment modalities for leiomyomas, and develop a postoperative teaching plan for the woman undergoing a surgical intervention?
2. Differentiate between structural and dysfunctional abnormal uterine bleeding?
3. Discuss the nurse's role when caring for the patient who will undergo a hysterectomy?

Ovarian Tumors

Because the ovary is composed of many different tissue types, growths or tumors involving the ovary may be of various types. Interestingly, more than 50 different types of ovarian tumors have been identified. Two of the most common types of ovarian tumors are follicular cysts and corpus luteum cysts, which are included in this discussion.

 Nursing Insight— Understanding about ovarian cysts

Ovarian cysts affect women of all ages; the vast majority of them are considered functional, or physiologic. Most disappear within a few weeks without treatment. Ovarian cysts occur most often during the childbearing years and typically represent a normal process. A dermoid cyst is an abnormal cyst that usually affects younger women; it may range in size from 1 cm (less than a half inch) up to 45 cm (17 inches) in diameter. A dermoid cyst is usually a benign tumor (2% are malignant) sometimes referred to as a mature cystic teratoma. Originating from a totipotential germ cell, the cyst is similar to those present on skin tissue and can contain fat and occasionally bone, hair, and cartilage. A dermoid cyst can cause the ovary to twist ("torsion") and produce severe abdominal pain.

FOLLICULAR CYSTS

A follicular cyst is the most common growth that occurs on the ovary. It develops during the first half of the menstrual cycle, called the "follicular phase." This type of ovarian cyst, termed a "functional" or "simple" cyst, forms when ovulation does not occur. Instead, the developing dominant follicle continues to grow and evolves into a large, fluid-filled cyst that contains a high concentration of estrogen. The follicular cyst can also form from one of the smaller follicles that failed to regress after another ovarian follicle gained dominance. Follicular cysts usually produce no symptoms and disappear spontaneously within a few months. However, approximately one-fourth of women with follicular cysts report symptoms such as pain or the sensation of a heavy, achy feeling in the pelvis.

The diagnosis is generally made on the basis of symptoms and bimanual examination. Ultrasonography may be used to confirm the findings and rule out pregnancy. Expectant management ("watch and wait") and a repeat examination in 6 to 10 weeks is the treatment of choice unless symptoms worsen. The majority of follicular cysts resolve after two to three menstrual cycles without

intervention. On occasion, oral contraceptive pills are prescribed to hasten cyst resolution (ACOG, 2007).

CORPUS LUTEUM CYSTS

A corpus luteum cyst forms from the corpus luteum during the second half, or luteal phase, of the menstrual cycle. The woman with a corpus luteum cyst may experience menstrual irregularity (e.g., delayed menses), although most often, the cyst regresses and disappears spontaneously within one or two menstrual cycles. The cyst may, however, fill with fluid or blood and persist on the ovary. Less commonly, the cysts rupture and can cause severe abdominal pain from the associated bleeding. When this occurs, surgical removal of the cyst may be necessary.

Polycystic Ovary Syndrome

Polycystic ovary syndrome (PCOS), also called Stein-Leventhal syndrome, is one of the most common endocrine disorders in reproductive-age women, affecting 1 in 15 women of childbearing age (Speroff & Mishell, 2007). The disorder occurs when an endocrine imbalance results in elevated levels of estrogen, testosterone, and luteinizing hormone (LH) and a decreased secretion of follicle-stimulating hormone (FSH). Multiple follicular cysts develop on one or both ovaries and produce excessive amounts of estrogen. Clinical findings associated with PCOS include obesity, hirsutism, acne, and infertility. Menstrual irregularity, which occurs in approximately 75% of women with PCOS, may be the first presenting symptom suggestive of the disorder. Women with this condition often have insulin resistance and are at an increased risk for developing type 2 diabetes mellitus (Speroff & Mishell, 2007). There is also an increased risk for coronary artery disease, hypertension, cancer (e.g., endometrial, ovarian, breast), and dyslipidemia. PCOS is often diagnosed during adolescence, and the prevalence of the disorder in Mexican Americans is twice that of other ethnic groups (ACOG, 2009b; DuRant, Leslie, & Critch, 2009; Lindenbaum, 2010).

 Optimizing Outcomes— **With lifestyle modifications to improve PCOS**

Diet, exercise, and weight loss are considered the best first-line interventions to improve PCOS. An increase in exercise combined with dietary change has been shown to reduce diabetes risk comparable to or better than medication. Weight control improves many aspects of the condition, leading to more regular menstrual cycles, reduced androgen levels, lowered lipid levels, and better glucose metabolism. To achieve weight loss, a low-fat, high-fiber diet with low-glycemic-index carbohydrates is recommended. Typically, women with PCOS have unique challenges achieving and maintaining healthy weights. Because they consume less energy metabolizing their food, they often require a lower-calorie diet than other women to lose weight. Obese women with PCOS should follow a hypocaloric diet (500 kcal/d deficit) that reduces the glycemic load. Reducing alcohol consumption is another way to decrease caloric intake. Moderate physical activity combined with muscle-strengthening exercises improves insulin sensitivity and helps to limit the loss of lean muscle mass. Cognitive behavior therapy, which involves teaching problem-solving skills and enhancing and reframing perceptions, may be useful in helping women with PCOS to overcome the barriers to adopting lifestyle changes needed to improve health (ACOG, 2009b; DuRant, Leslie, & Critch, 2009; Fan et al., 2008; Hoeger, 2007; Lindenbaum, 2010; Nelson, 2009).

Medical treatment of patients with PCOS usually depends on the presenting signs and symptoms. For women who are not attempting to conceive, combination low-dose hormonal contraceptives are the usual treatment because they inhibit LH and decrease testosterone levels. Oral contraceptives may also lessen acne and hirsutism. If pregnancy is desired, medications to induce ovulation, such as clomiphene citrate (Clomid) are usually prescribed. Insulin medications for type 2 diabetes such as metformin hydrochloride (Glucophage) are used to lower insulin, testosterone, and glucose levels, which, in turn, can reduce symptoms of acne, hirsutism, abdominal obesity, and other symptoms associated with PCOS (ACOG, 2007, 2009b; Lindenbaum, 2010; Neal, Formyduval, & Taylor, 2009; Speroff & Mishell, 2007).

Nurses can counsel women with PCOS about their chronic disorder and the potential long-term effects on their health. A holistic approach to care encompasses a variety of lifestyle strategies, such as diet, exercise, and weight loss along with prescribed medications, when needed, to achieve good clinical outcomes and a better quality of life. Referrals for resources including cognitive behavior therapy, counseling for issues concerning body image and self-esteem, and support groups and nutritional information may be appropriate as well (DuRant, Leslie, & Critch, 2009; Lindenbaum, 2010).

Ovarian Cancer

Ovarian cancer is the leading cause of gynecological deaths and the fourth most common cause of cancer deaths in women, resulting in 16,000 deaths annually. Ovarian cancer accounts for about 3% of all cancers in women, and a woman's risk of getting invasive ovarian cancer during her lifetime is approximately 1 in 71. About two-thirds of women with ovarian cancer are 60 or older, and it is slightly more common in Caucasian women than in African American women (American Cancer Society [ACS], 2009a).

Although the cause is unknown, there are identified risk factors, including nulliparity, pregnancy later in life, obesity (body mass index of at least 30), the presence of *BRCA1* and *BRCA2* genes, a personal history of breast cancer, and a family history of breast, ovarian, or colorectal cancer. Associative causes include the use of fertility medications, exposure to asbestos, genital exposure to talcum powder, a high-fat diet, and childhood mumps infection. Pregnancy and oral contraceptive use provide some protection against ovarian cancer, and the use of postmenopausal estrogen may increase the risk (ACS, 2009a).

Unfortunately, the signs and symptoms of ovarian cancer are often vague until late in development. Ovarian cancer should be considered in any woman over age 40 who has complaints of vague abdominal or pelvic discomfort or enlargement, back pain, indigestion, inability to eat normally, feeling full after eating only a small amount, a sense of bloating, constipation, urinary incontinence of recent onset, or unexplained weight loss. Enlargement of the abdomen due to accumulation of fluid (ascites) is the most common sign. Since ovarian cancer is a rapidly growing neoplasm, the diagnosis is often not made until the cancer has metastasized (ACOG, 2002; ACS, 2009a; Goff, Mandel, et al., 2007).

Ovarian cancer is rarely diagnosed early. In fact, nearly 70% of women with ovarian cancer have already experienced metastatic spread outside of the pelvis by the time of the initial diagnosis. Methods for mass screening and early detection have not been successful, and currently an annual bimanual examination is recommended. Tests that are used most frequently to screen for ovarian cancer include transvaginal sonography, which can be used to determine the size, location, and quality (e.g., fluid filled, solid) of the mass and serum CA-125 antigen levels (ACOG, 2002; ACS, 2009a).

---

 where research and practice meet:
HER LIFESTYLE Mneumonic for Recognizing PCOS

Neal, Formyduval, and Taylor (2010) developed HER LIFESTYLE, a tool designed to aid health-care providers in recognizing and managing PCOS in their adolescent patients. The mnemonic can be incorporated into clinical practice to assist with educational efforts about lifestyle modification and its positive effects on PCOS. Specifically, the mnemonic includes the following:

H—Hirsutism (discuss treatment options for this sensitive issue)
E—Education (educate about potential complications of PCOS, treatment options, lifestyle modifications)
R—Reassure (reassure that options are available to help manage PCOS)
L—Lose weight (to decrease symptoms and risk factors associated with PCOS)
I—Irregular periods (consider PCOS as a possible cause of irregular periods)
F—Fertility (impaired fertility, a complication of PCOS, can be devastating)
E—Exercise (include regular exercise in lifestyle changes)
S—Skin (assess for skin changes [e.g., acne, acanthosis nigricans]), consider treatment options
T—Talk (take time to talk with adolescent patients with PCOS; changes now can affect future health)
Y—Youth (consider the patient's developmental stage and present concerns)
L—Long-term consequences (stress what may happen without treatment; assess personal perception of risk)
E—Eating plan (encourage a high-fiber, low-fat diet; assess progress with each visit)

Optimizing Outcomes— **Biomarkers for epithelial ovarian cancer**

CA-125 is a serum protein that is higher in many women with epithelial ovarian cancer. In premenopausal women with symptoms, a CA-125 measurement is frequently not useful because elevated levels of the protein are associated with a variety of common benign conditions (e.g., uterine leiomyomata, PID, endometriosis, pregnancy). In post-menopausal women with a pelvic mass, a CA-125 measurement may be helpful in predicting a higher likelihood of a malignant tumor than a benign tumor, although a normal CA-125 measurement alone does not rule out ovarian cancer. Human epididymis protein 4 (HE4) is a secreted glycoprotein expressed in normal glandular epithelium of the reproductive tract. HE4 has been validated as a serum tumor marker for epithelial ovarian cancer (EOC), and it has recently been cleared by the FDA as a monitoring tool for patients diagnosed with EOC. A new ovarian cancer blood test, called OVA1, has also recently gained FDA approval. The OVA1 biomarker panel can help assess the likelihood of malignancy of an ovarian tumor before surgery and facilitate decisions about referral to a gynecological oncologist (ACOG, 2002; ACS, 2009a; Moore & MacLaughlan, 2009).

A strong family history of breast cancer may be caused by an inherited mutation in the *BRCA-1* or *BRCA-2* gene. Since alterations in these genes have been detected in women with ovarian cancer, screening women with the BRCA mutations can be performed to determine whether they carry these genes. Interestingly, these mutations also increase the risks for primary peritoneal carcinoma and fallopian tube carcinoma (ACOG, 2002; ACS, 2009a).

Laparotomy is performed for surgical confirmation and clinical staging, which provides direction to the treatment and prognosis of the cancer. The preferred treatment for ovarian cancer is surgical removal and usually requires a hysterectomy with bilateral salpingo-oophorectomy. After surgery, chemotherapy (administered intravenously and intraperitoneally), sometimes combined with immunotherapy, is used to treat any remaining cancer. Radiation therapy may be used as a palliative measure, although it is not typically used as a treatment option for ovarian cancer (ACOG, 2008c; Goff, Matthews, et al., 2007; Hordern, 2007).

 Optimizing Outcomes— **Enhancing ovarian cancer awareness**

Nurses can help promote women's awareness and understanding of their bodies by empowering them with information about specific symptoms that may be associated with ovarian cancer. The Geoff Symptom Index was developed to aid in the early identification of women with potential ovarian cancer. The tool focuses on symptoms most often seen among women who were later diagnosed with ovarian cancer. The easy-to-administer symptom index includes the following symptoms: bloating, pelvic or abdominal pain, difficulty eating or feeling full quickly, and urinary urgency or frequency. Scientists note that the frequency and/or number of symptoms are correlated with the diagnosis of ovarian cancer, and women who experience any of these symptoms on a daily basis for more than a few weeks should be counseled to contact their women's health-care specialist. Recently, the Ovarian Cancer National Alliance issued Interim Practice Guidance for the diagnosis of ovarian cancer. Posted online, these guidelines represent the first time that ovarian cancer diagnostic protocols have been made available to the public. In conjunction with the Gynecologic Cancer Foundation, a Symptom Diary, designed to help women measure the persistency and severity of their symptoms, is also available at http://www.ovariancancer.org/diary (Fife, 2007; Goff, Mandel, et al., 2007; Hellwig, 2007).

Endometrial Cancer

In the United States, cancer of the endometrium is the most common gynecological malignancy. According to estimates from the ACS (2009b), for the year 2009, approximately 42,000 new cases of cancer of the uterine corpus (body) were diagnosed. The estimates include both endometrial cancers and uterine sarcomas (which are rare and represent 2% of uterine body cancers). Most uterine malignancies arise within the inner lining of the uterus and are adenocarcinomas that develop from overgrowth (hyperplasia) of the endometrium. Uterine cancer is rarely found in women under age 40; approximately 70% of all cases are found in women in the 50–69 age group. The average chance of a woman being diagnosed with endometrial cancer during her lifetime is about 1 in 40. Currently, there are over 500,000 survivors of endometrial cancer living in this country. Interestingly, this cancer is more common in Caucasian women, but African American women are more likely to die from it (ACOG, 2005, 2007; ACS, 2009b).

 Nursing Insight— *Estrogen and endometrial cancer*

There is an established relationship between unopposed (i.e., absence of progesterone) exogenous estrogen and uterine cancer. Progesterone inhibits the growth of cells stimulated by estrogen and causes them to enter a more mature secretory state. Postmenopausal women who receive estrogen therapy without progesterone have much higher rates of uterine cancer.

Ethnocultural Considerations— **Endometrial cancer in African American women**

The lifetime mortality risk for Caucasian women with uterine cancer is 2.8% (risk for disease) and 0.48% (risk for death), as compared with African American women, whose risk for developing this condition is 1.7% and whose risk for dying from the condition is 0.73%. The 5-year survival rate for Caucasian women older than 65 years is 80.8%; for African American women in the same age group, the 5-year survival rate is 53.3%. It is unclear whether the high mortality in African American women is a result of delayed treatment, lack of access to care, or a higher likelihood of cancers with more serious prognostic characteristics. It is known, however, that of women with endometrial cancer, only 52% of African American women older than 50 years have the condition confined to the uterus at the time of the original surgery, as compared with 73% of Caucasian women older than 50 years (ACOG, 2008c; Ries et al., 2004).

The exact cause of uterine cancer is not known. However, risk factors have been established. These include unopposed estrogen therapy, nulliparity or low parity, early menarche (before age 12), late menopause (after age 55), therapy with tamoxifen (an anti-estrogen medication used in the prevention and treatment of breast cancer), infertility, diabetes, gallbladder disease, PCOS, a history of ovarian granulosa-theca cell tumors, hypertension, diabetes mellitus, a high-fat diet (which increases the levels of circulating estrogen), and obesity. Factors associated with a lower risk for endometrial cancer include multiparity, use of combination oral contraceptives, use of an intrauterine device, and menopausal estrogen therapy combined with progesterone therapy for women who have a uterus. A genetic syndrome known as hereditary nonpolyposis colon cancer has also been associated with both endometrial and ovarian cancer (ACOG, 2005, 2007; ACS, 2009b).

Endometrial cancer is slow growing, and over 75% of the neoplasms are adenocarcinomas that develop from endometrial hyperplasia. Most women are symptomatic in the early stages of this cancer, a factor that leads to early diagnosis and, frequently, successful treatment. There are no effective screening methods to detect endometrial cancer. Instead, women and their health-care providers must rely on signs and symptoms of the condition. For postmenopausal women, the cardinal symptom is vaginal bleeding; perimenopausal women may experience heavy or prolonged menstruation or spotting or bleeding between menses. Other symptoms for women in all age groups include pelvic pain, dyspareunia, and weight loss (ACOG, 2005, 2009a; ACS, 2009b).

Pelvic examination may reveal a uterine enlargement or mass. A patient who has abnormal vaginal bleeding should have an endometrial biopsy. Fractional curettage, a procedure that involves a scraping of the endocervix and the endometrium to obtain tissue for histological evaluation, may also be performed. Other diagnostic tests that may be conducted include hysteroscopy (examination of the uterus through an endoscope) and transvaginal ultrasound. If invasive endometrial cancer is present, systematic surgical staging is performed. The workup may also include chest radiography, abdominal computed tomography (CT) scan, MRI, cystoscopy, proctoscopy, liver function tests, renal function tests, bone scans, and serum testing for the presence of cancer antigen 125 (CA-125, released by some endometrial and ovarian cancers) to determine the extent of metastasis (ACOG, 2005, 2009a; ACS, 2009b).

Endometrial cancer is staged based on its location and extension into surrounding tissue and distant metastases. Treatment involves total abdominal hysterectomy along with removal of the ovaries, fallopian tubes, and local lymph nodes. Following the surgery, radiation therapy, chemotherapy, or hormone therapy may be prescribed, depending on the clinical findings. When diagnosed and treated early, survival rates are good. For all cases of endometrial cancer, the relative 5-year survival rate is approximately 83%; for cancers treated at an earlier stage, the 5-year survival rate exceeds 92% (ACOG, 2007; ACS, 2009b).

Now Can You— **Discuss ovarian tumors and endometrial cancer?**

1. Differentiate between ovarian follicular cysts and corpus luteum cysts?

2. Develop a holistic nursing plan of care for a woman with a diagnosis of polycystic ovary syndrome?

3. Develop an ovarian cancer awareness educational program for women?

4. Discuss the major risk factors for endometrial cancer, and identify the primary presenting symptom?

Diseases of the Vulva

The external female genital organs, or vulva, include all visible structures that extend externally from the mons pubis to the perineum. The vulvar tissue is richly supplied with sweat and sebaceous glands, and some areas contain hair follicles as well. The vulvar region supports a moist environment that contains increased concentrations of skin bacteria.

Symptoms of vulvovaginal disorders are common, often chronic, and can significantly interfere with a woman's sexual function and sense of well-being. Obtaining a detailed health history is an essential tool in the patient assessment, and it is important to remember that systemic conditions such as Crohn's disease can cause vulvar symptoms. Vulvar pruritus, or itching, is the most frequent symptom, and women often delay evaluation because they self-treat with readily available vaginal preparations. Other commonly reported symptoms in the vulvar region include a sensation of burning, the presence of a lump or sore, vaginal discharge, a rash, and pain. Frequently encountered vulvar conditions include vaginal infections, Bartholin's gland abscess, parasites, molluscum contagiosum, and vulvar warts (ACOG, 2008d).

VAGINAL INFECTIONS

Vaginal infections can produce vulvar symptoms. Candidiasis (yeast infection) often is associated with intense itching and tissue irritation. Women who are immunocompromised, diabetic, overweight, or receiving long-term antibiotic therapy are especially susceptible to vulvar yeast infections that may be resistant to treatment. Because the infection may stem from multiple types of yeast or include bacterial organisms, it is important to perform an appropriate diagnostic evaluation (ACOG, 2008d).

BARTHOLIN'S GLAND ABSCESS

The Bartholin's glands, also known as the greater vestibular or vulvovaginal glands, are located deep within the posterior portion of the vestibule near the posterior vaginal introitus (Fig. 4-6).

A & P review **The Bartholin's Glands**

The vestibule is essentially an oval-shaped space enclosed by the labia minora. It contains openings to the urethra and vagina, the Skene's glands, and the Bartholin's glands. This area of a woman's anatomy is extremely sensitive to chemical irritants. The Bartholin's glands secrete a clear mucus that moistens and lubricates the vagina during sexual arousal. ◆

Bartholin's cysts are the most common benign lesions of the vulva. Obstruction of the Bartholin duct leads to enlargement and formation of a cyst. The cyst may cause

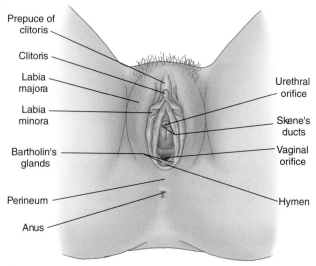

Figure 4-6 Female external genitalia (Dillon, P. M. (2007). *Nursing health assessment: A critical thinking approach* (2nd ed., p. 612). Philadelphia, F. A. Davis)

Figure 4-7 Molluscum contagiosum (Venes, D. (Ed.). (2009). *Taber's cyclopedic medical dictionary* (p. 1498, 21st ed.). Philadelphia: F. A. Davis)

no symptoms, but if it enlarges or becomes infected, the woman frequently experiences pain, dyspareunia, and an awareness of a tender mass in the area. When symptomatic, incision and drainage provides temporary relief. Because Bartholin's cysts tend to recur, a permanent opening for drainage may be recommended. Rarely, the abscess is caused by gonorrhea. Bartholin's abscesses are highly unusual in postmenopausal women and should be evaluated to rule out malignancy (ACOG, 2008d).

PARASITES

Lice or mites may infect the vulva. Intense itching of the skin that contains hair follicles is characteristic of infestation. Scabies, a dermatitis caused by the itch mite *Sarcoptes scabiei,* produces areas of excoriation composed of scaly papules and insect burrows. Scabies is transmitted by person-to-person contact or through infested bedding and clothing. The itching tends to worsen at night. Scabies spreads on the skin by fingernail contamination. Diagnosis is made by microscopic examination of skin scrapings to detect the presence of the mite, its eggs, or its excretions (Venes, 2009).

 Nursing Insight— Formulating appropriate nursing diagnoses for patients with scabies

Nursing diagnoses for patients with scabies usually focus on Impaired Skin Integrity related to the presence of invasive parasites and the development of pruritus and Deficient Knowledge regarding the communicable nature of the infestation, possible complications, therapy, and self-care needs related to a lack of information or misinterpretation.

MOLLUSCUM CONTAGIOSUM (SEED WART)

Molluscum contagiosum is a rash composed of small, dome-shaped papules with a central crater filled with a cheesy (caseous) material (Fig. 4-7). The lesions of molluscum contagiosum are caused by a pox virus. In adults, transmission is primarily sexual; in children, transmission is nonsexual and via fomites, substances that adhere to and transmit infection (Venes, 2009).

VULVAR CONDYLOMATA

A condyloma (plural: *condylomas, condylomata*) is a growth that resembles a wart on the skin or mucous membrane, usually of the genitals or anus. Vulvar condylomata, also known as "warts," "genital warts," and "venereal warts," are caused by certain strains of the human papillomavirus, different from those that produce cervical lesions. Condylomata can appear as small, thickened growths or large cauliflower-like masses on the vulva, along the perineum, or in and around the anus. The benign growths can be treated with chemicals, cryosurgery, electrosurgery, or laser vaporization. None of the treatments are fully successful, however, and recurrence is common. Despite removal of the lesions, surrounding tissues continue to harbor the human papillomavirus. Condylomata may be spread by physical contact with an area containing a wart, and the spread of a wart from one labium to the other by autoinoculation is possible (ACOG, 2008d; Venes, 2009). (See further discussion about human papillomavirus in Chapter 5.)

 Nursing Insight— Premalignant and malignant vulvar lesions

Most vulvar cancer is squamous in origin. Because the vulva is covered with skin, any malignancy that appears elsewhere on the skin can also occur on the vulva. *Vulvar intraepithelial neoplasia* (VIN) is a cancer precursor often associated with human papillomavirus. The most common symptom of VIN is persistent itching; localized burning and/or skin thickening or discoloration (e.g., red, pink, lighter, or darker) in the affected area may also be present. Biopsy is needed for diagnosis. Women who have a history of genital warts and who smoke have an increased risk of developing vulvar cancer. *Invasive vulvar cancer* is the presence of a malignant lesion that breaks through the cellular basement membrane. This type of cancer occurs most often in older (70+ years) women, and in the United States it is responsible for 5% of all female genital malignancies. Treatment involves surgical excision (vulvectomy) and inguinal lymphadenectomy (ACOG, 2008d; ACS, 2009c).

Melanoma is the second most common type of invasive vulvar malignancy, but it is extremely rare, accounting for less than 5% of all vulvar cancers. Most melanomas are located on the labia minora or clitoris and are blue-black in color. They have a jagged or fuzzy border, and the lesions may be raised or ulcerated. Although the condition may affect women of all ages, vulvar melanoma is more common in older (70+ years) women, and over 90% occur in Caucasian women. Biopsy is needed for diagnosis, and treatment involves surgical excision and in some situations inguinal lymphadenectomy (ACOG, 2008d; ACS, 2009c).

Paget disease is another rare neoplasm of the vulva. It also occurs more commonly in older (70+ years) women. Symptoms include intense vulvar itching and soreness, usually of long duration. Lesions of Paget disease are thick, often leading to an impression of leukoplakia. The affected area may also be red, moist, and elevated; biopsy is necessary for diagnosis. Treatment consists of surgical excision (ACOG, 2008d; ACS, 2009c).

THE NURSE'S ROLE IN PROMOTING VULVAR HEALTH

Nurses should be aware of common vulvar irritants and allergens (see Box 4-3) so that they can provide appropriate patient counseling and offer strategies for promoting and maintaining a healthy vulvar environment to reduce the risk of irritation and infection. Nurses can also teach women to wear cotton underwear, keep the vulvar area clean and dry, avoid douching, and perform monthly vulvar self-examination.

Box 4-3 **Common Vulvar Irritants and Allergens**

Adult or baby wipes

Antiseptics (e.g., povidone iodine, hexachlorophene)

Body fluids (e.g., semen, saliva)

Colored or scented toilet paper

Condoms (lubricant or spermicide containing)

Contraceptive creams, jellies, foams, nonoxynol-9, and lubricants

Dyes

Emollients (e.g., lanolin, jojoba oil, glycerin)

Laundry detergents, fabric softeners, and dryer sheets

Rubber products (including latex)

Sanitary products, including tampons and pads

Soaps, bubble bath and salts, shampoos, and conditioners

Tea tree oil

Topical anesthetics (e.g., benzocaine, lidocaine, dibucaine)

Topical antibacterials (e.g., neomycin, bacitracin, polymyxin)

Topical antimycotics (e.g., imidazoles, nystatin)

Topical corticosteroids

Topical medications, including trichloroacetic acid, 5-fluorouracil, and podofilox or podophyllin

Vaginal hygiene products, including perfumes and deodorants

Source: ACOG, 2008d.

Family Teaching Guidelines...
Performing Vulvar Self-examination

To prepare for vulvar self-examination, the woman places a flashlight and mirror within easy reach. She washes her hands, removes clothing from the waist down, and sits comfortably on the floor or bed, with a pillow support behind her back. The following steps should then be performed:

1. While bending her knees, she leans backward and allows her knees to fall slightly apart to expose the genital area. The mirror and flashlight should be positioned for optimal visualization.
2. External inspection of the genital area includes visualizing the labia, the clitoris, the urethral meatus, the vaginal opening, and the anal opening.
3. Using her fingers, the woman should gently spread the labia and inspect the vaginal vault. The vaginal walls should be pink and contain small folds or ridges called rugae.
4. The vaginal discharge should be evaluated at this time as well. Normal vaginal discharge is clear to cloudy and white, with a slightly acidic odor; it may be thick or thin, depending on the timing of the examination with regard to the menstrual cycle.
5. Findings that need to be reported to the health-care provider include the presence of sores or growths on the labia or vaginal walls, an unpleasant odor to the vaginal discharge, and tissue redness. Sores, redness, abnormal growths, malodorous or excessive vaginal discharge, and itching may indicate irritation or infection.

Source: Vulval Pain Society, 2008.

 Now Can You— **Discuss conditions of the vulva?**

1. Describe signs, symptoms, and treatment modalities for a Bartholin gland cyst?
2. Discuss signs and symptoms of vulvar carcinoma, and identify populations at greatest risk for development of this type of cancer?
3. Teach a patient how to perform vulvar self-examination?

summary points

◆ Menstrual disorders, such as amenorrhea, irregular bleeding, and dysmenorrheal, constitute some of the most common reproductive problems in women.

◆ Endometriosis is a chronic condition characterized by the presence of endometrial glands and tissue outside the uterus.

◆ Uterine leiomyomas are the most common solid pelvic tumors in women and the leading indication for hysterectomy.

◆ Dysfunctional uterine bleeding is defined as noncyclic menstrual blood flow that is derived from the endometrium.

◆ Ovarian cysts affect women of all ages, although they occur most often during the childbearing years and typically represent a normal process.

◆ Polycystic ovary syndrome occurs when an endocrine imbalance results in elevated levels of estrogen, testosterone, and luteinizing hormone and a decreased secretion of follicle-stimulating hormone.

◆ Ovarian cancer is the leading cause of gynecological deaths and the fourth most common cause of cancer deaths in women.

◆ In the United States, cancer of the endometrium is the most common gynecological malignancy, and approximately 70% of all cases are found in women in the 50–69 age group.

◆ Nurses can promote vulvar health by teaching women about strategies such as the avoidance of common vulvar irritants and how perform vulvar self-examination.

review questions

Multiple Choice

1. The nurse is aware that secondary amenorrhea may be caused by:
A. Lactation
B. Crohn's disease
C. Congenital absence of the vagina
D. Polycystic ovary syndrome

2. During patient teaching, the nurse explains that primary dysmenorrhea is related to:
A. Pregnancy
B. Leiomyoma
C. Perimenopause
D. Prostaglandins

3. When providing counseling for a patient with a diagnosis of endometriosis, the nurse explains that:
A. Consuming a high-fat diet may help to minimize symptoms.
B. Medical treatment is designed to reduce the amount of estrogen in the body.
C. Laparoscopic surgical removal of the lesions results in a permanent cure.
D. Infertility is a rare complication of the condition.

4. The nurse explains to a patient with a diagnosis of abnormal uterine bleeding that thermal balloon ablation is a technique developed to:
A. Restore fertility
B. Destroy the uterine lining
C. Treat uterine cancer
D. Open blocked fallopian tubes

5. Nurses can teach women about strategies to promote vulvar health, such as:
A. Performing monthly vulvar self-examination
B. Using scented toilet paper
C. Douching once a week
D. Wearing synthetic underwear

REFERENCES

Ailawadi, R. K., Jobranpufra, S., Kataria, M., Gurates, B., & Bulun, S. E. (2004). Treatment of endometriosis and chronic pelvic pain with letrozole and norethindrone acetate: A pilot study. *Fertility and Sterility, 81*(2), 290–296.

American Cancer Society (ACS). (2009a). *What are key statistics about ovarian cancer?* Retrieved March 10, 2010, from http://www.cancer.org/docroot/cri/content/cri_2_4_1x_what_are_the_key_statistics_for_ovarian_cancer_33.asp

American Cancer Society (ACS). (2009b). *Detailed guide: Endometrial cancer.* Retrieved March 11, 2010, from http://www.cancer.org/docroot/CRI/content/CRI_2_4_1x_What_is_Endometrial_Cancer.asp?sitearea=

American Cancer Society (ACS). (2009c). *Detailed guide: Vulvar cancer.* Retrieved March 11, 2010, from http://www.cancer.org/docroot/CRI/content/CRI_2_4_1X_What_is_vulvar_cancer_45.asp?sitearea=

American College of Obstetricians and Gynecologists (ACOG). (2000). *Management of anovulatory bleeding* (Practice Bulletin No. 14, pp. 1049–1056). Washington, DC: Author.

American College of Obstetricians and Gynecologists (ACOG). (2002, December). The role of the generalist obstetrician–gynecologist in the early detection of ovarian cancer (ACOG Committee Opinion No. 280). *Obstetrics and Gynecology, 100*(6), 1413–1416.

American College of Obstetricians and Gynecologists (ACOG). (2005). *Management of endometrial cancer* (Practice Bulletin No. 65, pp. 1258–1269). Washington, DC: Author.

American College of Obstetricians and Gynecologists (ACOG>. (2007). *Women's health care: A resource manual.* (3rd ed.). Washington, DC: Author.

American College of Obstetricians and Gynecologists (ACOG). (2008a). *Treatment of urinary tract infections in non-pregnant women* (Practice Bulletin No. 91, pp. 10–12). Washington, DC: Author.

American College of Obstetricians and Gynecologists (ACOG). (2008b). *Alternatives to hysterectomy in the management of leiomyomas* (Practice Bulletin No. 96, pp. 388–397). Washington, DC: Author.

American College of Obstetricians and Gynecologists (ACOG). (2008c). Intraperitoneal chemotherapy for ovarian cancer (ACOG Committee Opinion No. 396). *Obstetrics and Gynecology, 111*(3), 249–251.

American College of Obstetricians and Gynecologists (ACOG). (2008d). *Diagnosis and management of vulvar skin disorders* (Practice Bulletin No. 93, pp. 370–379). Washington, DC: Author.

American College of Obstetricians and Gynecologists (ACOG). (2009a). Choosing the route of hysterectomy for benign disease (ACOG Committee Opinion No. 444). *Obstetrics and Gynecology, 114*(5), 1156–1158.

American College of Obstetricians and Gynecologists (ACOG). (2009b). *Polycystic ovary syndrome* (Practice Bulletin No. 108, pp. 936–948). Washington, DC: Author.

American Society for Reproductive Medicine (ASRM). (2006). Endometriosis and infertility. *Fertility and Sterility, 86*(4), 156–160.

Audebert, A., Backstrom, T., Barlow, D.H., Benagiano, G., Brosens, I., Buhler, K., Donnez, J., Evers, J., Pellicer, A., & Mettler, L. (1992). Endometriosis 1991: A discussion document. *Human Reproduction, 7*(3), 432–435.

Bazot, M., Detchev, R., Cortez, A., Amouyal, P., Uzan, S., & Darai, E. (2003). Transvaginal sonography for the prediction of location of deep pelvic endometriosis. *Human Reproduction, 18*(8), 1686–1692.

Bertelsen, L., Mellemkjaer, L., Frederiksen, K., Kjaer, S. K., Brinton, L. A., Sakoda, L. C., van Valkengoed, I., & Olsen, J. H. (2007). Risk for breast cancer among women with endometriosis. *International Journal of Cancer, 120*(6), 1372–1375.

Bloski, T., & Pierson, R. (2008). Endometriosis and chronic pelvic pain: Unveiling the mystery behind this complex condition. *Nursing for Women's Health, 12*(5), 382–395.

Brankin, C. A., & Cackovic, M. (2010). Oral contraceptives for the treatment of pain associated with endometriosis. *Contemporary OB-GYN, 55*(3), 42–43.

Centers for Disease Control and Prevention (CDC). (2005). *Toxic shock syndrome.* Retrieved February 20, 2010, from http://www.cdc.gov/ncidod/dbmd/diseaseinfo/toxicshock_t.htm

Centers for Disease Control and Prevention (CDC). (2006a). *Sexually transmitted diseases treatment guidelines.* Retrieved February 15, 2010, from http://www.cdc.gov/std/treatment/2006/vaginal-discharge.htm#vagdis2

Centers for Disease Control and Prevention (CDC). (2006b). *Women's reproductive health: Hysterectomy.* Retrieved March 1, 2010, from http://www.cdc.gov/reproductivehealth/WomensRH/Hysterectomy.htm

Chopin, N., Ballester, M., Borghese, B., Fauconnier, A., Foulot, H., Marlartic, C., & Chapron, C. (2006). Relation between severity of dysmenorrhea and endometriosis. *Acta Obstetricia et Gynecologica Scandinavica, 85*(11), 1375–1380.

Coughlin, G., & Secor, M. (2010). Bacterial vaginosis: Update on evidence-based care. *Advance for Nurse Practitioners, 18*(1), 41–45.

Crosignani, P., Olive, D., Bergqvist, A., & Luciano, A. (2006). Advances in the management of endometriosis: An update for clinicians. *Human Reproduction Update, 12*(2), 179–189.

Day Baird, D., Dunson, D. B., Hill, M. C., Cousins, D., & Schectman, J. M. (2003). High cumulative incidence of uterine leiomyoma in African American and Caucasian women: Ultrasound evidence. *American Journal of Obstetrics & Gynecology, 188*(7), 100–107.

Deglin, J., & Vallerand, A. (2009). *Davis's drug guide for nurses* (11th ed.). Philadelphia: F. A. Davis.

Denny, E., & Mann, C. H. (2007). Endometriosis-associated dyspareunia: The impact on women's lives. *Journal of Family Planning and Reproductive Health Care, 33*(3), 189–193.

Dunican, K. (2008). OTC product: Vagisil Screening Kit for vaginal infections. *Journal of the American Pharmacists Association, 48*(2), e33.

DuRant, M. E., Leslie, N. S., & Critch, E. A. (2009). Managing polycystic ovary syndrome: A cognitive behavioral strategy. *Nursing for Women's Health, 13*(4), 293–300.

Elkins, B. L., & Mayeaux Jr., E. J. (2010). Bacterial vaginosis: Diagnosis and therapy. *Female Patient, 35*(3), 42–46.

Falagas, M. F., Betsil, G. I., & Athansion, S. (2006). Probiotics for prevention of recurrent vulvovaginal candidiasis: A review. *Journal of Antimicrobial Chemotherapy, 58*(9), 266–272.

Fan, A. Z., Russell, M., Naimi, T., Li, Y., Liao, Y., Jiles, R., & Mokdad, A. H. (2008). Patterns of alcohol consumption and the metabolic syndrome. *Journal of Clinical Endocrinology & Metabolism, 93*(10), 3833–3838.

Fife, A. (2007). Ovarian cancer: This "silent killer" does make noise. *Clinician Reviews, 17*(9), 10–16.

Fothergill, R., & Sulak, P. J. (2010). Ovulatory heavy menstrual bleeding. *Female Patient, 35*(3), 15–19.

Fraser, I. S., Critchley, H. O., Munro, M. G., & Broder, M. (2007). A process designed to lead to international agreement on terminologies and definitions used to describe abnormalities of menstrual bleeding. *Fertility & Sterility, 87*(3), 466–476.

Goff, B. A., Mandel, L. S., Drescher, C. W., Urban, N., Gough, S., Schurman, K. M., Patras, J., Mahony, B.S., & Andersen, M. R. (2007). Development of an ovarian cancer symptom index: Possibilities for earlier detection. *Cancer, 109*(2), 2031–2042.

Goff, B. A., Matthews, B. J., Larson, E. H., Andrilla, C. H., Wynn, M., Lishner, D. M., & Baldwin, L. M. (2007). Predictors of comprehensive surgical treatment in patients with ovarian cancer. *Cancer, 109*(10), 2031–2042.

Goodman, P., Herman, J., Murdaugh, C. L., Moneyham, L. D., & Phillips, K. D. (2007). Role of decision-making in women's self-diagnosis and management of vaginitis. *Women's Health Care, 6*(2), 57–63.

Guo, S. W., & Wang, Y. (2006). The prevalence of endometriosis in women with chronic pelvic pain. *Gynecologic & Obstetric Investigation, 62*(3), 54–58.

Hatcher, R. A., Trussell, J., Nelson, A., Cates, F., Stewart, F., & Kowal, D. (Eds.). (2008). *Contraceptive technology* (19th ed.). New York: Ardent Media.

Hellwig, J. P. (2007). Ovarian cancer: Considering symptoms. *Nursing for Women's Health, 11*(2), 123.

Helming, M. B. (2009). Three generations and counting: The many health threats of DES. *Advance for Nurse Practitioners, 17*(8), 27–30.

Hoeger, K. M. (2007). Obesity and lifestyle management in polycystic ovary syndrome. *Clinical Obstetrics and Gynecology, 50*(1), 277–294.

Hordern, B. (2007). Finding ovarian cancer early: What to look for. *Clinical Advisor, 10*(5), 99–103.

Huntington, A., & Gilmour, J. A. (2005). A life shaped by pain: Women and endometriosis. *Journal of Clinical Nursing, 14*(9), 1124–1132.

Keehbauch, J. A., & Nystrom, J. (2007). Diagnosis and management of abnormal uterine bleeding. *Female Patient, 32*(7), 38–40.

Koumans, E. H., Sternberg, M., Vruce, C., McQuillan, G., Kendrick, J., Sutton, M., & Markowitz, L. E. (2007). The prevalence of bacterial vaginosis in the United States, 2001–2004; Associations with symptoms, sexual behaviors, and reproductive health. *Sexually Transmitted Diseases, 34*(11), 864–869.

Lindenbaum, C. (2010). Polycystic ovarian syndrome: Where genetics and environment collide. *Advance for Nurse Practitioners, 18*(2), 20–27.

Moore, R. G., & MacLaughlan, S. (2009). A novel approach for the risk assessment of a pelvic mass for ovarian cancer. *Female Patient, 34*(9), 31–37.

National Cancer Institute (NCI). (2009). *Vaginal cancer.* Retrieved February 16, 2010, from http://www.cancer.gov/cancertopics/pdq/treatment/vaginal/HealthProfessional/

Nelson, A. L. (2009). Metabolic syndrome in women with polycystic ovary syndrome. *Female Patient, 32*(8), 15–22.

Nelson, A. L., & Baldwin, S. (2008). Menstrual disorders and related concerns. In R. Hatcher et al. (Eds.), *Contraceptive technology* (19th ed., pp. 451–469). New York: Ardent Media.

Neal, D. D., Formyduval, A. M., & Taylor, J. S. (2010). HER LIFESTYLE: A mnemonic for addressing polycystic ovary syndrome in adolescents. *Nursing for Women's Health, 13*(6), 473–478.

Ninia, J. G. (2007). Pelvic congestion syndrome. *Female Patient, 32*(8), 41–49.

Nyirjesy, P., & Sobel, J. D. (2005). Advances in diagnosing vaginitis: Development of a new algorithm. *Current Infectious Disease Reports, 7*(16), 458–462.

Pirotta, M. V., & Garland, S. M. (2006). Genital *Candida* species detected in samples from women in Melbourne, Australia, before and after treatment with antibiotics. *Journal of Clinical Microbiology, 44*(6), 3213–3217.

Ries, L. A. G., Eisner, M. P., Kosary, C. L., Hankey, B. F., Miller, B. A., Clegg, L., Mariotto, A., Feuer, E.J., & Edwards, B. K. (Eds.). *SEER cancer statistics review, 1975–2001.* Bethesda, MD: National Cancer Institute. Retrieved March 9, 1010, from http://seer.cancer.gov/csr/1975_2001/

Sadovsky, R. (2007). Managing first-time and recurrent UTIs. *Clinical Advisor, 9*(5), 46–51.

Sampson, J. A. (1940). The development of the implantation theory for the origin of peritoneal endometriosis. *American Journal of Obstetrics and Gynecology, 40*(6), 549–557.

Scolaro, K. L., Lloyd, K. B., & Helms, K. L. (2008). Devices for home evaluation of women's health concerns. *American Journal of Health-System Pharmacists, 65*(4), 299–314.

Sheary, B., & Dayan, L. (2005). Clinical practice. Recurrent vulvovaginal candidiasis. *Australian Family Physician, 34*(9), 147–150.

Shippen, E. R., & West, W. J. (2004). Successful treatment of severe endometriosis in two premenopausal women with an aromatase inhibitor. *Fertility and Sterility, 81*(5), 1395–1398.

Sinaii, N., Cleary, S. D., Younes, N., Ballweg, M., & Stratton, P. (2002). High rates of autoimmune and endocrine disorders, fibromyalgia, chronic fatigue syndrome and atopic diseases among women with endometriosis: A survey analysis. *HumanReproduction, 17*(10), 2715–2724.

Smith, O. W. (1948). Diethylstilbestrol in the prevention and treatment of complications of pregnancy. *American Journal of Obstetrics and Gynecology, 56*(3), 821–834.

Society of Obstetricians and Gynaecologists of Canada. (2005). SOGC clinical guidelines: Uterine fibroid embolization (UFE). *International Journal of Gynaecology and Obstetrics, 89*(3), 305–318.

Song, A. H. (2007). Global endometrial ablation devices: Minimally invasive surgical alternatives to hysterectomy. *Female Patient, 32*(7), 46–50.

Speroff, L., & Fritz, M. A. (2005). *Clinical gynecologic endocrinology and infertility* (7th ed.). Philadelphia: Lippincott Williams & Wilkins.

Speroff, L., & Mishell Jr., D. R. (2007). Polycystic ovary syndrome: Management and contraception. *Dialogues in Contraception, 11*(1), 5–7.

Spies, J. B., Myers, E. R., Worthington-Kirsch, R., Mulgund, J., Goodwin, S., & Mauro, M. (2005). The FIBROID registry: Symptom and quality-of-life status 1 year after therapy. *Obstetrics and Gynecology, 106*(6), 1309–1318.

Stern, J. L. (2007). *Cancers and treatments: Vagina.* Retrieved February 18, 2010, from http://womenscancercenter.com/info/types/typehome.html

Stern, L. (2009). Assessing excessive menstrual bleeding. *Clinical Advisor, 12*(1), 25–37.

U.S. Food and Drug Administration (FDA). (2009). *FDA approves Lysteda to treat heavy menstrual bleeding.* Retrieved March 5, 2010, from http://www.fda.gov/NewsEvents/Newsroom/PressAnnouncements/2009/ucm190551.htm

Venes, D. (2009). *Taber's cyclopedic medical dictionary* (21st ed.). Philadelphia: F. A. Davis.

Vermund, S. H., & Allen, K. L. (2009). Douching is a remediable risk factor for sexually transmitted infections. *The Female Patient, 34*(7), 37–39.

Vulval Pain Society. (2008). *How to perform a vulval self-exam.* Retrieved March 9, 2010, from http://vulvalpainsociety.org/index.php?page=self-examination

Watson, C., & Ng, G. (2008). Not that itch again: Dealing with recurrent vulvovaginal candidiasis. *Nursing for Women's Health, 12*(3), 215–223.

White, D., Vanthuyne, P., Wood, M., & Ayres, J. (2004). Zafirlukast for severe recurrent vulvovaginal candidiasis: An open label pilot study. *Sexually Transmitted Infections, 80*(2), 219–222.

Wolfe, J. (2006). Polycystic ovary syndrome: Case study decision tree. *Women's Health Care, 5*(7), 19–31.

Woodson, S. A. (2007). Chronic pelvic pain: Can you guess the cause? *Nursing for Women's Health, 11*(2), 200–204.

Wysocki, S. (2008). Vaginal pH as an OTC screening tool for vaginitis. *Advance for Nurse Practitioners,17*(20), 29–35.

 For more information, go to http://davisplus.fadavis.com/

Promoting Reproductive Health Through an Understanding of Sexually Transmitted Diseases

Shelton M. Hisley, PhD, RNC, WHNP-BC

We may run, walk, stumble, drive, or fly, but let us never lose sight of the reason for the journey, or miss a chance to see a rainbow on the way.

—Gloria Gaither

LEARNING TARGETS *At the completion of this chapter, the student will be able to:*

◆ Discuss signs and symptoms, modes of transmission, and treatment options for the most common sexually transmitted diseases (STDs).

◆ Identify various safer sex strategies.

◆ Describe the nurse's role in STD counseling and education.

Introduction

This chapter focuses on sexually transmitted diseases (STDs). Information regarding signs, symptoms, modes of transmission, and treatment options for various STDs is presented, along with a discussion of the nurse's role in promoting reproductive health. STDs encompass more than 25 infectious organisms that cause reproductive tract infections that are primarily transmitted by close, intimate contact. Nurses are perfectly situated to provide evidence-based, culturally sensitive STD counseling and education that facilitates understanding of these potentially lethal health threats and empowers women to make informed choices in their intimate relationships.

In many clinical settings, the terms *sexually transmitted disease* and *sexually transmitted infection* are used interchangeably. "Sexually transmitted disease" is the accepted subject heading in the PubMed database, and *STD* is also the term used by the Centers for Disease Control and Prevention (CDC) (Royer & Cerf, 2009). According to the CDC (2006b), an important component of STD health care is that providers use language that is understandable to patients. Owing to the fact that stigma associated with an STD can be a barrier to appropriate diagnosis and treatment (Royer & Zahner, 2009), some clinicians use the term STI instead of STD because discussing an infection with a patient may be less embarrassing than discussing a disease (Marrazzo et al., 2007).

In addition to the short-term emotional and physical distress usually associated with a reproductive tract infection, many serious long-term effects may also result from many of the STDs. Potential complications include fallopian tube blockage with resultant infertility, an increased risk of ectopic pregnancy, chronic pelvic pain, an increased risk of liver cancer and serious liver disease, and death. Women suffer more long-term reproductive consequences from STDs than do men, and women are more likely than men to acquire an infection from any single sexual encounter. Unfortunately, owing to the asymptomatic nature of many STDs, treatment is often delayed, and this factor increases the likelihood of more serious long-term consequences (Adler, 2007; Johnson-Mallard & Lengacher, 2007).

The incidence of several STDs has increased over the past few years. In late 2009, the CDC released STD Surveillance Data for the year 2008. According to the findings, Chlamydia remains the most commonly reported infectious disease in the United States. The rate of this infection has increased by 9.2% as compared to the 2007 data; however, it is important to note that the increase could be related to factors such as improved screening

where research and practice meet:
Exploring young women's beliefs about the terms *sexually transmitted disease* and *sexually transmitted infection*

It is unknown whether patients understand what their health-care provider means when using the terms *sexually transmitted disease* and *sexually transmitted infection*, and recent research (Royer, 2008) suggests that some female patients may be more familiar with the terms *sexually transmitted disease* or *STD*.

Royer and Cerf (2009) conducted a survey to determine whether young women differentiate between the terms *sexually transmitted disease* and *sexually transmitted infection* and, if so, whether their reasons were consistent with those of health-care providers. A total of 302 women aged 18 to 24 completed a survey that measured beliefs about STDs and whether they considered the terms *sexually transmitted disease* and *sexually transmitted infection* to be interchangeable. Fifty-seven percent responded that *sexually transmitted disease* and *sexually transmitted infection* do *not* mean the same thing; 28% believed that *STD* and *STI do* mean the same thing; and 15% responded that they did not know. The investigators concluded that while a majority of the young women do differentiate between the two terms, their rationale for doing so is not consistent with the rationale used by health-care providers. Based on the findings, the researchers suggested that professionals clarify their use of the terms *sexually transmitted disease* and *sexually transmitted infection* when talking with patients as a strategy to improve health communication and to improve STD health care.

methods and testing. Rates of gonorrhea have dropped from the 2007 data, with approximately 111 cases per 100,000 individuals. Similarly to Chlamydia, gonorrhea continues to be under-diagnosed and under-reported. Syphilis is on the comeback, with an increase of 18%, as compared to the 2007 data. Interestingly, at one point, this disease was once on the verge of elimination, but there have been increasing numbers of reported cases since 2001. Much of the increase has occurred among men who have sex with men and is attributed to increased rates of unsafe sexual practices (CDC, 2009a).

Nursing Insight— The National Health Initiative addresses sexually transmitted diseases

Several *Healthy People 2010* National Health Goals specifically focus on STDs:

- Reduce the proportion of adolescents and young adults with *Chlamydia trachomatis* infections from baselines of 12% (females) and 15% (males) to a target of 3%.
- Reduce new cases of gonorrhea to an incidence of no more than 19 new cases/100,000 people from a baseline of 123/100,000.
- Reduce primary and secondary syphilis to an incidence of no more than 0.2 cases/100,000 people from a baseline of 3.2 per 100,000.
- Reduce genital herpes to an incidence of no more than 14% from a baseline of 17%.
- Reduce pelvic inflammatory disease to an incidence of no more than 5% of women aged 15 through 44 from a baseline of 8% (U.S. Department of Health and Human Services [USDHHS], 2000).

Nurses can help the nation to meet these goals by providing education about methods of preventing STDs and information about how to recognize the signs and symptoms of these illnesses. Nurses can design studies and engage in research to provide evidence-based practice strategies for issues such as teaching women about safer sex practices, teaching youth about the methods of transmission of infection and the long-term consequences of the diseases, and ways that health professionals can increase STD awareness in their practice settings.

HIV/AIDS

In the years since acute HIV infection was first described, research has identified the cellular mechanisms that accompany its clinical presentation. HIV most commonly enters the host through percutaneous or genital routes. Once the virus has penetrated the mucosal epithelium, it infects macrophages, CD4+ T cells, and dendritic cells and spreads to the systemic lymph nodes within 2 days after infection. Within 3 days, it is detectable in the plasma. Plasma viremia then results in dissemination to various body organs, including the brain and spleen (Kahn & Walker, 1998; Swan, 2009).

Infection with HIV leads to a progressive disease that results in AIDS. The AIDS epidemic has in some way touched everyone's life, and the health profession has been affected profoundly. Many individuals living in the United States remain ignorant of the fact that AIDS affects men, women, and children and has reached epidemic proportions in many areas. Because HIV infection can remain asymptomatic for years, infected women can unknowingly harbor and transmit the virus. Women who are infected with HIV have special gynecological health needs that must be assessed and addressed (Marrazzo et al., 2007).

In this country, more and more young people, especially women, are contracting HIV. Most women are infected during sex with an HIV-infected man or while using HIV-contaminated syringes for the injection of drugs such as heroin, cocaine, and amphetamines. According to the CDC (2009b), approximately 56,300 individuals were newly infected with HIV in 2006. In 2007, the estimated number of persons diagnosed with AIDS was 37, 041. This is a higher estimate than those made in previous years and underscores the need to keep HIV prevention at the top of the public health agenda. In the United States, women ages 15 to 44 years represent one of the fastest growing segments of the epidemic. It is important to note that women are more likely than men to acquire HIV at any one contact (CDC, 2009b; Swan, 2009).

Ethnocultural Considerations— HIV disparities in the United States

According to the CDC, African American females are severely and disproportionately affected by HIV infection. In 2006, the HIV diagnosis rate for African American females (56.2) was more than 19 times the rate for Caucasian females (2.9). The rate for Hispanic women was 15.1, more than 5 times that for Caucasian females. Among American Indians/Alaska Natives, the rate for females (4.6) was nearly twice the rate for Caucasian females (CDC, 2008a).

Today, AIDS is the leading cause of death among young women in most of the world. The majority of women contracted the disease by exposure to infected men. The ratio of infected men and women worldwide approaches 1:1. Both sexual activity and IV drug use play major roles in current transmission statistics.

RISK FACTORS

Lifestyle behaviors that place a woman at risk for contracting HIV are listed in Box 5-1. When obtaining the patient history, it is important to routinely inquire about symptoms that may be associated with HIV. Although primary HIV infection is typically asymptomatic, women may describe nonspecific flulike discomforts such as fever, headache, night sweats, malaise, muscle aches, nausea, diarrhea, weight loss, sore throat, skin rash, and lymphadenopathy (Marrazzo et al., 2007).

 Nursing Insight— Current investigations in HIV prevention

In early 2009, the National Institutes of Health (NIH) published promising findings from a multisite clinical trial of topical products designed to reduce the risk of HIV. One product, a vaginal microbicide known as PRO 2000/5, is a vaginal gel applied before sex. The trial sites were in four African countries and also in the United States. When women used the PRO 2000/5 gel plus condoms, they had 30% fewer HIV infections than those offered only condoms or condoms plus a placebo gel. Reported adherence to the gel was very high, at 81%.

DETECTION, TESTING, AND DOCUMENTATION

Detecting HIV is a primary step in prevention of the virus. The CDC (2006a) recommends opt-out HIV testing for all patients in all health-care settings, including pregnant women. (*Opt-out testing* is defined as performing HIV screening after notifying the patient that the test will be performed and that the patient may elect to decline or defer testing. Assent is inferred unless the patient declines testing. *Opt-in testing* means that testing is offered and the patient is required to actively give permission before it can occur.) This latest guideline represents a major change from previous recommendations, which encouraged opt-in testing and suggested that providers consider HIV prevalence and individual risk factors when making recommendations for HIV testing to patients. The American College

---

Box 5-1 Risk Factors for HIV Infection

- Current or past history of drug use, especially IV drug use
- History of prostitution
- Frequent sexual intercourse with multiple partners
- Engaging in sexual intercourse under the influence of drugs
- Engaging in sexual intercourse with men who also have sex with men
- Residing in an area with a high prevalence of HIV infection (e.g., rural South and Northeast U.S.)
- Having received a blood transfusion or blood products before 1985

Source: CDC, 2009c.

---

of Obstetricians and Gynecologists (ACOG) supports routine screening for women aged 19 to 64 years and recommends screening for patients at high risk, including adolescents who are, or ever have been, sexually active. The latest guidelines are aimed at improving access to HIV testing across the country and increasing the number of individuals who are tested each year. It is estimated that up to 25% of persons infected with HIV are unaware of their status, and universal testing may identify more of them (ACOG, 2007; CDC, 2006a; Glynn & Rhodes, 2005; Swan, 2009).

 Optimizing Outcomes— **With CDC-endorsed HIV testing**

The CDC (2006) has published the following recommendations for HIV testing:
Patients in all health care settings:

- Perform HIV screening on every patient after informing the patient that testing will be performed unless the patient declines (opt-out testing).
- Screen patients at highest risk for HIV at least annually.
- General consent for medical care should be sufficient to encompass consent for HIV testing; no separate written consent should be required.
- Prevention counseling should not be required with HIV testing.

Pregnant women:

- Include HIV screen in routine prenatal testing for all pregnant women.
- Screening should be on an opt-out basis.
- General consent for medical care should be sufficient to encompass consent for HIV testing; no separate written consent should be required.
- Repeat HIV testing in the third trimester is recommended.

It is important for the nurse to assess the patient's level of understanding to ensure that she is aware of the legal, emotional, and medical implications of a positive or negative HIV test before she takes the test. Pregnancy is not encouraged for women who are HIV-positive; contraceptive counseling should be offered to HIV-positive women who do not desire pregnancy. Post-test counseling centers on telling the patient her test results, explaining the meaning of the results, and reinforcing infection prevention measures. Women should be advised that if they have been exposed in the past 6 months, they should be retested. All pre-and post-test counseling should be documented on the patient's chart.

 Be sure to— Conform to HIPAA regulations

If the HIV test results are to be placed on the patient's medical record, they are then available to everyone who accesses the chart. The patient must be advised of this policy before testing. Health-care facilities must have policies in place to safeguard patient information from inadvertent or inappropriate breaches of confidentiality. In some clinical settings, HIV-related information is maintained in a separate chart and a code is assigned for HIV test results. In other facilities, HIV-related information is removed from the medical record before it is released. Federal regulations set forth in the Health Insurance Portability and Accountability

Act (HIPAA) also provide specific rules for what information may be shared with other practitioners and agencies with and without an individual's permission. Results of HIV testing may need to be recorded and stored in a certain way. It is incumbent upon nurses to be familiar with the legal requirements that exist in the particular practice setting (ACOG, 2007; Marrazzo et al., 2007).

HIV infection is usually diagnosed via the HIV-1 and HIV-2 antibody tests. A schema for HIV screening in women is presented in Figure 5-1. Antibody testing is first performed with a sensitive screening test such as the enzyme-linked immunoassay (ELISA) (also called enzyme immunoassay [EIA]), which detects serum antibodies to HIV. Reactive screening tests are then confirmed by an additional test such as the Western blot or, less commonly, an immunofluorescence assay (IFA). If a positive antibody test is confirmed by a supplemental test, the woman is infected with HIV and is capable of infecting others. These diagnostic tests are very reliable; false-positive and false-negative results are rare. In general, seroconversion for HIV in adolescents and adults occurs from 6 to 12 weeks after transmission of the virus; HIV antibodies are detectable in at least 95% of patients within 3 months after infection (CDC, 2006a).

 Nursing Insight— Home testing for HIV

Patients who are reluctant to visit a care provider for testing can purchase a home collection kit at a pharmacy and collect their own finger-prick blood sample. The sample is then mailed to a lab and the patient may call for anonymous results and telephone counseling a few days later (Marrazzo et al., 2007).

Methods of rapid testing for HIV antibodies use a blood sample obtained by finger stick, venipuncture, or an oral fluid sample. The rapid tests can help to reduce unrecognized infections by improving access to testing in both clinical and nonclinical settings and increase the proportion of those tested who learn their results. Rapid testing facilitates patients receiving their test results the same day, usually at the encounter where the test specimen was collected. Like the conventional HIV EIAs, the rapid HIV tests are screening tests that require confirmation if reactive. Although false negatives are rare, they may occur in an individual who has been acutely infected but who has not yet developed HIV antibodies. All of the rapid tests are interpreted visually and require no instrumentation (Greenwald, Burstein, Pincus, & Branson, 2006; Swan, 2009).

Currently, no cure is available for HIV. Current standard of care for HIV is highly active antiretroviral therapy (HAART), a combination of oral antiretroviral agents that inhibit different targets of the virus (Marrazzo et al., 2007). The use of antiretroviral agents has been demonstrated to be effective in maintaining the health of HIV-positive women and in reducing or preventing the perinatal transmission of the virus. A number of opportunistic infections often accompany HIV infection. Information and current guidelines about management are available at the CDC AIDS Prevention hotline (1-800-CDC-INFO [232-4636]) and at their Web site, http://www.cdc.gov/hiv/.

SPECIAL CONCERNS FOR HIV-POSITIVE WOMEN

Women who are HIV positive may experience a number of psychosocial issues. They are often primary caregivers who bear the burden of responsibility for the care of their children. The illness presents major challenges in keeping appointments, receiving adequate rest, and complying with medication regimens. Other immediate needs may involve housing and financial difficulties, and in many situations, other family members are infected as well.

Gynecological problems are also a major concern. Owing to the immunocompromised state, vulvovaginal candidiasis, genital warts caused by human papillomavirus (HPV), and genital herpes lesions are more common and more severe in HIV-infected women. Menstrual problems such as heavy bleeding may require hormonal intervention to address the anemia and lessen the discomfort. However, because the relationship between HIV and menstrual disruption is unclear, all menstrual irregularities should be investigated (ACOG, 2007; Marrazzo et al., 2007).

 Across Clinical Settings: **Reducing HIV-related occupational risks for health-care providers**

There are three routes of transmission for HIV: direct sexual contact, perinatal transmission from the HIV-infected mother to her fetus or newborn, and direct inoculation with contaminated blood products, needles, or syringes. All health-care providers who may come in contact with

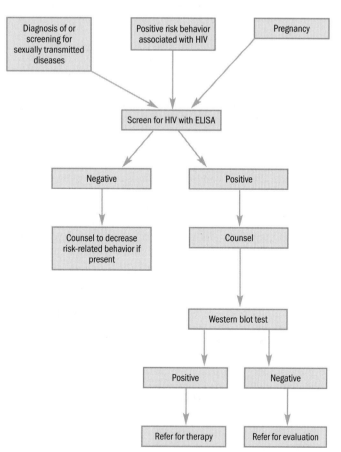

Figure 5-1 Screening for HIV in Women

contaminated blood products, needles, or syringes in any acute care, long-term care, or home care settings are at risk for occupational exposure to HIV. To address this risk, the CDC developed standard precautions, a set of principles to be used in the care of all patients at all times. To minimize personal risk, all health-care workers should consistently comply with the precautions.

 Now Can You— Discuss aspects of HIV infection?

1. Identify six risk factors for HIV infection?
2. Describe what is meant by "opt-out" HIV testing recommended by the CDC?
3. Discuss special concerns for HIV-positive women?

Chlamydia Trachomatis

Chlamydia trachomatis infection is the most common bacterial sexually transmitted disease in the United States and the leading cause of preventable infertility and ectopic pregnancy. Other potential complications include pelvic inflammatory disease (PID) and Fitz-Hugh-Curtis syndrome (infection of the liver capsule). Approximately 1.1 million cases were reported to the CDC (2009d) in 2007, and more than half occurred in women 15 to 25 years old. The reported rate of Chlamydia infection for women substantially exceeds the rate for men, primarily due to increased detection of asymptomatic infection in women through screening. It is estimated that 1 in 10 adolescent girls tested for Chlamydia is infected. Teenage girls tend to have the highest rates of Chlamydial infection. *C. trachomatis* is widespread geographically and is highly prevalent among economically disadvantaged young women (CDC, 2009d; Hackett, 2010; Hoover, Tao, & Kent, 2008; Ravin, 2007).

 Optimizing Outcomes— Teaching patients about STD prevention

Nurses can teach patients about strategies to prevent or decrease the transmission of Chlamydia and other STDs: practicing abstinence from sexual intercourse or sharing a mutually monogamous relationship with a partner who has been tested and is known to be uninfected and correctly and consistently using latex condoms, and avoiding condoms lubricated with the spermicide Nonoxynol-9 (N-9), an agent that has been associated with disruption of the genital epithelium, which may increase the risk for the transmission of infection.

The majority (75%) of Chlamydial infections are asymptomatic, especially in women. Only about 30% of those infected have a mucopurulent cervical discharge; other symptoms include spotting or postcoital bleeding and dysuria. Infected women who use oral contraceptives may report breakthrough bleeding. Chlamydia infection of the cervix causes inflammation that produces microscopic ulcerations, which may increase the risk for contracting HIV (Marrazzo et al., 2007; Weber-LaShore & Biro, 2009). The CDC and the U.S. Preventive Services Task Force (USPSTF) recommend annual screening for Chlamydia in

all sexually active women aged 25 years and younger. Chlamydia infection can be diagnosed using several different testing methods, such as culture, direct immunofluorescence, nucleic acid hybridization, and EIA, all of which require a pelvic examination to collect cervical epithelial cells. The nucleic acid amplification test (NAAT), which can detect Chlamydia from a cervical or vaginal swab (self- or clinician-collected) or urine sample (first few drops of the stream), is considered to be the most sensitive and specific test (CDC, 2009d; Hoover & Tao, 2008; USPSTF, 2001; Weber-La-Shore & Biro, 2009).

 Optimizing Outcomes— Recognizing and addressing barriers to screening for Chlamydia

Although Chlamydia screening is considered a priority preventive service, it remains underutilized by health-care providers. Barriers to screening include a lack of awareness that patients are sexually active and at risk for STDs, a lack of reimbursement for the time required to conduct patient testing and counseling, and a lack of knowledge that screening can be performed without a pelvic examination. Strategies to change provider behavior include the use of computerized reminders, placement of Chlamydia collection swabs alongside Pap test collection materials, and the practice of performing routine Chlamydia screening with other laboratory testing (CDC, 2009d; Christiansen-Lindquist, Tao, Hoover, Frank, & Kent, 2009; Hackett, 2010).

Unlike viruses, the Chlamydia bacterium is susceptible to antibiotics. The recommended antibiotic options for treatment of *C. trachomatis* include doxycycline 100 mg orally twice a day for 7 days or azithromycin 1 gm orally, given in a single dose. Alternatives are ofloxacin 300 mg orally two times a day for 7 days or erythromycin ethylsuccinate 800 mg orally four times a day for 7 days. In general, the erythromycin-based regimens are inferior to the other medications and should be used as a second-line therapy (CDC, Workowski, & Berman, 2006b; CDC, 2009d; Marrazzo et al., 2007).

Gonorrhea

Gonorrhea is caused by the gram-negative intracellular diplococcal bacterium *Neisseria gonorrhoeae*. Approximately 650,000 new cases of gonorrhea occur each year, making it the second most commonly reported STD in the United States. Similar to Chlamydia, gonorrhea is prevalent in the adolescent population and disproportionately affects minority groups. The rate of gonorrheal infections in African American women is 18 times higher than in Caucasian women (CDC, 2006b; Marrazzo et al., 2007; Weber-LaShore & Biro, 2009).

 Nursing Insight— *The magnitude of Chlamydial and gonorrheal infections in young women*

In 2008, there were more than 1.5 million total cases of Chlamydia and gonorrhea reported to the CDC, making them the two most commonly reported infectious diseases in the United States. Adolescent girls and young women are especially hard hit by these two diseases. The largest number of reported cases of both Chlamydia and gonorrhea in 2008 was among girls between 15 and 19 years of age, followed closely by young women 20 to 24 years of age. Because patients with gonorrhea are often co-infected with Chlamydia, dual treatment may be indicated (CDC, 2009a; Weber-LaShore & Biro, 2009).

In men, symptoms usually consist of dysuria and penile discharge. Women, however, are commonly asymptomatic. When present, symptoms are frequently less specific than in males but may include abnormal vaginal discharge, irregular menses, postcoital bleeding, low backache, and urinary frequency and dysuria.

The USPSTF recommends annual screening of all sexually active women 25 years old and younger; the CDC supports these recommendations. Gonorrhea is most often tested through government screening programs (CDC, 2009a; USPSTF, 2005). Testing methods include culture, nucleic acid hybridization, and NAAT. Either cervical swab or urine can be used as the specimen for NAAT.

The recommended therapies for gonorrhea include cefixime 400 mg orally single dose or ceftriaxone 125 mg IM single dose. Other treatment options include the following three synthetic broad-spectrum antibiotics known as "quinolones": ciprofloxacin 500 mg orally single dose, ofloxacin 400 mg orally single dose, or levofloxacin 250 mg orally single dose. However, these medications should be avoided in persons who may have acquired their infection outside the United States or in California or Hawaii, where rates of quinolone resistance are considerable (CDC, 2006b; Marrazzo et al., 2007). Sex partners also require treatment. Health professionals should consult the CDC's Web site (http://www.cdc.gov/std/treatment) for frequent updates regarding treatment recommendations.

 Optimizing Outcomes— With home screening for *C. trachomatis* and *N. gonorrhoeae*

Graseck, Secura, Allsworth, Madden, and Peipert (2010) recently conducted a study to compare the acceptability of home screening with clinic-based screening for two STDs (*C. trachomatis* and *N. gonorrhoeae*). In a telephone interview, women (ages 14–45 years) were given a choice of no-cost screening with vaginal swabs for self-collection mailed to their home (detailed instructions and a pre-addressed and stamped specimen mailer were included in the kit) or screening that was available without an appointment at area family planning clinics. The participants were much more likely to choose to screen for STDs at home than at a clinic or with their own medical provider. The researchers concluded that future interventions to increase screening rates in young women should consider alternative screening strategies such as home-based or patient-controlled testing.

Pelvic inflammatory disease (PID) develops in up to 40% of untreated women with cervical gonorrhea and may progress to a systemic infection. Patients with gonorrhea who have oral sex should be evaluated and treated for pharyngeal gonorrhea as necessary. Rectal testing for Chlamydia and gonorrhea may improve case-finding for both STDs; recent research (Barry, Kent, Philip, & Klausner, 2010) revealed that among women, rectal infections were as common as

genital infections. Maternal transfer of both gonorrhea and Chlamydia may occur during childbirth, causing neonatal eye infection (ophthalmia neonatorum), scalp abscess at the site of fetal monitors, rhinitis, or anorectal infection (Marrazzo et al., 2007).

Trichomoniasis

Caused by the protozoan *Trichomonas vaginalis*, trichomoniasis is the most common curable STD in the United States. An estimated 5 million new cases occur in this country each year. Infection with trichomoniasis has been shown to increase the risk of HIV transmission. Although infection with *T. vaginalis* may be asymptomatic, it often produces a profuse frothy gray or yellow-green vaginal discharge with a foul odor. Erythema, edema, and pruritus of the external genitalia may be present, and the patient may report dysuria and dyspareunia. Upon examination, small red ulcerations in the vagina or on the cervix ("strawberry cervix") may be observed. The pH of the vaginal discharge is usually higher (more alkaline) than normal (CDC et al., 2006b; Marrazzo et al., 2007; Sorvillo, Smith, Kerndt, & Ash, 2001; Weber-LaShore & Biro, 2009).

Microscopic evaluation is used to confirm trichomoniasis. Microscopic examination of the vaginal secretions on a wet prep reveals the motile trichomonad parasites. *T. vaginalis* can also be detected by performing the rapid trichomoniasis test (results available in 10 minutes) or by performing the Affirm VP III test (results available in 45 minutes). The most sensitive and specific method of diagnosis of trichomoniasis is by performing a vaginal culture (CDC et al., 2006b; Weber-LaShore & Biro, 2009).

Nursing Insight— *The vaginal wet mount*

A wet mount, also known as a "wet-prep" or "wet smear," is frequently used in the clinical setting to diagnose three of the most common vaginal infections: bacterial vaginosis, trichomoniasis, and yeast (candidiasis). To perform this test, the clinician inserts a speculum and uses a moist cotton swab to take a sample of the discharge from the posterior vaginal fornix. The discharge is then placed on a glass slide and viewed under a microscope. Alternately, a dry swab may be used: The sample is placed in 1 mL of saline, mixed, and placed on a slide, or a drop of saline is placed on a slide and the sample is added to it.

The slide may be warmed briefly (to increase motility of the trichomonads). A cover slip is then applied and the slide is promptly viewed.

Metronidazole (Flagyl), the medication of choice for trichomoniasis, is associated with a 95% cure rate. Metronidazole may be administered as a single dose—2 g orally—or 500 mg orally twice daily for 7 days. Alternately, tinidazole (Tindamax) 2 g orally single dose may be used, and this medication is recommended for the treatment of metronidazole-resistant *T. vaginalis* infections. Partners should be simultaneously treated, and patients should be counseled to use condoms to prevent future infections and to avoid drinking alcohol until 24 hours after completing metronidazole therapy and 72 hours

(3 days) after completing tinidazole therapy. Combining these medications with alcohol ingestion may produce a reaction characterized by flushing, nausea, vomiting, headache, and abdominal cramps (CDC et al., 2006b; Deglin & Vallerand, 2009; Marrazzo et al., 2007; Weber-LaShore & Biro, 2009).

 Now can you— **Discuss Chlamydia, gonorrhea, and trichomoniasis?**

1. Explain why infection with *Chlamydia trachomatis* poses such a danger to young women?
2. Identify the U.S. population that is at highest risk for infection with gonorrhea?
3. Describe patient education that should accompany metronidazole therapy?

Pelvic Inflammatory Disease (PID)

Pelvic inflammatory disease (PID) is an acute infection of the uterus and fallopian tubes, which, if left untreated or unresolved, results in scarring, adhesions, or blockage of the fallopian tubes. A number of different organisms (e.g., *Escherichia coli*, *Mycoplasma hominis*) are usually involved, but the most common causative agents are *Chlamydia trachomatis* (> 50%) and *Neisseria gonorrhoeae*. In the United States, PID accounts for nearly 180,000 hospitalizations every year, and 1 in 7 reproductive-aged American women reports having received treatment for PID. Since PID may be caused by many organisms and encompasses a wide spectrum of pathological processes, the infection may be acute, subacute, or chronic. The two greatest reproductive consequences of acute PID are infertility and tubal pregnancy resulting from scarring of the fallopian tubes (Marrazzo et al., 2007).

 Nursing Insight— Recognizing risk factors for pelvic inflammatory disease

When taking a sexual history, nurses should be aware of certain factors—such as a history of multiple sexual partners, a new partner in the last 6 months, lower age at first intercourse, and lower economic status—that place women at increased risk for PID. Age constitutes another risk factor: Adolescents have the highest incidence of PID of any age group, and 70% of all cases of PID occur in women under age 25. Women who use intrauterine devices (IUDs) are also at increased risk if they have more than one sexual partner or if their partner has other sexual partners, because they are at higher risk for an STD (Marrazzo et al., 2007).

Symptoms of PID can range from none to severe abdominal, uterine, and ovarian pain and tenderness; abnormal bleeding; nausea; and vomiting. The infected individual may also experience extreme tenderness when the cervix is moved on examination ("cervical motion tenderness"; the "chandelier sign"). Fever, chills, and an elevated white blood cell (WBC) count and erythrocyte sedimentation rate (ESR) may also be present.

PID can be treated on an outpatient basis, but hospitalization may be necessary, depending on the individual case. For patients treated on an outpatient basis,

reexamination within 48 to 72 hours is a crucial part of therapy. Combined drug therapy is advised, especially at the initiation of treatment, because the full spectrum of all organisms involved is often unknown. The CDC provides specific guidelines for PID treatment (http://www.cdc.gov/std/treatment/2006/pid.htm). Also, a PID Teaching Module for physicians, advanced practice nurses, and physician assistants is available at http://www2a.cdc.gov/STDTraining/Ready-To-Use/Manuals/PID/pid-notes-2009.pdf.

Human Papillomavirus (HPV)

Human papillomavirus (HPV), which causes genital warts (also called condylomata acuminata), is a DNA virus transmitted by skin-to-skin contact. There are more than 100 viral types currently identified, and of these, more than 30 types can infect the genital area. Approximately one-half of all HPV genital infections occur in young women and men between the ages of 15 and 24 years. The majority of HPV infections are asymptomatic, unrecognized, or subclinical. Genital HPV infection can cause warty growths in the vagina or on the vulva, perineum, or anal area. The growths can be single or multiple, and they are soft and fleshy and usually painless. Other strains of HPV infect the cervix and remain unnoticed until findings from a routine Pap smear reveal the presence of the virus. Certain viral types are associated with the growth of abnormal cervical cells, which can lead to cancer of the cervix (CDC et al., 2006b; Mayeaux, 2007; Schmidt, 2007).

 Optimizing Outcomes— **HPV prevention and testing**

Strategies for prevention of HPV include sexual abstinence, confining sexual intimacy to a long-term monogamous relationship, and prophylactic vaccination. A vaccine against HPV types 6, 11, 16, and 18 first became available in 2006 and is recommended for all females, ages 9 to 26 years (Advisory Committee on Immunization Practices, 2009; ACOG, 2006). Although testing is available based on HPV-DNA in cervical cells, routine screening is not recommended except in specific circumstances following an abnormal Pap test (CDC et al., 2006b; Nelson, 2007).

Several topical chemical agents are available for the treatment of external genital warts. These include trichloroacetic acid (TCA) and podophyllin (provider administered) and podofilox 0.5% (Condylox) and imiquimod (Aldara), both of which are patient administered. Cryotherapy (freezing), CO_2 laser surgery, electrosurgery, and surgical removal are other treatment options, depending on the severity of the lesions and resistance to treatment (CDC et al., 2006b; Marrazzo et al., 2007).

When clinician-administered agents are used, the nurse should stress the importance of returning for regular treatment until the lesions have resolved. Once the warts have responded to therapy, no special follow-up is necessary. Owing to the risk of sequelae from cervical cancer, regular Pap smears are crucial for all women with documented HIV infection. Nurses should also encourage tobacco cessation to reduce the risk of HPV and neoplasia (Marrazzo et al., 2007).

Herpes Simplex Virus (HSV) 1 and 2

Herpes simplex virus 1 and 2 (HSV-1 and HSV-2), also known as human herpes virus 1 and 2 (HHV-1 and HHV-2), are members of the herpes virus family *Herpesviridae* that infect humans. Both HSV-1 and HSV-2 are transmitted horizontally during close contact with an infected person who is shedding virus from the skin, often in saliva or in genital secretions. Although transmission occurs most often when lesions are present, viral shedding and transmission can also occur in the absence of visible sores. HSV-1 is usually transmitted during childhood via nonsexual contacts. It is most commonly associated with cold sores or fever blisters on the mouth or face. Genital HSV-1 may result from oral–genital sexual contact with a person infected with oral HSV-1. Genital HSV-1 is unlikely to recur, and treatment may only be needed in persons with initial symptoms (Xu et al., 2006).

HSV-2 is primarily a sexually transmitted disease. HSV-2 is associated with genital lesions, although, depending on sexual practices, HSV-1 and HSV-2 are not exclusively associated with the respective sites. HSV-2 occurs more frequently in women than in men, which most likely results from the greater incidence of male-to-female transmission. HSV-infection rates are significantly higher among African Americans (46%) than among Caucasians (18%). Although HSV infection is not a reportable disease, it is estimated that 50 million Americans are infected with genital herpes (CDC et al., 2006b; Winer & Richwald, 2007).

Most infected persons have no or only minimal signs or symptoms from HSV-1 or HSV-2 infection. If symptoms develop during the first HSV-2 outbreak, they usually appear within 2 weeks after exposure and can be very pronounced. Owing to the fact that the body has not had an opportunity to develop antibodies, symptoms that result from a primary HSV infection are usually much more severe than with subsequent outbreaks (CDC et al., 2006b; Gardner, 2006).

 Nursing Insight*— *Recognizing signs and symptoms of HSV infection

Symptoms of HSV-2 infection are similar to those that occur with the flu—malaise, muscle aches, and headache. Other symptoms include dysuria and the development of multiple fluid-filled, blister-like lesions, which can be extremely tender and persist for 2 to 3 weeks (Fig. 5-2). Before the appearance of the lesions, the patient may experience a period of prodromal symptoms characterized by skin sensitivity and nerve pain in the area where the lesions will appear. Reddening of the skin frequently follows these symptoms. The lesions form pustules and ulcers that dry up, crust over, and then heal without scarring. The woman may also experience itching, inguinal tenderness, vulvar edema, and a heavy watery or purulent vaginal discharge. In some instances, women with "chronic yeast infections" are actually experiencing herpes outbreaks that go undiagnosed because the typical herpetic lesions are not present (CDC et al., 2006b; Gardner, 2006).

Typically, recurrent outbreaks are less severe than the primary infection and usually involve localized symptoms with less severe lesions that last 5 to 7 days. The prodromal characteristic genital tingling sensation is common

Figure 5-2 Herpes Vulvovaginitis

with recurrence. The virus then enters a latent stage in the nerves at the base of the spine, only to reactivate when the patient's immune system is weakened. The lesions may occur along any skin surface supplied by that particular distribution (e.g., vulva, vagina, cervix, urethral meatus, buttocks). Because transmission of the virus is most likely during an active outbreak, patients should abstain from sexual contact during this time. However, viral transmission may occur at any time when the infected individual is producing and releasing ("shedding") the virus, and some individuals shed virus between active outbreaks (Gardner, 2006).

In most situations, a diagnosis of HSV is suspected based on the patient history and physical examination. HSV can be confirmed by obtaining a viral culture from the exudate swabbed from the vesicular (blister) lesion. Testing for the presence of HSV-2 antibodies in capillary blood or serum (i.e., HSV glycoprotein G-specific antibodies, IgG by immunoblot [HerpeSelect]) is also available for clinical use. However, screening of the general population is not indicated (CDC et al., 2006b; Nelson, 2007).

The goal of treatment for herpes is to hasten healing and reduce symptoms. Several oral antiviral medications (e.g., acyclovir [Zovirax], valacyclovir [Valtrex], famciclovir (Famvir]) are available and may be used for primary or recurrent episodes or as daily suppressive therapy. The medications do not eradicate the infection, nor do they alter subsequent risk, frequency, or recurrences once the medication has been stopped. When indicated, acyclovir may be administered intravenously for 5 to 7 days for severe symptoms (CDC et al., 2006b; Nelson, 2007).

 Optimizing Outcomes— **Teaching women about HSV infection**

Providing counseling and education are essential components of holistic care for women with herpes infections. Nurses should offer information about the etiology, signs, symptoms, modes of transmission, treatment options, and the possibility of suppression therapy to prevent partner transmission. It is important to advise women about the times when transmission is most likely and the need to avoid sexual contact beginning with the onset of prodromal symptoms until all lesions have healed. Some experts recommend the consistent use of condoms for all individuals with genital herpes. Nurses can help women explore potential precipitating factors in the reactivation of the latent herpes virus. Triggers may include stress, menstruation, febrile illnesses, chronic illnesses, and ultraviolet light. Some patients find that keeping a personal diary provides insights about precipitating events for their herpetic outbreaks.

 Complementary Care— *Measures to reduce HSV discomforts and outbreaks*

For many women, certain comfort measures and dietary changes are useful in decreasing HSV symptoms and the frequency and severity of HSV outbreaks. Comfort measures may include warm sitz baths with baking soda or oatmeal, the use of cotton underwear, the use of a hair dryer (on the cool setting) to enhance drying of the lesions, the application of compresses containing peppermint oil and clove oil to the lesions, and the application of cool, wet, black tea bags or tea tree oil applied to the lesions. Oral analgesics including aspirin or ibuprofen may help relieve pain. Dietary strategies center on consumption of a diet rich in vitamin C, B-complex vitamins, zinc, and calcium and the daily use of kelp powder and sunflower seed oil as well as the amino acid l-lysine, which is thought to suppress the herpes simplex virus (Gardner, 2006; Stonehouse & Studdiford, 2007).

Syphilis

One of the oldest known sexually transmitted diseases, syphilis is caused by the spirochetal bacterium *Treponema pallidum*. It is believed that the organism is transmitted through microscopic abrasions that can occur during sexual intercourse. Kissing, biting, and oral–genital sex may also be modes of transmission. Congenital syphilis occurs via maternal–fetal transmission. Syphilis cannot be contracted through toilet seats, daily activities, hot tubs, or sharing eating utensils or clothing. Left untreated, syphilis can cause severe systemic disease and death. In 2008, there were 13,500 reported cases of primary and secondary syphilis, and this figure represents the highest number of

cases since 1995 and an increase over 2007, when there were 11,466 reported cases. Less than a decade ago, syphilis was on the verge of elimination. However, syphilis reemerged as a public health threat in 2001, and rates of infection have steadily increased since then (CDC, 2009a).

Although the majority of reported syphilis cases in the United States occur among men who have sex with men, rates among women have increased each year since 2004. In 2008, the syphilis rate among women increased 36% from the previous year (1.1 cases per 100,000 females in 2007, as compared with 1.5 cases in 2008). The syphilis rate among African American women increased to 7.6 cases per 100,000 in 2008, up from 5.5 reported cases in 2007. Also, the rate of reported syphilis cases among Hispanics (4.7 per 100,000) was double that of Caucasian (2.2 per 100,000) (CDC, 2009a).

 Optimizing Outcomes— **Through targeted syphilis screening efforts**

The CDC (2009a) and the USPSTF (2009) recommend that persons at increased risk for syphilis infection (i.e., all men who have sex with men) be tested at least annually for syphilis and that all pregnant women be screened for syphilis at the first prenatal visit to avoid transmission to their infants.

Syphilis is a complex disease with several stages. Different manifestations occur depending on the stage of the disease. In the primary stage, approximately 10 to 90 days after the initial exposure, a painless ulcer (chancre) appears at the point of contact, which is usually the genitalia. Lymphadenopathy may also be present. The lesion may persist for 4 to 6 weeks and usually resolves on its own without treatment (CDC, 2009a).

Secondary syphilis occurs 6 weeks to 6 months after the appearance of the chancre. During this stage, patients may have fever, a sore throat, weight loss, skin rash on the trunk and extremities (Fig. 5-3), headache, generalized malaise, mucous patches on the genitals or in the mouth, lymphadenopathy, alopecia, and the appearance of moist, flat warts in the genital and anal areas (condylomata lata). If left untreated, the symptoms resolve within 2 to 10 weeks. Approximately one-third of infected individuals will then develop tertiary syphilis (CDC, 2009a; Marrazzo et al., 2007).

Tertiary syphilis usually occurs 1 to 10 years after the initial infection, although in some cases systemic symptoms may not appear until 30 to 50 years later. This stage is characterized by the formation of gummas (soft, tumorlike

Figure 5-3 Secondary Syphilitic Rash on Chest and Palms

balls of inflammation). Other manifestations of tertiary syphilis include neuropathic joint disease (degeneration of joint surfaces), neurosyphilis, and cardiovascular syphilis. It is estimated that approximately 20% to 30% of untreated individuals with syphilis develop tertiary syphilis (CDC, 2009a).

 Nursing Insight— *Understanding the entity termed "latent syphilis"*

Latent syphilis is defined as having serological proof of infection without signs or symptoms of the disease. Latent syphilis may be "early" or "late." By definition, early latent syphilis is having the infection for greater than 2 years but without clinical evidence of the disease. This stage is treated with a single intramuscular injection of a long-acting penicillin. Late latent syphilis requires 3 weekly intramuscular injections of a long-acting penicillin (CDC, 2009a).

Effective tests and treatments for syphilis were developed during the 20th century. Microscopy of fluid from the primary or secondary lesion using darkfield illumination is highly accurate in detecting *T. pallidum*. Screening tests include the Rapid Plasma Reagin (RPR) and Venereal Disease Research Laboratory (VDRL). When positive, the tests should be followed up by a more specific treponemal test. Tests based on monoclonal antibodies and immunofluorescence, including treponema pallidum hemagglutination assay (TPHA) and fluorescent treponemal antibody absorption (FTA-ABS) are more specific tests. Tests based on ELISAs are also used to confirm results of the simpler screening tests for syphilis. Neurosyphilis is diagnosed via analysis of the cerebrospinal fluid. Because there is some evidence that the incidence of neurosyphilis is higher in HIV patients, some experts recommend that all HIV-positive individuals have a lumbar puncture to assess for asymptomatic neurosyphilis (CDC, 2009a).

Penicillin, in the form of penicillin G, is the treatment of choice for syphilis, and the specific regimen and duration depends on the length of infection. Doxycycline and tetracycline may be used as alternative treatments for individuals who are allergic to penicillin (CDC, 2009a). For the most current treatment guidelines, health professionals may visit the CDC Web site at http://www.cdc.gov/mmwr/preview/mmwrhtml/rr5511a1.htm.

 Be sure to— Teach patients about the possibility of a Jarisch-Herxheimer reaction

The Jarisch-Herxheimer reaction occurs when large quantities of toxins are released into the body as bacteria, typically spirochetal bacteria, die during treatment with antibiotics. Death of the bacteria and the associated release of endotoxins occur more quickly than the liver and kidneys can remove the toxins. Fever, chills, headache, myalgia, and exacerbation of skin lesions are the hallmarks of this acute reaction. In syphilis, the duration is usually only a few hours but can persist for much longer with other diseases. Treatment, aimed at reducing symptoms, centers on the use of analgesics and antipyretics.

 Now Can You— **Discuss PID, HPV, HSV, and syphilis?**

1. Identify six risk factors for PID?
2. Describe strategies for HPV prevention?
3. Discuss the nurse's role in teaching women about HSV infection?
4. Differentiate among the primary, secondary, and tertiary stages of syphilis?

Hepatitis

Hepatitis is the leading cause of liver cancer and the most common reason for liver transplantation. In the United States, an estimated 1.2 million individuals are living with chronic hepatitis B virus (HBV) and 3.2 million persons are living with chronic hepatitis C virus (HCV). Many are unaware that they are infected. Each year, an estimated 25,000 persons become infected with the hepatitis A virus (HAV), 43,000 with hepatitis B, and 17,000 with hepatitis C (CDC, 2010).

 Nursing Insight— *Hepatitis A virus*

Formerly known as "infectious hepatitis," hepatitis A is an acute infectious disease of the liver caused by HAV. Every year, approximately 10 million people worldwide are infected with the virus, and the incidence of infection is highest in developing countries and in regions with poor hygiene standards. HAV causes no clinical signs and symptoms in over 90% of infected children, and since the infection confers lifelong immunity, the disease is of no special significance to the indigenous population. In the United States, HAV is primarily contracted by susceptible young adults, the majority of whom are infected with the virus during trips to countries with a high incidence of the disease. There is no specific treatment for HAV. Hepatitis A can be prevented by vaccination, good hygiene, and sanitation (Connor, 2005; Ryan & Ray, 2005; Steffen, 2005; Thiel, 1998).

HEPATITIS B VIRUS (HBV)

In 2007, an estimated 43,000 persons in the United States were newly infected with HBV. The highest incidence of HBV occurs in persons aged 20 to 49 years, and the virus is 50 to 100 times more contagious than HIV. It causes liver disease and can be fatal. Each year, approximately 6,000 Americans die from complications resulting from HBV infection (CDC, 2009e).

Hepatitis B virus is a species of the genus *Orthohepadnavirus*, which is a part of the *Hepadnaviridae* family of viruses. This virus causes the disease hepatitis B. The incubation period from the time of exposure to the onset of symptoms is 6 weeks to 6 months. HBV is found in highest concentrations in blood and in lower concentrations in other body fluids such as semen, vaginal secretions, and wound exudates. Although heterosexual intercourse is the predominant mode of transmission, HBV may also be spread through blood-to-blood contact. Blood-to-blood contact can occur through the sharing of razors, toothbrushes, and manicure tools, as well as through contaminated instruments used for dental procedures, tattooing, and body piercing. Vertical transmission occurs when a pregnant woman passes the virus to her fetus. HBV is not spread through food or water, sharing eating utensils, breastfeeding, hugging, kissing, hand holding, coughing, or sneezing (CDC, 2009e; Holloway & D'Acunto, 2006).

 Optimizing Outcomes— Identifying populations at increased risk for HBV

Nurses should be aware of certain factors that place men, women, children, and intimate partners at increased risk for HBV. Taking a detailed patient history can help nurses to identify these individuals, who include (CDC 2009e):

* Infants born to infected mothers
* Sex partners of infected persons
* Sexually active persons who are not in a long-term (> 6 months) mutually monogamous relationship
* Men who have sex with men
* Injection drug users
* Household contacts of persons with chronic HBV infection
* Health-care and public safety workers at risk for occupational exposure to blood or blood-contaminated body fluids
* Hemodialysis patients
* Residents and staff of facilities for developmentally disabled persons
* Travelers to countries with intermediate or high prevalence of HBV infection

Signs and symptoms of infection with HBV are often absent, especially in children under age 5 years and in newly infected immunosuppressed adults. However, it is estimated that up to 50% of persons older than 5 years have initial signs and symptoms of the infection, such as fever, fatigue, loss of appetite, nausea, vomiting, abdominal pain, dark-colored urine, clay-colored stools, joint pain, and jaundice. On average, symptoms appear from 60 to 150 days after exposure to HBV and last for several weeks (CDC, 2009e).

 Nursing Insight— Acute and chronic HBV infection

Acute HBV infection ranges from asymptomatic or mild disease to fulminate hepatitis (rare). The disease is more severe among older adults (> 60 years). The risk for chronic infection varies according to the age at infection and is greatest among young children: Approximately 90% of infants and 25% to 50% of children (ages 1–5 years) will remain chronically infected with HBV. The vast majority (> 95%) of adults with HBV infection recover completely and do not become chronically infected. Approximately 25% of those who become chronically infected during childhood and 15% of those who become chronically infected after childhood die prematurely from cirrhosis or liver cancer, and the majority remain asymptomatic until the onset of cirrhosis or end-stage liver disease. In the United States, chronic HBV infection results in an estimated 2,000 to 4,000 deaths each year (CDC, 2009e).

Individuals at high risk for contracting HBV should be screened on a regular basis. The USPSTF (2004) recommends that all women should be screened for HBV at the first prenatal visit, regardless of whether they have been tested previously, and screening should be repeated later in the pregnancy for women with high-risk behaviors. No routine screening is recommended for the general population. Testing for HBV is complex. There are a number of different markers identified in a blood test, some of which indicate active infection, chronic carrier state, or past infection (American Academy of Pediatrics & ACOG, 2007; CDC, 2009e; USPSTF, 2004).

 Optimizing Outcomes— With vaccines for hepatitis B prevention

Two single-antigen vaccines (Engerix-B and Recombivax HB) and three combination vaccines are licensed in the United States. The combination vaccines include the following: Comvax (combined hepatitis B-*Haemophilus influenzae* type b [Hib])—cannot be administered before age 6 weeks or after age 71 months); Pediarix (combined hepatitis B, diphtheria, tetanus, acellular pertussis [DtaP], and inactivated poliovirus [IPV] vaccine)—cannot be administered before age 6 weeks or after age 7 years; and Twinrix (combined hepatitis A and hepatitis B vaccine—recommended for persons age 18+ years who are at risk for both HAV and HBV). The vaccination schedule most often used for children and adults is three intramuscular injections; the second and third doses administered 1 and 6 months after the first dose. After a person has been exposed to HBV, appropriate prophylaxis (i.e., hepatitis B vaccine), given as soon as possible but preferably within 24 hours, can effectively prevent infection. Although persons who have already been infected with HBV will receive no benefit from vaccination, there is no risk to a previously infected person who receives the vaccination (CDC, 2009e).

The CDC (2009e) Advisory Committee on Immunization Practices has published recommendations for hepatitis B vaccination. At-risk individuals who should receive HBV vaccination are presented in Box 5-2. The Advisory Committee has also determined that adults who receive care in health-care, evaluation, and treatment settings should also receive HBV vaccination. Specific settings are presented in Box 5-3.

There is no specific therapy for acute hepatitis B infection; treatment is supportive. Several antiviral drugs (adefovir dipivoxil [Preveon, Hepsera], interferon alfa-2b [Peg-Intron], pegylated interferon alpha 2-a [Pegasys], lamivudine [Epivir], entecavir [Baraclude], telbivudine [Tyzeka]) are used for treatment of chronic infection. Individuals with chronic HBV infection require medical evaluation and regular monitoring to determine whether the disease is progressing and to identify liver damage or hepatocellular carcinoma (cancer of the liver) (CDC, 2009e).

HEPATITIS C VIRUS (HCV)

Largely unknown to the American public, hepatitis C virus (HCV) infection is the most common chronic bloodborne infection in the United States. According to the CDC (2009f), approximately 3.2 million persons are chronically infected. Previously known as "non-A, non-B hepatitis," up to 85% of individuals infected with HCV will progress to chronic viral hepatitis.

Box 5-2　Individuals Who Should Be Vaccinated Against Hepatitis B

- All infants, beginning at birth
- All children aged <19 years who have not been vaccinated previously
- Susceptible sex partners of hepatitis B surface antigen (HbsAg)–positive persons
- Sexually active persons who are not in a long-term, mutually monogamous relationship (e.g., >1 sex partner during the previous 6 months)
- Persons seeking evaluation or treatment for an STD
- Men who have sex with men
- Injection drug users
- Susceptible household contacts of HbsAg-positive persons
- Health-care and public safety workers at risk for exposure to blood or blood-contaminated body fluids
- Persons with end-stage renal disease, including predialysis, hemodialysis, peritoneal dialysis, and home dialysis patients
- Residents and staff of facilities for developmentally disabled persons
- Travelers to regions with intermediate or high rates of endemic HBV infection
- Persons with chronic liver disease
- Persons with HIV infection
- All other persons seeking protection from HBV infection—acknowledgment of a specific risk factor is not a requirement for vaccination

Source: CDC, 2009e.

Box 5-3　Settings Where Hepatitis B Vaccination Should Be Administered to All Adults Who Receive Care

- STD treatment facilities
- HIV testing and treatment facilities
- Facilities providing drug-abuse treatment and prevention services
- Health-care settings targeting services to injection drug users
- Correctional facilities
- Health-care settings targeting services to men who have sex with men
- Chronic hemodialysis facilities and end-stage renal disease programs
- Institutions and nonresidential day-care facilities for developmentally disabled persons

Source: CDC, 2009e.

HCV is primarily spread through blood-to-blood contact and less efficiently through semen, saliva, or urine. As with HBV, transmission of HCV can potentially occur through blood contact with shared needles, razors, and toothbrushes. Persons at risk for HCV include those with STDs such as hepatitis B and HIV and those with multiple sex partners, a history of blood transfusions, or a history of IV drug use. Currently, no vaccine for HCV infection is available (CDC, 2009f).

Newly acquired HCV infection is often asymptomatic. When symptoms occur, however, they may include fever, fatigue, dark-colored urine, clay-colored stools, abdominal pain, anorexia, nausea, vomiting, joint pain, and jaundice. Approximately 20% to 30% of individuals newly infected with HCV experience fatigue, abdominal pain, poor appetite, or jaundice. The average time period from exposure to symptom onset (if any) is 4 to 12 weeks (CDC, 2009f).

 Nursing Insight— *Progression of acute HCV infection to chronic HCV infection to death*

Of every 100 persons infected with HCV, approximately 75 to 85 will develop chronic infection; 60 to 70 will develop chronic liver disease; 5 to 20 will develop cirrhosis over a period of 20 to 30 years; and 1 to 5 will die from the consequences of chronic infection (e.g., liver cancer or cirrhosis). Chronic HCV infection, the leading indication for liver transplantation in this country, accounts for an estimated 8,000 to 10,000 deaths in the United States each year (CDC, 2009f).

According to the CDC (2009f), certain individuals and populations should be tested for HCV infection (Box 5-4). Blood tests that may be performed to test for HCV infection include screening tests for antibody to HCV (e.g., EIA, enhanced chemiluminescence immunoassay [CIA], recombinant immunoblot assay [RIBA]), qualitative tests to detect presence or absence of the virus, and quantitative tests to detect the amount of virus. The CDC provides a table on interpretation of HCV test results for health professionals, available at http://www.cdc.gov/hepatitis/HCV/PDFs/hcv_graph.pdf.

Following diagnosis, HCV-infected patients should be evaluated for the presence of chronic liver disease and determination of the need for hepatitis B vaccination. Combination therapy with pegylated interferon and ribavirin is the treatment of choice for individuals with chronic hepatitis C. According to the CDC (2009f), success rates are improved with the addition of polymerase and protease inhibitors to standard pegylated interferon/ribavirin combination therapy.

 Optimizing Outcomes— **With holistic nursing care for women with chronic hepatitis**

Nurses can empower women with chronic hepatitis infection by providing education and counseling about strategies to optimize health, reduce the transmission of infection, and communicate concerns with intimate sexual partners. Referrals to local resources such as professional

---

Box 5-4　Testing for HCV Infection

The CDC (2009f) recommends that the following individuals are at increased risk for HCV infection and should undergo testing:

- Persons who have ever injected illegal drugs, including those who injected only once many years ago
- Recipients of clotting factor concentrates made before 1987
- Recipients of blood transfusions or solid organ transplants before July 1992
- Patients who have ever received long-term hemodialysis treatment
- Persons with known exposures to HCV (e.g., health-care workers after needle sticks involving HCV-positive blood, recipients of blood or organs from a donor who later tested HCV-positive)
- All persons with HIV infection
- Patients with signs or symptoms of liver disease (e.g., abnormal liver enzyme tests)
- Children born to HCV-positive mothers (to avoid detecting maternal antibody, testing should not be performed prior to 18 months of age)

counselors and peer support groups may also be of benefit. Nurses can teach women about the importance of maintaining a high level of personal hygiene with measures such as performing strict hand washing after toileting and ensuring the careful disposal of all tampons, sanitary pads, and bandages. Patients can also be taught to avoid sharing razor blades, toothbrushes, needles, and manicure implements and to promptly clean blood spills with soap and water. Non-HBV-vaccinated male sexual partners should consistently use latex condoms. Nutritional strategies may include the consumption of a low-protein, low-fat diet; avoidance of protein or amino acid supplements; the use of an antioxidant formula vitamin supplement; and the avoidance of alcohol and tobacco. Patients are also advised to avoid medications that are hepatotoxic (e.g., Tylenol) (Holloway & D'Acunto, 2006).

HEPATITIS D VIRUS (HDV)

Hepatitis D virus (HDV) is a single-stranded circular RNA molecule with some double-stranded attachments. HDV infection can only occur in a person already infected with HBV; a person can be infected by HBV and HDV simultaneously or by HBV first. Infection with HDV is clinically indistinguishable from other forms of hepatitis. After exposure, the incubation period is 21 to 45 days. Up to 90% of cases of HDV are asymptomatic, but when present, symptoms include jaundice, fatigue, abdominal pain, confusion, pruritus, anorexia, nausea, vomiting, and joint pain (Kellogg-Spadt, 2009).

Serum testing is complex and includes assays for serum HDAg, serum HDV RNA, anti-HDV antibody, and tissue markers for HDV infection. Transmission of HDV occurs through body fluids, including blood, semen, vaginal fluids, and saliva. Perinatal transmission is rare. Nurses can teach women to reduce their risk of contracting HDV through the avoidance of illicit IV drugs and the consistent practice of safer-sex strategies (e.g., latex condoms during vaginal, anal, and oral sex). Women may also wish to consider vaccination against hepatitis B (Kellogg-Spadt, 2009).

 Now Can You— **Discuss aspects of viral hepatitis?**

1. Identify populations at greatest risk for infection with HBV?
2. Identify seven settings where hepatitis B vaccination should be administered to adults who receive care?
3. Explain how the hepatitis virus may be transmitted?

Chancroid, Lymphogranuloma Venereum, Granuloma Inguinale, and Pthirus Pubis (Pubic Louse)

Although they occur less commonly, STDs including chancroid, lymphogranuloma venereum, granuloma inguinale, and pubic lice may be identified in the clinical setting.

CHANCROID

Caused by the gram-negative streptobacillus *Haemophilus ducreyi*, infection with chancroid begins with a small bump (usually on the labia majora) that quickly develops into a painful ulcer with a base that is covered with a gray or yellow-gray material. Symptoms include dysuria and dyspareunia. Inguinal adenopathy is present in approximately one-third of infected individuals. The diagnosis is made via special culture media. Treatment consists of a single oral dose (1 g) of azithromycin (Zithromax), a single intramuscular dose (250 mg) of ceftriaxone (Rocephin), oral ciprofloxacin (Cipro) (500 mg bid) for 3 days, or oral erythromycin (E-Mycin, E.E.S.) (500 mg tid) for 7 days (CDC et al., 2006b).

LYMPHOGRANULOMA VENEREUM

Lymphogranuloma venereum (LGV) is caused by the bacterium *Chlamydia trachomatis*. Primarily an infection of the lymphatics and lymph nodes, LGV gains entrance through breaks in the skin or via the mucous membranes. The primary infection produces a self-limited, painless genital ulcer at the contact site approximately 3 to 12 days after exposure. Owing to its hidden location, women frequently are unaware of its presence. The second stage, which usually occurs from 10 to 30 days later, involves the lymph nodes and lymphatic drainage pathways. Localized symptoms include cervicitis, perimetritis, salpingitis, and lymphadenitis; systemic symptoms include fever, decreased appetite, and malaise. The diagnosis is based on clinical suspicion, epidemiological information, and the exclusion of other causes, along with *C. trachomatis* testing. Serological testing is also available. LGV is treated with doxycycline (Vibramycin) 100 mg orally bid for 21 days or erythromycin base (E-base, Robimycin) 500 mg orally qid for 21 days (CDC et al., 2006b).

GRANULOMA INGUINALE

Granuloma inguinale (also known as "donovanosis") is a genital ulcerative disease caused by the intracellular gram-negative bacterium *Klebsiella granulomatis*. The disease commonly produces painless, progressive, beefy-red ulcerative lesions; regional lymphadenopathy is absent. The lesions most commonly occur on the labia or perineum. The diagnosis is made based on the patient's sexual history, absence of inguinal lymphadenopathy, and identification of the lesions. Tissue biopsy may be used to aid in the diagnosis. Granuloma inguinale is treated with doxycycline (Vibramycin) 100 mg orally bid for at least 3 weeks and until all lesions have completely healed. Alternative regimens include azithromycin (Zithromax) (1 g orally once per week × 3 weeks, ciprofloxacin (Cipro) (750 mg orally bid × 3 weeks) or trimethoprim-sulfamethoxazole (Bactrim) (one double-strength [160 mg/800 mg] tablet orally bid × 3 weeks) (CDC et al., 2006b).

PTHIRUS PUBIS

Lice are parasitic insects that can be found on the head and body, including the pubic area. Human lice survive by feeding on human blood. Lice infestations are primarily spread by close person-to-person contact. Lice move by crawling—they are unable to hop or fly. The Pthirus pubis (pubic louse, "crab" louse) is very short (1.1 to 1.8 mm in length) and crablike in appearance (Fig. 5-4). Pubic lice are typically found attached to hair in the pubic area but can sometimes be found on coarse hair in the eyebrows, eyelashes, beard, mustache, chest, or armpits. Pubic lice are usually spread through sexual contact and are most common in adults. Although they do not transmit disease, secondary bacterial infection can occur from scratching of the skin. Pubic lice and nits (eggs) may be large enough to be seen with the naked eye, although a magnifying lens may be necessary to find them (CDC, 2008b).

⑤ Optimizing Outcomes— **Through prevention and control of pubic lice**

The nurse counsels infected women about strategies to help prevent and control the spread of pubic lice. Patients are taught to (CDC, 2008b):

- Ensure that all sexual contacts are examined and all infested persons are treated.
- Avoid sexual contact until treatment and reevaluation have been completed.
- Machine wash all clothing and bedding in hot (at least 130°F) water and machine dry on the high heat drying cycle. Clothing and items that are not washable can be dry-cleaned or sealed in a plastic bag and stored for 2 weeks.
- Avoid the sharing of clothing, bedding, and towels.
- Avoid the use of fumigant sprays or fogs—these products can be toxic if inhaled or absorbed through the skin.

A lice-killing lotion containing 1% permethrin or a mousse containing pyrethrins and piperonyl butoxide can be used to treat pubic lice. These products are readily available over-the-counter without a prescription at a local drugstore. When used exactly according to the instructions listed on the package, these medications are safe and effective (CDC, 2008b).

The Nurse's Role in Fostering Reproductive Health Through STD Education and Counseling

When educating women about STDs, nurses should include basic information along with sexual decision-making skills. When dealing with adolescents, it is often helpful to discuss basic communication skills needed to negotiate in a relationship and how to operate from an internal value system rather than submit to peer pressure. Educating women about the workings of their bodies and encouraging them to be active participants in their own

Figure 5-4 Pubic Louse

health care enhances their personal control over their reproductive health. Nurses can empower women of all ages by providing them with specific strategies for making safe choices in their intimate relationships. When appropriate, teaching about strategies for "safer sex" provides guidance and serves to foster wellness and promote reproductive health (Box 5-5). During STD counseling, the nurse can emphasize that condoms offer the best protection against the transmission of disease and stress that intimate sexual contact should be avoided if the person or partner has any sore areas or visible lesions (Marrazzo et al., 2007).

During private counseling sessions, it is important to inquire about substance use and other high-risk behaviors that may increase the likelihood of exposure to an STD.

Box 5-5 Safer Sex Strategies for Sexual Intimacy and HIV and STD Prevention

STRATEGIES CONSIDERED TO BE SAFE
- Sexual fantasies
- Massage
- Hugging
- Body rubbing
- Dry kissing
- Masturbation without contact with the partner's semen or vaginal secretions
- Erotic conversation, books, movies, videos, or DVDs
- Eroticizing feet, fingers, buttocks, abdomen, ears, or other body parts
- All sexual activities when both partners are monogamous and known by testing to be free of HIV and other STDs

STRATEGIES WITH A LOW RISK, CONSIDERED TO BE POSSIBLY SAFE
- Wet kissing with no broken skin, cracked lips, or damaged mouth tissue
- Hand-to-genital touching or mutual masturbation
- Vaginal or anal intercourse using latex or plastic condom
- Oral sex on a woman using a latex or plastic barrier, such as a female condom, dental dam, or modified male condom (especially if the woman does not have a vaginal infection with discharge and is not menstruating)
- Oral sex on a man using a latex or plastic condom
- All sexual activities, when both partners agree to a monogamous relationship and trust each other

STRATEGIES CONSIDERED UNSAFE IN THE ABSENCE OF HIV TESTING AND TRUST AND MONOGAMY
- Blood contact of any kind, including menstrual blood
- Any vaginal or anal intercourse without a latex or plastic condom
- Oral sex on a woman without a latex or plastic barrier, such as a female condom, dental dam, or modified male condom, especially if she has a vaginal infection with discharge or is menstruating
- Semen in the mouth
- Oral–anal contact
- Sharing sex toys or douching equipment
- Any sex that causes tissue damage or bleeding (e.g., rough vaginal or anal intercourse, rape, fisting)

Source: Marrazzo et al., 2007.

A woman who drinks heavily or who practices binge drinking may not remember the details of sexual encounters that took place while intoxicated. A history of injected drug use increases the risk for infection with hepatitis and HIV; women who smoke have a higher rate of cervical cancer (Marrazzo et al., 2007; Ravin, 2007).

 Nursing Insight— *Contraceptive choice and safer sex*

Nurses should recognize that women who use nonbarrier contraceptive methods (e.g., oral contraceptive pills [OCPs], IUDs, subdermal hormonal implants) usually choose these methods for the freedom involved. Thus it is important to inform oral contraceptive users that the "pill" may cause changes in the cervix and in the immune system that increase susceptibility to HIV infection. Women who are in new or nonmonogamous relationships should be encouraged to use a barrier method along with the OCP, IUD, or subdermal hormonal implant.

The nurse should approach the counseling sessions with sensitivity and awareness that the individual may feel uncomfortable with sharing personal information about the sexual history or STD infection in the past. When possible, partners should be included in discussions concerning reproductive health issues.

 Optimizing Outcomes— **Reducing the likelihood of STD transmission and progression of disease**

To promote health maintenance and safety and reduce the likelihood of STD transmission, nurses can teach women:

- How to use condoms (male and female, if appropriate) properly
- How to perform a genital self-examination
- To avoid the sharing of personal care items, such as toothbrushes and razors
- To take all prescribed antibiotics, even if symptoms resolve
- To abstain from sexual intercourse until both partners have completed treatment (to prevent reinfection)
- To return for evaluation, as indicated, after treatment has been completed

Nurses should also inquire about vaginal douching, a common practice among women in the United States. Findings from a 2001 survey (Sutton, Bruce, & Sternberg, 2006) showed that approximately 22% of women douche, with the prevalence highest among African American women (50%). To date, no study has shown that douching is in any way beneficial to a woman's reproductive health or that it decreases the risk for contracting an STD. In fact, women who douche are at increased risk for STDs, especially if they are less educated, are economically disadvantaged, have more sexual partners, have higher-risk sexual partners, or have a past history of pelvic inflammatory disease. Owing to their biological and behavioral vulnerability to STDs, at-risk adolescents may experience even greater risks associated with douching (Martino & Vermund, 2002; Vermund & Allen, 2009).

 Nursing Insight— *Douching and STIs*

Douching increases the risk for STDs by washing away the resident lactobacilli, which increase vaginal acidity, thereby creating an inhospitable environment for pathogens. The lactobacilli also adhere to epithelial cells that prevent pathogen adherence. Without a preponderance of beneficial lactobacilli, the vaginal acidity decreases and pathogens can more readily adhere to the vagina (Schwebke, 2000). Younger women who douche and are more sexually active may be at an especially high risk for contracting an STD; the risk with douching may not be as great for older women (Vermund & Allen, 2009).

Nurses who work with women of all ages can provide counseling about the harmful effects of douching. The information should be presented in a patient-centered, nonjudgmental manner that is appropriately attuned to the patient's age, culture, sexual orientation, and developmental level. When appropriate, engaging the support of influential family members (e.g., mothers, sisters, mothers-in-law) may also be of benefit in effecting the desired behavioral change (Vermund & Allen, 2009).

Nursing diagnoses for women with STDs are developed after careful consideration of all patient assessment data, the plan of treatment, and specific directives from the health-care provider. One appropriate diagnosis, for example, may focus on the threat to physiological functioning: "Acute Pain/Impaired Tissue Integrity related to effects of the infection process/excoriation of pruritic areas/hygiene practices." Another may address the emotional dimensions of the diagnosis: "Anxiety/Situational Low Self-Esteem/Disturbed Body Image related to perceived effects on intimate relationships and long-term sequelae of infection," or "Social Isolation and Impaired Social Interaction related to perceived effects on relationships with others if the STD status is not known." A nursing diagnosis that addresses educational needs is "Deficient Knowledge related to transmission/prevention/reinfection/management of infection or safer sex behaviors."

Nursing interventions center on the use of therapeutic communication to foster nonjudgmental, culturally appropriate discussion to facilitate learning and understanding. Providing emotional support is an essential component of care. The nurse assesses the patient's (and partner's, if appropriate) level of knowledge about the infection and uses this information to develop an individualized teaching plan. Emphasis is placed on the use and importance of safe sexual practices and, depending on the treatment regimen, the need to complete all prescribed medication and return for further evaluation. Referral to support groups may be appropriate.

In some situations, the patient may confide that she is too embarrassed to reveal information about the STD to her intimate partner and ask for guidance. The nurse can assist her by offering strategies, such as role-playing, for approaching the partner and sharing the information. It is important to emphasize that although this is a difficult topic for discussion, most individuals would rather know about the possibility that they are infected rather than not know. Exploring ways of communicating sensitive information is an important nursing intervention that can strengthen the therapeutic relationship, enhance adherence with the treatment plan, and improve STD case finding.

" What to say" — *Exploring strategies for communicating STD infection information*

When counseling the patient about how she may approach her intimate partner about her STD, the nurse may suggest that she use statements such as "I care about you and I want you to know that I am concerned about your health. I want you to know that I am undergoing treatment for an STD—and you need to be evaluated as well."

Now Can You— **Describe the nurse's role in promoting reproductive health?**

1. Identify eight "safer sex" strategies?
2. Explain patient teaching about the practice of douching?
3. Formulate three potential nursing diagnoses for a woman with an STD?
4. Discuss aspects of patient education and counseling about STDs?

summary points

◆ STDs encompass more than 25 infectious organisms that cause reproductive tract infections.

◆ Potential complications of STDs include infertility, ectopic pregnancy, chronic pelvic pain, liver disease, liver cancer, and death.

◆ Chlamydia, the most commonly reported infectious disease in the United States, is the leading cause of preventable infertility and ectopic pregnancy.

◆ Once on the verge of elimination, syphilis has reemerged as a common STD.

◆ In the United States, women represent one of the fastest growing segments of the HIV epidemic.

◆ Gonorrhea and Chlamydia are prevalent in the adolescent population and disproportionately prevalent in minority groups.

◆ Infection with *Trichomonas vaginalis* increases the risk of HIV transmission.

◆ Pelvic inflammatory disease is most often caused by the organisms *Chlamydia trachomatis* and *Neisseria gonorrhoeae*.

◆ Hepatitis is the leading cause of liver cancer and the most common reason for liver transplantation.

◆ In the area of reproductive health promotion, an important nursing role centers on education about STDs, safer sex strategies, and actions to reduce the likelihood of STD transmission.

review questions

Multiple Choice

1. Self-care measures that reduce the transmission of STDs include:
   A. Withdrawal of the penis before ejaculation
   B. Douching immediately after sexual intercourse
   C. Use of barrier methods of contraception
   D. Mutual masturbation

2. Strategies for safer sex that avoid contact with bodily fluids include:
   A. Erotic massage
   B. Oral–genital stimulation
   C. Careful anal intercourse
   D. Consensual sharing of sex toys

3. Factors that place women at increased risk for HIV infection include:
   A. History of premenstrual syndrome
   B. History of prostitution
   C. History of a seizure disorder
   D. History of an ectopic pregnancy

4. The most common STD that frequently produces no signs or symptoms in women is:
   A. Chancroid
   B. Herpes
   C. Chlamydia
   D. Syphilis

5. The first sign of syphilis is a sore that is:
   A. Painful
   B. Filled with clear fluid
   C. Itchy and scaly
   D. Painless

REFERENCES

Adler, S. (2007). The importance of routine STD screening. *Clinical Advisor, 10*(6), 35–40.

Advisory Committee on Immunization Practices, Vaccines for Children Program. (2009). *ACIP provisional recommendations for HPV vaccine.* Retrieved March 20, 2010, from http://www.cdc.gov/vaccines/recs/provisional/downloads/hpv-vac-dec2009-508.pdf

American Academy of Pediatrics and the American College of Obstetricians and Gynecologists. (2007). *Guidelines for perinatal care* (6th ed.). Washington, DC: Author.

American College of Obstetricians and Gynecologists (ACOG). (2006, September). ACOG Committee Opinion No. 344: Human papillomavirus vaccination. *Obstetrics and Gynecology, 108*(4), 699–705.

American College of Obstetricians and Gynecologists (ACOG). (2007). *Women's health care: A resource manual* (3rd ed.). Washington, DC: Author.

Barry, P. M., Kent, C. K., Philip, S. S., & Klausner, J. D. (2010). Results of a program to test women for rectal Chlamydia and gonorrhea. *Obstetrics and Gynecology, 115*(4), 753–759.

Centers for Disease Control and Prevention (CDC). (2006a). Revised recommendations for HIV testing of adults, adolescents, and pregnant women in health-care settings. *MMWR Recommendations and Reports, 55*(RR14), 1–17.

Centers for Disease Control and Prevention (CDC), Workowski, A., & Berman, S. M. (2006b). *Sexually transmitted diseases treatment guidelines, 2006. Morbidity and Mortality Weekly Report, 55*(RR-11), 1–94.

Centers for Disease Control and Prevention (CDC). (2008a). *HIV and AIDS in the United States: A picture of today's epidemic.* Retrieved March 20, 2010, from http://www.cdc.gov/hiv/topics/surveillance/pdf/us_media.pdf

Centers for Disease Control and Prevention (CDC). (2008b). *Pubic "crab" lice.* Retrieved April 2, 2010, from http://www.cdc.gov/lice/pubic/index.html

Centers for Disease Control and Prevention (CDC). (2009a). *Sexually transmitted diseases surveillance, 2008.* Retrieved March 18, 2010, from http://www.cdc.gov/std/stats08/main.htm

Centers for Disease Control and Prevention (CDC). (2009b). *Basic statistics.* Retrieved March 20, 2010, from http://www.cdc.gov/hiv/topics/surveillance/basic.htm

Centers for Disease Control and Prevention (CDC). (2009c). *AIDS in the United States by geographic distribution.* Retrieved March 20, 2010, from http://www.cdc.gov/hiv/resources/Factsheets/geographic.htm

Centers for Disease Control and Prevention (CDC). (2009d). Chlamydia screening among sexually active young female enrollees of health plans—United States, 2000–2007. *MMWR Morbidity and Mortality Weekly Report, 58*(14), 362–365.

Centers for Disease Control and Prevention (CDC). (2009e). *Hepatitis B information for health professionals.* Retrieved March 24, 2010, from http://www.cdc.gov/hepatitis/HBV/HBVfaq.htm#treatment

Centers for Disease Control and Prevention (CDC). (2009f). *Hepatitis C information for health professionals.* Retrieved April 4, 2010, from http://www.cdc.gov/hepatitis/HCV/index.htm

Centers for Disease Control and Prevention (CDC). (2010). *Viral hepatitis.* Retrieved March 22, 2010, from http://www.cdc.gov/hepatitis/

Christiansen-Lindquist, L., Tao, G., Hoover, K., Frank, R., & Kent, C. (2009). Chlamydia screening of young sexually active, Medicaid-insured women by race and ethnicity, 2002–2005. *Sexually Transmitted Diseases, 36*(10), 642–646.

Connor, B. A. (2005). Hepatitis A vaccine in the last-minute traveler. *American Journal of Medicine, 118*(Suppl. 10A), 58S–62S.

Deglin, J. H., & Vallerand, A. H. (2009). *Davis's drug guide for nurses* (11th ed.). Philadelphia: F. A. Davis.

Gardner, J. (2006). What you need to know about genital herpes. *Nursing 2006, 36*(10), 26–27.

Glynn, M., & Rhodes, P. (2005). *Estimated HIV prevalence in the United States at the end of 2003.* Abstract presented at the National HIV Prevention Conference, 2005, Atlanta.

Graseck, A. S., Secura, G. M., Allsworth, J. E., Madden, T., & Peipert, J. F. (2010). Home screening compared with clinic-based screening for sexually transmitted infections. *Obstetrics and Gynecology, 115*(4), 745–752.

Greenwald, J. L., Burstein, G. R., Pincus, J., & Branson, B. (2006). A rapid review of rapid HIV antibody tests. *Current Infectious Disease Reports, 8*(11), 125–131.

Hackett, K. M. (2010). Chlamydia screening. *Advance for Nurse Practitioners, 18*(2), 16.

Holloway, M., & D'Acunto, K. (2006). An update on the ABCs of viral hepatitis. *Clinical Advisor, 9*(6), 26–40.

Hoover, K., & Tao, G. (2008). Missed opportunities for Chlamydia screening of young women in the United States. *Obstetrics & Gynecology, 11*(5), 1097–1102.

Hoover, K., Tao, G., & Kent, C. (2008). Low rates of both asymptomatic Chlamydia screening and diagnostic testing of women in U.S. outpatient clinics. *Obstetrics & Gynecology, 112*(4), 891–898.

Johnson-Mallard, V., & Lengacher, C. A. (2007). STD health communication intervention. *Women's Health Care, 6*(8), 27–31.

Kahn, J. O., & Walker, B. D. (1998). Acute human immunodeficiency virus type 1 infection. *New England Journal of Medicine, 339*(1), 33–39.

Kellogg-Spadt, S. (2009). Hepatitis D: Implications for sexuality. *American Journal for Nurse Practitioners, 13*(10), 39–40.

Marrazzo, J. A., Guest, F., & Cates, Jr., W. (2007). Reproductive tract infections, including HIV and other sexually transmitted infections. In R. Hatcher, J. Trussell, A. Nelson, W. Cates Jr., F. Stewart, & D. Kowal (Eds.), *Contraceptive technology* (19th ed., pp. 499–557). New York: Thomson Reuters.

Martino, J. L., & Vermund, S. H. (2002). Vaginal douching: Evidence for risks or benefits to women's health. *Epidemiologic Review, 24*(2), 109–124.

Mayeaux, E. J., Jr. (2007). External genital warts: An update. *Female Patient, 32*(12), 33–35.

National Institutes of Health (NIH). (2009). *BufferGel and PRO 2000/5: Vaginal gels to prevent HIV infection in women.* Retrieved April 5, 2010, from http://clinicaltrials.gov/ct2/show/NCT00074425

Nelson, A. L. (2007). Sexually transmitted treatment guidelines, 2006: An update. *Forum, 5*(1), 2–5.

Ravin, C. R. (2007). Preventing STDs: Ask the questions. *Nursing for Women's Health, 11*(1), 88–91.

Royer, H. R., & Cerf, C. (2009). Young women's beliefs about the terms sexually transmitted disease and sexually transmitted infection. *Journal of Obstetric, Gynecologic, & Neonatal Nursing, 38*(6), 686–692.

Royer, H. R., & Zahner, S. (2009). Providers' experiences with young people's cognitive representations and emotions related to prevention and treatment of sexually transmitted infections. *Public Health Nursing, 26*(2), 161–172.

Ryan, K. J., & Ray, C. G. (Eds.). (2004). *Sherris medical microbiology* (4th ed., pp. 541–544). New York: McGraw-Hill

Schmidt, J. V. (2007). HPV vaccine: Implications for nurses and patients. *Nursing for Women's Health, 11*(1), 83–87.

Schwebke, J. R. (2000). Vaginal infections. In M. B Goldman & M. C. Hatch (Eds.), *Women and health.* San Diego: Academic Press.

Sorvillo, F., Smith, L., Kerndt, P., & Ash, L. (2001). *Trichomonas vaginalis*, HIV, and African-Americans. *Emerging Infectious Diseases, 7*(6), 38–49.

Steffen, R. (2005). Changing travel-related global epidemiology of hepatitis A. *American Journal of Medicine, 118*(10), 46–49.

Stonehouse, A., & Studdiford, J. (2007). Allergic contact dermatitis from tee tree oil. *Consultant, 47*(8), 781.

Sutton, M. Y., Bruce, C., & Sternberg, M. R. (2006). *Prevalence and correlates of vaginal douching among women in the United States, 2001–2002.* Paper presented at the National STD Prevention Conference, May 2006, Jacksonville, FL.

Swan, A. M. (2009). Acute HIV infection in primary care. *Advance for Nurse Practitioners, 17*(9), 49–54.

Thiel, T. K. (1998). Hepatitis A vaccination. *American Family Physician, 57*(7), 1500–1501.

U.S. Department of Health and Human Services (USDHHS). (2000). *Healthy People 2010: Understanding and improving health.* Washington, DC: U.S. Government Printing Office.

U.S. Preventive Services Task Force (USPSTF). (2001). Screening for Chlamydial infection: Recommendations and rationale. *American Journal of Preventive Medicine, 20*(3 Suppl.), 90–94.

U.S. Preventive Services Task Force (USPSTF). (2004). *Screening for hepatitis B virus infection.* Retrieved March 25, 2010, from http://www.ahrq.gov/clinic/uspstf/uspshepb.htm

U.S. Preventive Services Task Force (USPSTF). (2005). Screening for gonorrhea: Recommendation statement. *Annals of Family Medicine, 3*(3), 263–267.

U.S. Preventive Services Task Force. (2009). U.S. Preventive Services Task Force Reaffirmation Recommendation Statement: Screening for syphilis infection in pregnancy: *Annals of Family Medicine, 150*(5), 705–709.

Vermund, S. H., & Allen, K. L. (2009). Douching is a remediable risk factor for sexually transmitted infections. *Female Patient, 34*(7), 37–39.

Weber-LaShore, A., & Biro, F. M. (2009). Cervicitis and sexually transmitted infections in the adolescent population. *Female Patient, 34*(6), 34–36.

Winer, S., & Richwald, G. A. (2007). Genital HSV update. *Forum, 5*(2), 18–22.

Xu, F., Sternberg, M. R., Kottiri, B. J., McQuillan, G. M., Lee, F. K., Nahmias, A. J., et al. (2006). Trends in herpes simplex virus type 1 and type 2 seroprevalence in the United States. *Journal of the American Medical Association, 296*(8), 964–973.

Promoting Reproductive Health Through an Understanding of Cervical Cytology Screening, Human Papillomavirus, and Cervical Cancer

Shelton M. Hisley, PhD, RNC, WHNP-BC

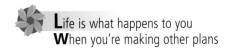

Life is what happens to you
When you're making other plans

—Betty Talmadge

LEARNING TARGETS *At the completion of this chapter, the student will be able to:*

◆ Describe the cervical epithelium and the process of metaplasia

◆ Discuss methods of cervical cytology screening

◆ Identify treatment options for various preinvasive conditions of the cervix

◆ Identify risk factors for human papillomavirus (HPV)

◆ Discuss the HPV–cervical cancer link

◆ Identify risk factors for cervical cancer

◆ Develop materials for patient education and counseling regarding cervical cytology screening, human papillomavirus, and cervical cancer

Introduction

This chapter, which explores cervical cytology screening, focuses on human papillomavirus (HPV) and its association with premalignant and malignant cervical disease. HPV is a nonenveloped, double-stranded DNA virus. It is the most common sexually transmitted disease in the United States. More than 40 HPV types that can infect the genital areas of males and females exist, and these HPV types can also infect the mouth and throat.

According to the Centers for Disease Control and Prevention (CDC) (2009a), approximately 20 million Americans are currently infected with HPV, and another 6 million people become newly infected each year. HPV is so common that at least 50% of all sexually active men

and women get it at some point in their lives. Around 1% of sexually active adults in the United States have genital warts at any one time, and each year approximately 12,000 American women get cervical cancer. HPV infection is known to be the primary cause of cervical cancer. Other cancers that may be caused by HPV include pharyngeal, vulvar, vaginal, penile, and anal (CDC, 2009a).

Although HPV has been recognized since 1907, it has only been within the past three decades that an understanding of the virus has evolved and its link to cervical and other cancers has been clearly established. The past 10 years have brought major advances in cervical screening technologies with the advent of liquid-based Pap tests and HPV testing. Most recently, two HPV vaccines have become available. The vaccines are indicated for the prevention of cervical cancer, genital warts, and dysplastic or precancerous cervical lesions caused by several of the HPV viruses types (American Cancer Society [ACS], 2010; CDC, 2009b; Howley, Yang, Spalholz, & Rabson, 1986; Moore & Seybold, 2007; National Association of Nurse Practitioners in Women's Health [NPWH], 2007; Wysocki, Reiter, & Berman, 2007).

The Cervix and the Cervical Transformation Zone

To enhance understanding about the uterine cervix and the cervical Pap test, it is important for the nurse to be knowledgeable about cervical cytology and the normal cellular changes that occur throughout a woman's life. The surface of the cervix and the canal that leads into the uterus—termed the "endocervical canal"—is composed of two types of cells: squamous epithelium and columnar epithelium.

A & P review Cervical Cell Types, the Squamocolumnar Junction, and the Transformation Zone

The cervix, which is typically 2.5 cm long, communicates with the endometrial cavity of the corpus uteri (uterine body) through the internal os and with the vagina through the external os. The vaginal portion (also called the exocervix, ectocervix, or portio vaginalis) is covered by stratified *squamous epithelium.* The squamous epithelium is smooth and light pink in appearance. The cervical canal is covered by *columnar epithelium,* which also forms endocervical glands, more correctly called "clefts." In young women, columnar epithelium can also be noted on the outer surface of the cervix around the external cervical os. The glandular tissue has a rough texture and is dark pink in color.

The area in which the squamous epithelium and the columnar epithelium come together on the cervix is called the *squamocolumnar junction (SCJ).* The SCJ is located where the more delicate, darker pink columnar cells that line the uterus meet the sturdier, lighter pink squamous epithelium of the vagina. Throughout the reproductive years, some columnar cells at the SCJ are replaced by squamous epithelium through a process termed squamous metaplasia. The area between the old and new SCJ is called the *transformation zone.* The size of the transformation zone varies from 2 to 15 mm. In most adult women, the squamocolumnar junction is not an abrupt meeting point but a zone containing irregular areas of glandular and squamous epithelium. This site undergoes continuous cell growth and replacement. The squamous type of cell replaces the columnar type of cell in a constant cycle of cell turnover, which is influenced by the female hormones. Metaplasia, which is a normal process of cell turnover, occurs most rapidly during adolescence and pregnancy. Cervical cancer usually develops in this area of rapid cell division. The immature cells undergoing the transformation from columnar to squamous tissue are especially vulnerable to events that can change the genetic material of the cells. These changes, or mutations, may result in the development of premalignant or malignant

cells (Teitelman, Stringer, Averbuch, & Witkoski, 2009; Wysocki et al., 2007). ◆

 Nursing Insight— *Natural migration of the transformation zone*

In infants and postmenopausal women, the transformation zone is located deep within the endocervical canal. In women of childbearing age, beginning at puberty, the transformation zone moves out of the endocervical canal and lies primarily on the ectocervix; this movement is termed *cervical ectopy.* Elevated hormone states that occur, for example, during pregnancy and with the use of hormonal contraception, may cause the transformation zone to become enlarged or more greatly exposed (Woodson, 2008).

Cervical Cancer Screening

DEVELOPMENT OF THE PAP TEST

Prior to the 1940s when the Pap test for cervical cytological screening became widely available, cervical cancer was the most common cause of cancer death in women in the United States. Over the last 30 years, the incidence of invasive cervical cancer has decreased by 50 percent. The ACS (2010) estimated that in 2009 around 11,270 new cases of invasive cervical cancer would be diagnosed, and around 4,070 American women would die from cervical cancer.

 Nursing Insight— *Origins of the Pap test*

The Pap test is named for Dr. George Papanicolaou, the physician who, along with Dr. Herbert Traut, developed the procedure in the 1930s. The Pap test is a cytological study used to detect cancer in cells that an organ has shed. Although used most often in the diagnosis and prevention of cervical cancers, the Pap test is also of value in detecting pleural or peritoneal malignancies and in the evaluation of cellular changes caused by radiation, infection, or atrophy. In women's health, the Pap test is a screening technique used to detect cervical cancer or cervical abnormalities that may progress to cancer. The test can detect 95% of all cervical cancers and precancerous abnormalities. In the years since World War II, the Pap test has become the most widely used cancer screening method in the world, and it is the most successful cancer screening technique in medical history. Pap screening reduced cervical cancer death rates by 74% between 1955 and 1992, and the rate continues to decline by about 2% each year (Venes, 2009).

 Nursing Insight— *Screening and early detection for cervical cancer*

The goal of screening for cervical cancer is to detect cervical cell changes and early cervical cancers before any symptoms develop. *Screening* refers to the use of tests (e.g., the Pap test) and exams to find a disease, such as cancer, in individuals who have no symptoms. *Early detection* means applying a strategy that results in an earlier diagnosis of cervical cancer than otherwise might have occurred. Screening tests offer the best chance to detect cervical cancer at an early stage when successful treatment is likely. Screening for cervical cancer is especially beneficial because it affords an opportunity to detect abnormal cell changes (precancers) so that they can be treated before they progress to cervical cancer (ACS, 2009a).

PAP TEST TECHNIQUES

The Pap test is usually a part of a routine pelvic examination. A sample of cervical epithelium is gathered from the squamocolumnar junction, which can often be visualized on the cervix. An adequate Pap test should contain both columnar cells and squamous cells, which indicates that the squamocolumnar junction was sampled. The Pap test is obtained before any digital examination of the vagina is performed and before any endocervical bacteriological specimens are collected. Prior to insertion, the vaginal speculum may be moistened with water or saline if necessary; no other lubricants are recommended. The examiner may use a large cotton-tipped applicator to remove excess cervical discharge before the cytological specimen is obtained (Teitelman et al., 2009).

Various sampling devices (e.g., spatula [paddle], cervix brush, plastic "broom") may be used (Fig. 6-1). When conventional Pap tests are performed, a single microscope slide, combining both the endocervical and ectocervical samples, or two separate glass slides can be used. The exocervix (outer area) is first sampled with the spatula (Fig. 6-2). This is done first to minimize the possibility of obscuring the cells with blood. The endocervix (inner area) is then sampled with the brush placed into the cervical os. The plastic "broom-like" brush is designed to simultaneously sample the endocervix and the exocervix. This device is inserted and rotated 360 degrees for a total of three to five times. If the patient has had a hysterectomy, the vaginal cuff (the portion of the vagina that remains open to the peritoneum following removal of the uterus) is sampled. The vaginal wall is usually not sampled unless the woman is approaching menopause, and in that case, a second sample may be obtained to evaluate the hormonal effects on vaginal tissue (ACOG, 2007; Policar, 2008).

The cytology sample is promptly transferred onto one or two thin glass slides and the sampling device is discarded. With this method of Pap testing, the most important consideration is rapid fixation. The slide should be

Figure 6-2 Taking a Cervical Smear (Source: From *Nursing Health Assessment: A Critical Thinking, Case Studies Approach,* 2nd ed., by P. M. Dillon, 2007, Philadelphia: F. A. Davis, p. 637.)

sprayed with a preservative within 5 seconds to prevent drying of the specimen (Bickley & Szilagyi, 2007; Dillon, 2007) (Fig. 6-3). Drawbacks of the conventional "slide method" of Pap test collection include the possibility of inadequate cellular sampling, the presence of artifacts (e.g., blood, discharge, lubricant) that obscure the cervical cells, the clinician's failure to properly "fix" the specimen in a timely manner, and inaccurate interpretation by the laboratory cytologist (ACOG, 2009a; Wysocki et al., 2007).

Today, the majority of cervical cytology screening performed in the United States uses a liquid-based process (e.g., ThinPrep Pap Test, BD SurePath Pap Test). With the liquid-based technique, exfoliated cells are collected from

Figure 6-3 A Cytology Brush and Spatula are Used for Specimens Obtained During a Conventional Pap Test. The Specimen Is Placed onto a Thin Glass Side and Immediately Sprayed with a Preservative (Fixative) (Source: From *Nursing Health Assessment: A Critical Thinking, Case Studies Approach,* 2nd ed., by P. M. Dillon, 2007, Philadelphia: F. A. Davis, p. 65.)

Figure 6-1 Tools for Pap Test (top to bottom): Cytobrush, Cervical Cytobroom, and Wooden Spatula (Source: From *Taber's Cyclopedic Medical Dictionary,* 21st ed., by D. Venes, 2009, Philadelphia: F. A. Davis, p. 1697.)

the transformation zone of the cervix and transferred to a vial of liquid alcohol-based preservative. The sample is then processed in the laboratory and a slide is produced for interpretation. With this method, almost all of the sample cells are transferred to the liquid preservative, and most of the contaminating blood, inflammatory cells, and debris are filtered out. However, heavy menstrual blood may limit the number of squamous cells available for interpretation. Prompt suspension of the cells in the liquid preservative eliminates the problem of air-drying artifact, a factor that can limit the interpretation of conventional cervical cytology (American College of Obstetricians and Gynecologists [ACOG], 2009a).

 Nursing Insight— Comparing the conventional Pap test with the liquid-based Pap test

In the conventional Pap test, cell samples are obtained from the vagina, cervix, and cervical canal and spread on a glass slide. In liquid-based Pap testing, cell samples are collected using a special brush that is immediately washed in an alcohol-based fluid. In the laboratory, a special machine filters out the cells from the solution and deposits them in a thin, uniform monolayer (a single layer of cells) on a glass slide. Analysis usually includes initial computer screening followed by slide review by a cytotechnologist. The liquid-based Pap test method removes contaminants such as blood and mucus, which frequently obscure cells in the conventional Pap test. The monolayer of cells is also easier to examine under the microscope, resulting in an increased rate of detection of abnormal cells. The disadvantage of the liquid-based method primarily centers on the increased cost incurred by the collection fluid and the continuing operation of the laboratory filtering machine.

With the liquid-based technology, between 50,000 and 70,000 diagnostic cells are available for screening; with the conventional process, approximately 4,000 to 300,000 cells are "smeared" onto a slide, where they often overlap or are obscured by non-cervical material. In addition, according to the laboratory-based cytotechnologists, the liquid-based tests are easier to read. Although the liquid-based cytology is more expensive than conventional cytology, it provides the added ability to test for HPV, gonorrhea, and Chlamydia from the same sample (ACOG, 2009a; Gupta, 2007).

" **What to say**" — *Informing patients of Pap test limitations*

Counseling patients about Pap test limitations constitutes a central role for nurses in women's health care. Nurses can advise about the limits of Pap test accuracy while reassuring them that the Pap test is the single most reliable method to detect preinvasive cancer of the cervix. However, there is no guarantee that any single Pap test will identify abnormal cells that may be present. Rescreening, when necessary, carries the burden of an additional expense, which may or may not be covered by insurance, whether funded by private, state, or federal sources (ACOG, 2009a; Gupton, 2007).

 Now Can You— **Describe normal cervical epithelium and the cervical Pap test?**

1. Identify the types of cells normally found in the cervix?
2. Define the terms *squamous metaplasia, squamocolumnar junction, and transformation zone*?
3. Describe the proper technique for obtaining a Pap test, and compare the liquid-based method with the conventional slide method?

INITIATION AND RECOMMENDED FREQUENCY OF CERVICAL CANCER SCREENING

Cancer of the cervix is usually a slow-growing neoplasm that is almost always caused by infection with the sexually transmitted disease human papillomavirus (HPV). (See later discussion of HPV in this chapter.) Screening for cervical cancer should begin at age 21 years, regardless of the woman's sexual history. Cervical neoplasia develops in susceptible individuals in response to infection with a high-risk type of HPV (i.e., types 12–14, 20, and 21). HPV causes carcinogenesis in the transformation zone of the cervix, where the process of squamous metaplasia replaces columnar epithelium with squamous epithelium. Squamous metaplasia is particularly active in the cervix during adolescence and early adulthood. HPV is commonly acquired by young women shortly after the initiation of vaginal intercourse, but in most situations the HPV is cleared by the immune system within 1 to 2 years without producing neoplastic changes. The risk of neoplastic transformation increases in women whose HPV infections persist. The recommendation to initiate cervical cancer screening at age 21 years regardless of the age of onset of sexual intercourse is based in part on the very low incidence of cancer in younger women. It is also based on the potential for adverse effects associated with follow-up of young women with abnormal cytology screening results (ACOG, 2009a).

 Nursing Insight— Potential adverse effects associated with cervical cancer screening in adolescents

Initiating cervical cancer screening in the adolescent population may result in increased anxiety, morbidity, and expense from the testing and overuse of follow-up procedures. The emotional impact of labeling an adolescent with both a sexually transmitted disease (i.e., HPV) and a potential precancer must be considered in light of the fact that the adolescent period is characterized by emerging sexuality and a heightened concern for self-image. Sexually active adolescents (i.e., females younger than 21 years) should be counseled and tested for STDs and educated about safer sex and contraception. These measures may be carried out without cervical cytology screening and, in the asymptomatic patient, without the use of a speculum (ACOG, 2009b; Wright et al., 2007).

Cervical cytology screening is recommended every 2 years for women aged 21 to 29 years, with either conventional or liquid-based cytology. Women aged 30 years and older who have had three consecutive cervical cytology test results that are negative for intraepithelial (potentially precancer) lesions and malignancy may be screened every 3 years. Women with the following risk factors may require more frequent cervical cytological screening (ACOG, 2009a):

* Women who are infected with HIV
* Women who are immunosuppressed (e.g., those who have received renal transplants)
* Women who were exposed to diethylstilbestrol (DES) in utero
* Women previously treated for cervical intraepithelial neoplasia (CIN) 2, CIN 3, or cancer

 Be sure to— Educate patients about strategies to optimize cervical cancer screening

Nurses can teach patients about strategies to optimize cervical cancer screening. In the ideal situation, the Pap test should be collected at midcycle. Patients should avoid intercourse, douching, or the use of vaginal medications for 24 to 48 hours prior to the test. The presence of infection (e.g., yeast) can cause vaginal inflammation and interfere with the test results. Over-the-counter vaginal creams, gels, foams, or suppositories used within 24 to 48 hours before the Pap test is obtained may interfere with the collection of an adequate cytological specimen.

CERVICAL CANCER SCREENING IN THE OLDER WOMAN

Cervical cancer tends to occur in midlife. It rarely develops in women younger than age 20. Most cases of cervical cancer and related deaths occur in women older than age 50. Almost 20% of women with cervical cancer are diagnosed over age 65. In fact, many older women do not realize that the risk of developing cervical cancer is still present as they age. Sadly, up to two-thirds of older women with cervical cancer have not received adequate Pap screening prior to their cancer diagnosis. Thus, all women with a cervix should continue to receive Pap test screening according to standard guidelines and their care provider's recommendations (ACS, 2010; Chase & Tewari, 2010; Gupton, 2007; Olbrys, 2010).

Currently, the ACS suggests that cervical cancer screening may be stopped in women aged 70 years or older if they have had three or more recent consecutive negative test findings and no abnormal test findings in the previous 10 years (ACS, 2009). The U.S. Preventive Services Task Force (USPSTF) (2007) recommends screening cessation in women older than 65 years with negative test results who are not otherwise considered to be high risk for cancer. ACOG has determined that it is reasonable to discontinue cervical cancer screening at either 65 years of age or 70 years of age in women who have three or more negative cytology test results in a row and no abnormal test results in the past 10 years (ACOG, 2009a). A summary of the current ACOG recommendations concerning cervical cancer screening is presented in Box 6-1. All expert groups are in agreement that cervical cancer screening can be discontinued in women who have had a hysterectomy if the surgery was performed for benign reasons and there is no past history of high-grade cervical lesions.

Box 6-1 Cervical Cancer Screening: ACOG Recommendations

The following ACOG recommendations for cervical cancer screening (2009) are based on good and consistent scientific evidence (Level A):

* Cervical cancer screening should begin at age 21 years. Screening before age 21 should be avoided because it may lead to unnecessary and harmful evaluation and treatment in women at very low risk of cancer.
* Cervical cytology screening is recommended every 2 years for women between the ages of 21 years and 29 years.
* Women aged 30 years and older who have had three consecutive negative cervical cytology screening test results and who have no history of CIN 2 or CIN 3, are not HIV infected, are not immunocompromised, and were not exposed to diethylstilbestrol (DES) in utero may extend the interval between cervical cytology examinations to every 3 years.
* Both liquid-based and conventional methods of cervical cytology are acceptable for screening.
* In women who have had a total hysterectomy for benign indications and have no prior history of high-grade CIN, routine cytology testing should be discontinued.
* Co-testing using the combination of cytology plus HPV DNA testing is an appropriate screening test for women older than 30 years. Any low-risk woman aged 30 years or older who receives negative test results on both cervical cytology screening and HPV DNA testing should be rescreened no sooner than 3 years subsequently.

 Be sure to— Document all communications concerning Pap tests

When Pap test results are received, it is essential that patients be promptly notified of abnormal results. Neglect to do so may result from a breakdown in communication between the care provider and the office staff or from poor follow-up efforts to contact patients. Documentation of test results and patient follow-up efforts is equally important. It is essential that information regarding efforts to report results, make treatment recommendations, and order appropriate follow-up, as well as efforts to obtain patient history and informed consent or informed refusal, be documented in the chart (Duffy, 2009).

 ***Across Care Setting:* Ensuring cervical cancer screening for medically underserved women**

In this country, all states are making cervical cancer screening more available to medically underserved women through the National Breast and Cervical Cancer Early Detection Program (NBCCEDP). The program provides free or low-cost breast and cervical cancer screening to women with no health insurance. The goal of NBCCEDP is to reach as many women in medically underserved communities as possible, including older women, women without health insurance, and women who are members of racial and ethnic minorities. Nurses can contact the Department of Health in their practice state for specific information regarding program location and eligibility requirements, or they may contact the CDC at 1-800-CDC-INFO, or visit the CDC Web site at www.cdc.gov/cancer/nbccedp.

INTERPRETING CERVICAL CYTOLOGY FINDINGS: THE BETHESDA SYSTEM TERMINOLOGY

The Bethesda System is the classification for abnormal cervical cytology and histology that is most commonly used today. First developed in 1988 under sponsorship of the National Institutes of Health (NIH), the updated 2001 Bethesda System terminology is used to describe the categories of epithelial cell abnormalities, including atypical squamous cells (ASC), low-grade or high-grade squamous intraepithelial lesions (LSIL or HSIL), and glandular cell abnormalities, including atypical glandular cells (AGC) and adenocarcinoma in situ (AIS). Histology diagnoses of abnormalities are reported as CIN Grades 1–3 (ACOG, 2008). The 2001 Bethesda System terminology is presented in Box 6-2.

 Optimizing Outcomes— **With the Bethesda System: A standardized approach for cytology/histology findings and interpretation to guide patient care**

Over the years, the Bethesda System has undergone a number of major changes in approach and terminology in attempts to standardize reporting systems worldwide and provide more information about what was actually identified in the cellular sample. Developed by major medical groups including the ACOG, the ACS, the Association of Reproductive Health Professionals (ARHP), and the American Society for Colposcopy and Cervical Pathology (ASCCP), the original guidelines have undergone review several times in past years in response to emerging data on the role of HPV in cervical cancer. The latest (2007) ASCCP consensus guidelines reflect evidence-based advances in the understanding of the natural history of HPV, its influence on the development of cervical dysplasia and cancer, and the role of Pap tests with a liquid-based sample (ACOG, 2008; Wright et al., 2007; Wysocki et al., 2007).

 Now Can You— **Discuss cervical cytology screening?**

1. Identify the appropriate time for initiation and recommended frequency for cervical cancer screening according to guidelines established by ACOG?
2. Explain why cervical cancer screening in the adolescent population is discouraged?
3. Teach a patient how to prepare for her Pap test and include three strategies intended to optimize the test results?

FOLLOW-UP FOR ABNORMAL CERVICAL CYTOLOGY SCREENING RESULTS

Depending on the result of the Pap test, further evaluation or treatment or both may be indicated. Reflex HPV DNA testing is an option for the management of an ASCUS Pap test result. Reflex HPV DNA testing is performed to determine whether HPV is present and if referral for colposcopy is indicated. Women of all ages with ASCUS Pap test results should be tested for HPV. The liquid-based Pap samples can be immediately tested for HPV if there is an ASCUS result. Women with an ASCUS Pap result who test positive for HPV should be referred for colposcopy with directed biopsy and endocervical sampling (ACOG, 2008; Wysocki et al., 2007).

Colposcopy

Colposcopy is a medical diagnostic procedure that uses a colposcope to provide an illuminated, magnified view of the cervix and the tissues of the vagina and vulva. The colposcope is a low-powered binocular microscope with a powerful light source mounted to allow visualization of the vagina and cervix during a pelvic examination. This instrument allows for a close-up view of the cervix and surrounding tissue for evaluation. The main goal of colposcopy is to prevent cervical cancer by the early detection and treatment of precancerous lesions.

❝ **What to say** ❞ — *Preparing the patient for colposcopy*

The nurse can do much to allay a patient's anxiety about colposcopy. The nurse may offer the following description of the procedure to help the patient understand what to expect:

Once you have emptied your bladder, I will assist you into position (dorsal lithotomy) for a pelvic examination. The clinician (colposcopist) will insert a vaginal speculum and most likely use cotton swabs to apply an acetic acid (vinegar) solution to the cervix. Abnormal areas turn white (acetowhite) and become more prominent in response to the acetic acid, allowing for improved visualization. Areas that turn white after the application of acetic acid or have an abnormal vascular pattern are often considered for biopsy. If no lesions are visible, an iodine solution (Schiller's or Lugol's solution) may be applied to the cervix and vagina to help highlight areas of abnormality. The colposcopist determines the

---

Box 6-2 The 2001 Bethesda System Terminology

SQUAMOUS CELL
- ASC
- Of undetermined significance (ASC-US) (the most minor form of cytological abnormality detected on the Pap test)
- Cannot exclude high-grade SIL*
- LSIL (encompasses HPV, mild dysplasia, and CIN1)**
- HSIL (encompasses HPV, moderate and severe dysplasia, CIS, and CIN 2 and CIN 3)
- Squamous cell carcinoma

GLANDULAR CELL
- AGC (a cytological abnormality of the glandular cells that line the endocervix or uterus)
- Atypical glandular cells, favors neoplasia
- Endocervical adenocarcinoma in situ
- Adenocarcinoma

* SIL: cytological abnormalities identified on the Pap test, classified as low-grade (LSIL) or high-grade (HSIL).
** CIN: cervical cancer precursor (confirmed by biopsy), divided into low-grade (CIN1) and high-grade (CIN2/3) (ACOG, 2008; Wysocki et al., 2007).

areas with the highest degree of visible abnormality and may obtain biopsies from these areas. A numbing medication (lidocaine) is used to diminish discomfort, especially if many biopsy samples are taken. Although not common, potential complications include bleeding and infection. To minimize the risk of infection, you should use a panty liner or sanitary napkin and avoid sexual intercourse until all vaginal bleeding or discharge has stopped. Your health-care provider may advise you to take a mild pain reliever such as ibuprofen approximately 30 minutes to 1 hour before the procedure and afterward as needed for cramping and discomfort. Be sure to promptly notify your health-care provider if you develop any signs of infection, such as fever, continued pain, bleeding, foul-smelling vaginal discharge, or painful urination (dysuria), or have any concerns. Also, it is a good idea to bring a support person with you.

Endocervical Sampling

Endocervical sampling is performed if the colposcopy is unsatisfactory (e.g., no lesions are identified, or the endocervical canal cannot be fully visualized) and in women who have follow-up colposcopy after treatment for CIN 2 or 3 with a positive endocervical margin. Endocervical sampling may be conducted either with vigorous endocervical brushing or by the traditional endocervical curettage (ECC), a procedure that uses a sharp, spoon-shaped instrument (curette). A small tissue sample is obtained and sent to a pathology lab for evaluation. Examination of the tissue allows for determination of whether abnormal lesions are located inside the endocervical canal; this information is an important determinant in the treatment plan (ACOG, 2008; ACOG, 2009a).

During the endocervical sampling procedure, which usually only takes a few minutes, the patient will most likely experience abdominal pain and menstrual-like uterine cramps. Endocervical sampling is not indicated in the pregnant patient. Monsel's Solution (Basic Ferric Sulfate Solution, a hemostatic agent) is applied with large cotton swabs to the surface of the cervix to control bleeding. This solution, which is mustard colored, turns black when exposed to blood. After the procedure, the Monsel's Solution is expelled naturally. The nurse can explain to the patient that she may experience a thin, coffee-ground-like vaginal discharge for several days after the procedure (ACOG, 2009a).

Optimizing Outcomes— Addressing abnormal Pap test results during pregnancy

The management of abnormal Pap test results during pregnancy takes into consideration the duration of the pregnancy, the woman's desire to maintain the pregnancy, and the degree of cellular abnormality. Colposcopy is used for diagnosis, and the primary goal of both cytology and colposcopy is to identify invasive cancer that requires treatment before or at the time of delivery. Cervical biopsies are safe and should be performed for suspected high-grade disease or cancer. Biopsy during pregnancy has not been linked to fetal loss or preterm birth. Endocervical sampling should not be performed. Unless invasive cancer is identified, treatment is postponed until after the pregnancy has ended (ACOG, 2008).

MANAGEMENT OF ABNORMAL CERVICAL CYTOLOGY/COLPOSCOPY FINDINGS

There are a number of ways to treat the lesions identified in a colposcopic examination; the treatment depends on the location and severity of the lesions. Four types of interventional techniques are available: cryosurgery, laser ablation, conization, and the loop electrosurgical excision procedure.

Cryosurgery

Cryosurgery (cryotherapy), a gynecological treatment that involves the freezing of cervical tissue, is performed in the office setting. The patient is assisted into a dorsal lithotomy position and a vaginal speculum is inserted. Cryo probes are placed over the abnormal areas on the cervix. Liquid nitrogen flows through the cryo probes at a temperature of approximately –50°C, making the metal cold enough to freeze and destroy the tissue. Cryosurgery is relatively painless and produces very little scarring. An "ice ball" forms on the cervix, killing the superficial abnormal cells. The most effective treatment result is obtained by a process of freezing for 3 minutes, allowing the area to thaw, and then refreezing for 3 more minutes. Throughout the procedure, the patient may experience slight cramping and/or a sensation of cold or heat. Cryosurgery effectively destroys all of the abnormal cervical tissue in over 85% of cases (ACOG, 2008).

> **" What to say "** — *Teaching patients about aftercare following cryosurgery*
>
> Offering explanations about what to expect following cryosurgery and alerting patients to danger signs constitutes an important nursing role. The nurse can counsel the patient that she:
>
> - may return to most normal activities the day following the cryosurgery;
> - will experience a foul-smelling watery vaginal discharge, caused by sloughing of the necrotic cervical tissue, for a few weeks;
> - should avoid inserting anything (tampons, douches) into the vagina and refrain from intercourse for at least 2 to 3 weeks;
> - should promptly call her health-care provider if she experiences any symptoms of infection (fever, vaginal bleeding heavier than a normal menstrual cycle, severe or increasing pelvic pain, foul-smelling or yellow-green vaginal discharge); and
> - should be sure to return for her follow-up appointment and comply with her health-care provider's recommendations for repeat Pap testing.

A long-term complication of cryosurgery concerns the migration of the squamocolumnar junction (the transformation zone—the area on the cervix where the outer squamous cells meet the inner glandular columnar cells). Following the procedure, the squamocolumnar junction migrates upward into the cervical canal. The relocation of the transformation zone may create the need for a more invasive procedure in the future if abnormal lesions occur that are not visible with the colposcope (i.e., the abnormal cells are located inside the endocervical canal). Although rare, cryosurgery may cause scarring of the cervix and lead to stenosis (narrowing) of the cervical opening, making future cervical cytology screening (Pap testing) and evaluation (colposcopy) difficult (ACOG, 2008).

Laser Ablation

Laser ablation (destruction) involves the use of a thin, high-energy beam of light precisely directed at the abnormal tissue to cause cell destruction through vaporization. Depending on the circumstances, the procedure may be performed in the office, or outpatient setting of the clinic or hospital. The technique uses a laser (mounted on a colposcope) to vaporize the transformation zone, where the abnormal cells are located. Advantages of laser ablation include rapid healing (3–4 weeks), minimal scarring, and no retraction of the transformation zone. Following laser ablation, patients may experience less vaginal discharge than with cryosurgery, but they may experience more discomfort immediately after the procedure. Vaginal spotting or bleeding may occur for several days after the surgery.

" What to say " — *Preparing the patient for cervical laser ablation*

Prior to the procedure, the nurse provides information, answers questions, and asks the patient to empty her bladder. The nurse may offer the following description of the procedure to help the patient understand what to expect:

- Medication will be given to decrease cramping and to numb the area to be treated.
- Everyone in the room will wear special glasses and surgical masks.
- Because laser burns or vaporizes cells, there will be a small amount of smoke present, and a smoke evacuator is used to remove the smoke from the air.

- The entire procedure (when done in the office or clinic) will take approximately 5 to 20 minutes, depending on the size of the abnormal area.
- Recovery time is minimal; most women leave within 20 minutes following the procedure.
- Some vaginal discharge is normal, but immediately report bleeding heavier than a menstrual period or yellow-green, foul-smelling discharge.
- A mild analgesic such as acetaminophen or ibuprofen may be taken as needed for pain, but severe abdominal pain should be reported immediately.
- Intercourse, douching, or the use of tampons should be avoided for 3 weeks.
- A fever above 100°F (38°C) should be reported immediately.
- Tub baths and showers may be taken, and you may return to work the day after the treatment.
- It is a good idea to ask a support person to accompany you to the appointment.
- Be sure to keep your follow-up appointment and follow your health-care provider's recommendations for repeat Pap testing.

Conization: Cold Knife Cone; Laser Conization; Loop Electrosurgical Excision Procedure (LEEP)

Conization of the cervix is defined as excision of a cone-shaped or cylindrical wedge from the uterine cervix that includes the transformation zone and all or a portion of the endocervical canal (Fig. 6-4). This procedure may be done when the lesion found on colposcopy extends into the endocervical canal and cannot be fully seen. Cold knife conization (CKC; also known as "cone biopsy") involves the use a scalpel without electrosurgical current; laser conization employs use of a laser for the excision of

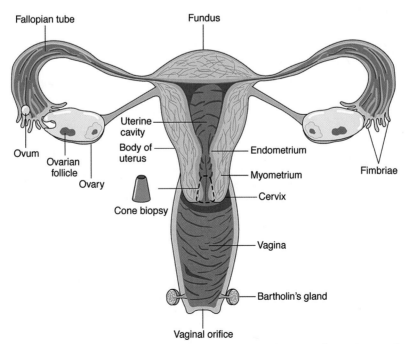

Figure 6-4 Cervical Conization (Source: From *Understanding Medical-Surgical Nursing,* 3rd ed., by L. S. Williams and P. D. Hopper, 2007, Philadelphia, F. A. Davis, p. 928.)

tissue. Cold knife and laser conization, which are usually performed in the hospital outpatient surgical center, may be done for diagnostic purposes, or for therapeutic purposes, to remove precancerous cells. Techniques for diagnostic and therapeutic conization are virtually identical. Depending on the circumstances and setting, patients may receive a local anesthetic with IV sedation, regional anesthesia, or general anesthesia. Potential complications of cervical conization include infection, bleeding, and cervical scarring or stenosis (narrowing); the procedure may also increase the risk of cervical incompetence and preterm birth (ACOG, 2008; Burkman, 2010; Shanbhag, Clark, Timmaraju, Bhattacharya, & Cruickshank, 2009).

Conization performed with electrosurgical loop is called the loop electrosurgical excision procedure (LEEP), or large loop excision of the transformation zone (LLETZ). LEEP uses a low-voltage electrical current to remove abnormal cervical tissue. With this procedure, the cervix is anesthetized with a local anesthetic, and a fine wire loop electrode is used to simultaneously remove and cauterize a portion of the cervix. The advantage of the electrosurgical loop procedure and other excisional techniques (e.g., CKC) over the ablative therapies (e.g., cryosurgery, laser vaporization) is that the tissue is removed, not destroyed. Thus, the tissue is available for evaluation by a pathologist. Also, the LEEP procedure is fast (20–30 minutes), virtually bloodless, and may be performed in the office. Following the procedure, healing is rapid, and there is only a mild vaginal discharge afterward. Patients may experience mild pain and cramping for the first few hours after the LEEP; the discomfort can be relieved by oral medications. Possible short- and long-term complications include bleeding, cervical stenosis, preterm birth, infertility, and loss of cervical mucus (ACOG, 2008; Burkman, 2010).

〝What to say〞 — *Preparing the patient for cervical conization*

An important nursing role in caring for the patient who will undergo cervical conization centers on education and support. Prior to the conization, the nurse answers questions and addresses concerns. The nurse may offer the following description of the procedure to help the patient understand what to expect:

- The procedure will take less than 1 hour.

- Some form of anesthesia will be used to control pain.

- Depending on the type of anesthesia to be used, nothing should be taken by mouth for 8 hours prior to the procedure (when IV sedation or general anesthesia is planned).

- The physician will first insert a vaginal speculum and then use a knife (CKC), laser, or heated loop (LEEP) to remove a cone-shaped section of tissue (containing any abnormal cells) from the cervix.

- Self-absorbable sutures may be placed in the cervix to control bleeding.

- Analgesics may be taken as needed for pain control after the conization.

- If the conization is performed in an outpatient surgery center, and depending on the type of anesthesia used, you may leave after you are fully awake, but someone must be with you to drive you home.

- If the conization is planned as an office procedure (LEEP), an electrosurgical dispersive pad (a gel-covered adhesive electrode that provides a safe return path for the electrosurgical current) will be placed on your thigh and removed after the procedure.

- Vaginal bleeding or discharge may be present for several days after the conization; a panty liner or sanitary napkin should be worn to protect clothing.

- Tampons, douches, and sexual intercourse should be avoided for 4 to 6 weeks.

- You should avoid lifting items heavier than 25 pounds for at least 1 week.

- Tub baths and showers may be taken as desired.

- Any signs of infection or other complications (e.g., fever, chills, foul-smelling discharge from the vagina, worsening abdominal pain, heavy vaginal bleeding [may not occur until about 1 week after the procedure, when the healing scar is shed from the cervix]) should be promptly reported to your health-care provider.

- It is important to return for the postoperative examination and to follow your health-care provider's recommendations for repeat Pap testing.

 Now Can You— **Discuss diagnostic/treatment modalities for abnormal cervical cytological screening results?**

1. Describe colposcopy, and explain how to prepare a patient for a colposcopic examination?
2. Discuss the importance of endocervical sampling?
3. Compare and contrast cervical cryosurgery, laser ablation, and conization, and provide patient teaching for each of these treatment modalities?

Human Papillomavirus

The human papillomavirus (HPV) is a DNA tumor virus that can infect cutaneous and mucosal surfaces, including the anogenital epithelium. Anogenital and cutaneous HPV infections are very common, but only a small fraction of genital infections actually progress to cancer. Cervical cancer, rarely found among women in celibate religious orders, has long been associated with intimate sexual activity. Owing to the rising epidemic of the sexually transmitted HPV infection, the average age of women with abnormal Pap test findings is declining steadily. HPV is most prevalent among the younger population of women, although it does occur with the same frequency in older women as well (Teitelman et al., 2009; Wysocki et al., 2007).

 Nursing Insight— *The papillomavirus–cancer link*

Many of the papilloma viruses cause papillomas. Papillomas are not cancers and are more commonly called warts. The most important risk factor in the development of cervical cancer is infection with a high-risk strain of HPV. The virus–cancer connection occurs as a result of alterations in the cervical cells that can lead to the development of CIN, which can then lead to cancer. HPV is passed from one individual to another during skin-to-skin contact. Although the virus is frequently transmitted during vaginal intercourse, anal intercourse, or oral sex, intercourse does not have to take place for HPV to be spread from one person to another. Skin-to-skin contact with an area of the body infected with HPV is the only requirement for transmission (ACS, 2010).

 where research and practice meet:
Incidence of HPV infection in new sexual relationships

According to a recent study, more than half (56%) of young adults who reported that they were involved in a new sexual relationship were infected with HPV; of those, nearly half (44%) were infected with an HPV type that causes cancer. The results also indicated a high probability of HPV transmission between partners. When one partner had HPV, the researchers observed that in 42% of couples, the other partner also had the infection. If one partner was infected with HPV, the other partner's chance of also being infected with the same HPV type increased more than 50 times. The researchers concluded that the study findings support the belief that HPV infection is very common among young adults and underscore the importance of prevention programs for HPV-associated diseases such as cervical cancer screening and HPV vaccination (Burchell, Tellier, Hanley, Coutlee, & Franco, 2010).

HPVs are a family of more than 100 virus types with a multitude of manifestations that include common warts, plantar warts, skin cancers, anal and genital warts, recurrent respiratory papillomatosis (a rare, benign infection of type HPV 6 or 11—it passes from mothers to neonates during vaginal childbirth), head and neck cancers, genital cancers, and cervical cancer (Hellwig, 2006; Moore & Seybold, 2007; Schmidt, 2007). Young men and women between the ages of 15 and 24 account for approximately half of all new HPV infections (Cates, Brewer, Fazekas, Mitchell, & Smith, 2006).

 Nursing Insight— *Maternal HPV and neonatal laryngeal papillomatosis*

Transmission to the infant of HPV type 6 or 11 is known to be possible during vaginal childbirth, but it is rare. Most experts believe that the risk of cesarean birth to both the mother and her infant exceeds the risk of neonatal genital warts or laryngeal papillomatosis (the presence of HPV 6– or 11–induced warts in the larynx or upper airway). However, cesarean birth may be indicated for women with genital warts if the pelvic outlet is obstructed or if vaginal birth would result in excessive bleeding. Once the maternal warts are no longer present, especially if the woman has had no detectable HPV lesions for 6 months or more, transmission of HPV to the infant during a vaginal birth becomes increasingly unlikely (ASCCP, 2010; CDC, 2006).

Of more than 100 known types of HPV, approximately 40 strains are believed to be capable of infecting the genital tract. HPV types 6 and 11 have been identified as "low risk." These are the types most likely to be associated with condylomata acuminata (genital warts), benign cervical changes, and low-grade cervical intraepithelial lesions. Important associations have been identified between HPV type 16 and squamous cell carcinoma and between type 18 and cervical adenocarcinoma. In fact, these two HPV strains together are responsible for approximately 70% of all cervical cancers. Many other HPV types (i.e., types 31, 33, 35, 39, 45, 51, 56, 58, 59, 68, 73) are considered to be "high risk" (they carry the potential to cause cervical cancer), and one or more of these particular types is detected in nearly every patient diagnosed with cervical cancer (Moore & Seybold, 2007). High-risk HPV produces no visible symptoms; instead, it is detected by DNA testing for the virus, or on the basis of abnormal Pap test results. HPV is the primary cause of cervical neoplasia, and persistent infection with high-risk types of HPV constitutes the most significant risk factor for cervical cancer (ACS, 2010; Moore & Seybold, 2007; Teitelman et al., 2009; Woodson, 2008).

HPV DNA TESTING

Most HPV infections produce no symptoms, and frequently a woman learns that she has been exposed to the virus only after undergoing a routine Pap test. Reflex HPV DNA testing, performed on a sample of vaginal or cervical cells collected during a pelvic examination, is most commonly performed on cells collected from residual preservative when liquid-based cytology is used. The HPV DNA test can often be performed on the same sample collected for the Pap test. HPV DNA testing assesses exfoliated cervical cells for the presence of 1 or more of 13 or 14 of the 15 to 18 potentially cancer-causing HPV types (ACOG, 2009a; Gupton, 2007).

 Optimizing Outcomes— **Through co-testing: A combination of cytology + HPV DNA testing**

Although the Pap test can detect cellular changes caused by high-risk types of HPV, it is not as sensitive as the HPV test, which specifically detects the viral DNA. DNA testing for HPV has gained widespread acceptance as an additional cervical cancer screening tool and as follow-up to abnormal changes detected with a Pap test. Today, there are several DNA HPV tests that can detect either the majority of the high-risk types of HPV or specific subtypes, such as HPV-16 and HPV-18. The tests are performed on cervical or vaginal cells collected through self-sampling or obtained by a health-care provider during a pelvic examination. Co-testing using the combination of cytology plus HPV DNA testing is an appropriate screening test for women older than 30 years. ACOG recommends that women 30 years or older be offered an HPV DNA test in addition to their Pap test and pelvic exam, and this recommendation is supported by various organizations, including the ACS, the National Institutes of Health (NIH), the ASCCP, the NPWH, and the American Medical Women's Association (AMWA). The HPV DNA test is not recommended for screening adolescents because infections with HPV are relatively common in this age group and often resolve without treatment or complications (ACOG, 2008; Duffy, 2008; Garfield, Gavaghan, Poret, & Ilika, 2010).

POTENTIAL MANIFESTATIONS OF HPV INFECTION

In women with HPV infection, abnormal findings on Pap screening are common. Of persons infected with HPV, only about 1% develop external genital warts, while approximately 10% develop cervical lesions. When present, HPV lesions most often occur on the posterior part of the vaginal introitus. Other locations include the buttocks, vulva, vagina, urethra, anus, and cervix. Four different types of genital warts have been identified (Box 6-3). It is possible to be infected with several different genotypes of HPV; some may be associated with a low risk, while others are associated with a high risk for the development of cervical cancer (ACOG, 2008; ACS, 2010; Moore & Seybold, 2007).

"What to say" — *Counseling patients about abnormal Pap test results and HPV*

It is incumbent upon the nurse to listen generously to patient concerns about HPV and cervical cancer and offer support in coping with abnormal or positive results. Nurses should be sensitive to the fact that sharing the results of an abnormal Pap test with a patient can evoke feelings of anxiety, fear, and difficulty assimilating the implications of the results. In this situation, the nurse may wish to include the following information:

Your abnormal Pap test result is not a diagnosis of a disease; it merely alerts us to the fact that there is a need for closer surveillance (e.g., more frequent testing) or further evaluation (e.g., colposcopy). Because it takes so long for cervical changes caused by HPV to develop into cancer, women who obtain Pap tests regularly are very unlikely ever to develop cervical cancer because there is plenty of opportunity to identify and treat the problem at an early stage (ASCCP, 2010; Woodson, 2008).

HPV is an elusive virus with a clinical course that is characterized by spontaneous regressions and recurrences. Once a woman contracts genital HPV, she may develop a latent HPV infection, a subclinical HPV infection, a clinical HPV infection (manifested by the appearance of warts and/or cervical changes), or regression of the HPV lesions (Box 6-4). For most women, HPV infection resolves without intervention. It is estimated that up to 70% of HPV infections clear in 1 year and 91% of infected women do not have detectable levels of cervical

---

Box 6-3 **Types of Genital Warts**

Condyloma acuminata are soft, moist, pink, red, or gray lesions that may occur singularly or in multiples. The warts occur on moist surfaces and often cluster to form a cauliflower shape.

Smooth papular warts are small dome-shaped papules that are usually skin colored. They occur on hair-bearing or non-hair-bearing skin and do not occur on mucosal tissue.

Keratotic genital warts have a thick layer and often look like "common" warts. They develop on hair-bearing or on non-hair-bearing skin and other non-skin tissues.

Flat warts are generally flat or slightly raised with flat tops. These lesions can occur on moist or on dry tissue (Wysocki et al., 2007).

Box 6-4 **Potential Manifestations of HPV Infection**

Following exposure to HPV, one or more of the following may occur (ASCCP, 2010):

Latent HPV infection: No detectable warts are present (i.e., undetectable by visual inspection, cytology, or HPV testing) and the person is noncontagious. However, because the virus can move from latency to "expressed" HPV disease (e.g., warts, cervical cell changes), there is no guarantee that the person will remain noncontagious indefinitely.

Subclinical HPV infection: Applies to changes in the skin cells of the lower genital tract that cannot be seen with the naked eye. The most common subclinical change is intraepithelial neoplasia of the cervix (cervical "precancerous change," dysplasia, CIN 1, 2, or 3) that can be seen following the application of vinegar (acetic acid) to the skin, followed by close examination (e.g., colposcopy magnification) of areas that turn white (acetowhitening). Although subclinical HPV may appear anywhere in the lower genital tract, acetowhitening is very nonspecific and often unrelated to HPV. Tissue biopsy must be used to confirm the diagnosis of HPV infection.

Clinical HPV: The presence of warts and precancerous changes on the external genitalia (vulvar and perianal intraepithelial neoplasia; cervical and other lower genital tract cancers) that can be seen with the naked eye. Common clinical manifestations of HPV are:

- Condyloma acuminata: Raised, cauliflower-appearing (papillary) warts. Most are caused by the low-risk HPV 6 or 11 and are generally found on the external vulva, although they may also appear in the vagina, cervix, and anus.
- Condyloma planum: "Flat" warts; although most are caused by HPV 16 or other high-risk types, they should be treated as genital warts and not as a true precancerous condition.
- High-grade intraepithelial neoplasia: "Precancerous" flat HPV lesions that may appear on the vulva and the perianal and anal canal area. They can be very white (due to thick layers of keratin) or red (due to an increased blood supply) or various shades of brown to dark gray (due to increased pigment).
- Cancer: HPV is the cause of virtually all cancers of the cervix, as well as about 80% of vaginal cancers and 90% of anal cancers. In any of these areas, the cancer may appear as a nodule, erosion, ulcer, or thickening.

Immune mediated regression:

- Most HPV lesions eventually resolve because of a host immune response to the virus. This is especially true for genital warts and CIN 1 because neither is truly precancer. Approximately 40%–50% of CIN 2 will resolve spontaneously; CIN 3 is considered a true cancer precursor, although some CIN 3 may resolve spontaneously to an immune-mediated regression.
- It is not known whether an immune-mediated regression clears that particular HPV type from the body completely or just suppresses it to the point where it is not likely to be contagious or cause HPV-induced disease in the future.

HPV infection after 2 years. It is unknown whether the virus is truly absent or is simply reduced to undetectable levels. For the remaining 10% of women, persistent infection with certain types of HPV constitutes the major risk factor for cervical cancer (Dunne & Markowitz, 2006; Frazer et al., 2006; Schmidt, 2007).

Nursing Insight— HPV and chronological age

HPV infections are most common in teenagers and women in their early 20s, with prevalence decreasing as women age. Most women will come in contact with HPV shortly after they become sexually active; by age 50, more than 80% of women will have had HPV at some time in their lives. In adolescents and young women, HPV infections and dysplasia (precancerous changes) are likely to resolve spontaneously. This finding suggests that HPV infections detected in older women are more likely to reflect persistent infections acquired in the past (ACOG, 2009a; ASCCP, 2010; Lara-Torre & Murchison, 2009).

The triggers that activate HPV and cause abnormal cell growth, as well as why some lesions heal on their own and others become precancerous, are not known. Cervical infections are caused by a group of about 15 oncogenic (cancer causing) types of HPV. Persistent infection with these viruses can lead to a precancerous condition. While the vast majority of cervical HPV infections (including those caused by the oncogenic types) heal through the body's natural immune response, some of them persist and can eventually progress to invasive cervical cancer. The strains most strongly associated with cervical cancer are types 16, 18, 31, and 45, and a few others, to a lesser degree. However, in most women with high-risk types of cervical HPV, cervical cancer will not develop (Kiviat, Hawes, & Feng, 2008; NPWH, 2007).

 Nursing Insight— *Routine clinical examinations for HPV are not performed with STD screening*

Couples who are contemplating a sexual relationship should always be encouraged to undergo STD testing prior to initiating intercourse. However, because HPV is so very common and most often undetectable, neither the CDC nor the American Medical Association recommends clinical examinations for HPV as a component of STD screening.

 Now Can You— **Discuss certain aspects of HPV?**

1. Identify the population at highest risk for contracting HPV?
2. Briefly discuss the link between HPV and cervical cancer?
3. Explain the process of "co-testing" and identify patients for whom this procedure is most appropriate?

THE NURSING ROLE IN REDUCING PATIENT RISK FOR CERVICAL CANCER

Currently, researchers continue to investigate factors that may promote the development of cervical cancer. The role and the progression of HPV-induced lesions into cancer have recently become clearer. Research has demonstrated that cigarette smoking interferes with women's ability to clear an HPV infection and is associated with an increased risk of new HPV infection, persistent HPV infection, and cervical cancer. Also, a dose–response relationship with the amount of tobacco consumed has been noted (Lindstrom et al., 2008; Oh, Ju, Franceschi, Quint, & Shin, 2008). Other potential factors that link HPV with cervical cancer include long-term oral contraceptive use, young age, nutritional deficiency, presence of other genital tract infections, and immunodeficiency, such as occurs with HIV infection. For women with a healthy immune system, it may take decades for cervical cancer to develop from an initial exposure to high-risk viral types (Moore & Seybold, 2007; NPWH, 2007; Wysocki et al., 2007).

 Optimizing Outcomes— **Identifying risk factors associated with HPV infection and HPV-related cervical disease**

To guide clinical HPV screening and educational efforts, nurses who work with women of all ages should be aware of certain risk factors that are associated with HPV infection and/or HPV-related cervical disease (Escobar & Orr, 2008), including the followoing:

* A sex partner more than 2 years older
* More than three lifetime sex partners
* A new sex partner in the last 12 months
* Illegal drug use in the last 12 months
* Engaging in intercourse while impaired by alcohol
* Never having been married

A recent review of the literature revealed that several studies have linked HPV and cervical cancer to intimate partner violence in women, likely because women victims are less able to successfully negotiate strategies for safer sex, such as condom usage and monogamy, with an abusive partner. Women who have sex with women (WSW) are also at risk of contracting HPV. Although less common than heterosexual transmission, woman-to-woman HPV transmission is possible. Many WSW also report a history of sexual encounters with men. WSW may be less likely to seek regular pelvic examinations and Pap tests, although these health-promoting practices are recommended for women regardless of their sexual partners' gender (Coker, 2007; Hutchinson, Thompson, & Cederbaum, 2006; Marazzo, Koutski, Kiviat, Kuypers, & Stine, 2001; Teitelman et al., 2009).

An important role for nurses in reproductive health promotion centers on counseling and education about strategies to enhance the immune system and reduce the risk for contracting HPV and other STDs. For example, the nurse can teach patients that refraining from smoking; limiting the use of alcohol; consuming a healthy, nutritious diet; and avoiding exposure to chemical and environmental hazards are health practices that enhance the strength of the immune system. Observing sexual abstinence or, if sexually active, consistently using condoms or receiving prophylactic HPV vaccination are other preventive strategies to reduce the risk for infection. The nurse can counsel women that they can lower their chance of getting HPV by remaining in a faithful relationship with one partner, by limiting the number of sex partners, and by choosing a partner who has had no or few prior sex partners (ASCCP, 2010; CDC, 2009).

 Optimizing Outcomes— **Heightening HPV awareness: The AWHONN "Be Confident!" campaign**

In January 2010, the Association of Women's Health, Obstetric and Neonatal Nurses (AWHONN) launched the "Be Confident!" campaign for adolescents and parents. The grant-funded program features brochures, posters, articles, and a public service announcement to educate adolescents and young women about HPV and encourage informed decisions about cervical health issues. Available in English and Spanish, the comic book–style posters and brochures are intended to encourage open discussions between young women and their parents and health-care providers. According to the organization, outreach to the Hispanic community constitutes a heavy emphasis of the campaign. Hispanic females have the highest incidence of cervical cancer among all groups of women and often experience disparities in access to cervical cancer screening and access to information related to cervical cancer screening and prevention (AWHONN, 2010). AWHONN is distributing the educational materials to health-care providers and community health settings; additional copies may be downloaded at www.awhonn.org/HPV.

The patient with genital warts may benefit from HPV counseling sessions that include her intimate partner. Meeting with both partners provides an opportunity for the couple to learn that HPV infection is common and probably shared between partners and affords the possibility for other STD evaluation and screening along with Pap screening. The nurse can again emphasize the importance of routine cytological screening for cervical cancer (CDC, 2006).

Optimizing Outcomes— **With condoms to reduce the risk of contracting HPV**

Latex condoms offer some protection against HPV, and consistent condom use appears to reduce the risk of HPV transmission by about 70%. However, condoms protect only those areas of skin that they cover—and many infected individuals have HPV in non-covered areas of their skin that come into contact with their partner's skin. Secretions may also be a source of HPV-infected skin cells that could come into contact with a partner's uncovered skin areas. Spermicides and condoms coated with spermicide are not effective in preventing HPV and may cause microscopic abrasions that facilitate transmission of HPV and other STDs. Because female condoms cover more of the female introital epithelium at risk for HPV, they may provide a more protective barrier for both partners. However, the female condom may also be more easily dislodged during intercourse (ASCCP, 2010).

"What to say" — *When discussing HPV with patients*

When discussing HPV, the nurse can be instrumental in dispelling various myths and misconceptions about genital HPV. Providing current, evidence-based information empowers the woman to make informed choices and decisions about her reproductive health. Depending on the situation, sharing the following information may be appropriate:

Genital HPV is very common. It is primarily transmitted through sexual contact involving genital skin, and penetrative intercourse is not required. The only way to entirely eliminate the possibility of being exposed to HPV is abstinence from any form of genital–genital or oral–genital contact. The lifetime likelihood of getting genital HPV is estimated at 75 to 90%, and the risk of exposure to HPV is estimated to be approximately 15 to 25% per partner. That is, for every sexual partner one has, there is up to a 25% chance of being exposed to some type of HPV. Because HPV rarely causes symptoms, most people who get HPV never know they have it— they do not develop genital warts, receive an abnormal Pap test result, or develop any other manifestations of HPV that they can identify. An HPV diagnosis does not necessarily mean that your partner has not been monogamous; it means only that the infection was contracted at some point in that person's life. HPV testing is not indicated for partners of persons with genital warts. An abnormal Pap test result does not necessarily mean that a woman is at high risk for cervical cancer. The abnormal result can be related to infection, local irritation, a low-risk HPV type, or a higher risk HPV type. Depending on the degree of abnormality, further evaluation or a follow-up Pap test obtained 3 months later may be rec ommended. Reflex HPV DNA testing may obviate the need for repeated Pap tests—and if no high-risk HPV types are identified, the Pap test may be repeated in 1 year. Only one in four cases of cervical lesions, if left untreated, will progress to cancer, and treatment is almost always successful in preventing cancer if the cells are discovered early. Undergoing routine Pap testing according to the recommendations of your health-care provider is an important preventive strategy (ASCCP, 2010; CDC, 2006).

HPV VACCINES

A vaccine (Gardasil) against HPV types 6, 11, 16, and 18 became available in 2006. Gardasil is the first HPV vaccine in the United States. The quadrivalent recombinant (non-live virus) vaccine is recommended for females ages 9 to 26 years. (The quadrivalent HPV vaccine may also be given to males ages 9 through 26 years to reduce their likelihood of acquiring genital warts; ideally the vaccine should be administered before potential exposure to HPV through sexual contact.) Vaccination consists of three intramuscular injections given over 6 months, with the second dose to be given 2 months after the first dose and the third dose given 6 months after the first dose. If the HPV vaccine schedule is interrupted, the vaccine series does not need to be restarted (ASCCP, 2010; CDC, 2009; Moore & Seybold, 2007; Wysocki et al., 2007).

The HPV vaccine is supplied in prefilled syringes for single use only and in single-use vials; the vials must be stored under refrigeration and protected from light. The vaccine is highly protective, especially when the vaccination occurs before sexual activity. Although the vaccine does not prevent infection with all types of HPV, it provides protection against the HPV types associated with 70% of cervical cancers (16, 18), and 90% of external genital warts (6, 11). However, if a woman has already been infected with HPV 16, 18, 6, or 11, the vaccine offers no protection, and only limited or no protection against the other HPV types. Hence, the protection afforded by the vaccine is lower in women who have had sex prior to vaccination. The quadrivalent vaccine has also been demonstrated to protect against vulvar and vaginal cancers (ASCCP, 2010; CDC, 2009; Moore & Seybold, 2007; Wysocki et al., 2007).

Cervarix is a bivalent vaccine that protects against HPV 16 and 18. Approved by the FDA in 2009, Cervarix also consists of three intramuscular injections given over 6 months; the second dose is given 1 month after the first dose and the third dose is given 6 months after the first dose (ASCCP, 2010; CDC, 2009; Moore & Seybold, 2007; Wysocki et al., 2007).

 Be sure to— Offer HPV vaccines to appropriate patients

It is important that an HPV vaccine be administered before people become sexually active. The CDC's Advisory Committee on Immunization Practices (CDC ACIP, 2009) recommends that Gardasil and Cervarix be routinely given to girls when they are 11 or 12 years old. However, Gardasil can be started as early as age 9 and can also be given to women 13 to 26 years old. Cervarix is approved for use in females 10 through 25 years of age. Although the vaccine series should begin before the initiation of sexual intercourse, a "catch-up" series is recommended for young women in the older age group who are already sexually active. HPV vaccines are not recommended for use in pregnant women, but pregnancy testing is not needed before vaccination. Completion of the HPV vaccine series should occur before pregnancy or after a pregnancy is complete. The HPV vaccines are contraindicated for persons with a history of immediate hypersensitivity to any vaccine component. The quadrivalent HPV vaccine (Gardasil) is contraindicated for persons with a history of immediate hypersensitivity to yeast. The bivalent HPV vaccine (Cervarix) in prefilled syringes is contraindicated for persons with an anaphylactic latex allergy. Because the HPV vaccines are not live vaccines, they may be administered either simultaneously or at any time before or after an inactivated or live vaccine. Syncope may occur after vaccination; to avoid patient injury related to a syncopal episode, the nurse should consider observing the patient for 15 minutes after the vaccination is administered. The most commonly reported adverse reactions to the vaccinations include pain, redness, and swelling at the injection site and fatigue, headache, muscle and joint aches, and gastrointestinal distress. Since the vaccines do not cover all of the HPV types that can cause cervical cancer, routine Pap test screening is still recommended for those who have been vaccinated against HPV (CDC, 2009; Markowitz et al., 2007; Rome & Hicks, 2009).

 Be sure to— Be knowledgeable about immunization laws in your practice state

Federal law does not explicitly require parental consent for immunizations such as the HPV vaccine. However, it does require that prior to administration the parent or guardian receive federally mandated vaccine information statements on any immunizations their children will receive. State law is the authority on whether parental consent is required. Minor consent laws are based on status (e.g., emancipated, married, in armed services, "mature" minor, pregnant, incarcerated) and services they are seeking (e.g., pregnancy-related care, family planning, and sexual health services) (Burns, Walsh, & Popovich, 2010; English, Shaw, McCauley, & Fishbein, 2008). It is essential that the health-care provider have an understanding of the laws in the particular practice state; this information is available at www.cahl.org.

 Be sure to— Comply with federal mandates regarding HPV vaccination for immigrant women

Although compulsory HPV vaccination is not currently mandated for any U.S. population, immigrant women aged 11–26 years are now required to receive the first injection (of the three doses) of the vaccine as a result of the 1996 Illegal Immigration Reform and Immigrant Responsibility Act. According to this law, immigrants applying for visas to enter the United States or to adjust their immigration status must receive the inoculations that the CDC ACIP recommends for U.S. residents (Hachey, Allen, Nothnagle, & Boardman, 2009).

 where research and practice meet: Identifying disparities in attitudes, acceptability, and beliefs about the HPV vaccine

Several epidemiological and behavioral studies have identified disparities in attitudes, acceptability, and beliefs about the HPV vaccine (Burns et al., 2010). Watts and colleagues (2009) found that acceptance of the HPV vaccine was high among Latina women for themselves and their daughters, and this was primarily motivated by the concern for cancer prevention. An investigation by Cates and colleagues (2009) discovered racial differences between African American and Caucasian in HPV knowledge in a rural Southern U.S. sample; Caucasian were significantly more informed about the HPV vaccine. African American were significantly less likely to perceive cervical cancer as a threat to their daughters' health and had lower intentions to vaccinate their daughters against HPV than whites. Based on their research, Gottlieb and Brewer (2009) concluded that the demographic factors of race and educational level were found to influence the use of information sources to learn about the HPV vaccine; this finding may be used to guide communication-based interventions for future research and practice. Other investigators (Brewer & Fazekas, 2007; Fazekas, Brewer, & Smith, 2008; Kahn et al., 2008; Marshall, Phillip, Don, & Peter, 2007) reported factors (i.e., lack of insurance or resources to pay for the vaccine, perception that the vaccine is unsafe, fear that receipt of the vaccine would encourage sexual behavior, and personal perception of being at low risk for HPV and cervical cancer) that may inhibit patients' intention to receive the HPV vaccine or parents' intention to have their child receive the HPV vaccine. These studies highlight the importance of the nurse's role in developing culturally appropriate health promotion programs that target vaccination education and outreach. To successfully accomplish this goal, nurses must seek the latest evidence-based information about vaccines, remain knowledgeable about current vaccination guidelines, and possess an awareness of various behavioral disparities that place some populations at greater risk than others (Burns et al., 2010; Theroux, 2008).

 Collaboration in Caring— *Securing funding resources for HPV vaccination*

Most health insurance plans cover the recommended HPV vaccines, although some plans may not cover any or all vaccines. The Vaccines for Children (VFC) program helps families of eligible children who may not otherwise have access to vaccines. The program provides vaccines at no cost to physicians who serve eligible children. Children younger than 19 years of age are eligible for VFC vaccines if they are Medicaid eligible, American Indian, Alaska Native, or have no health insurance. "Underinsured children" who have health insurance that does not cover vaccination can receive VFC vaccines through Federally Qualified Health Centers or Rural Health Centers (CDC, 2009). For more information about the program, nurses may visit the CDC Web site at www.cdc.gov/vaccines/programs/vfc/.

AWHONN supports HPV vaccination for the prevention of cervical cancer along with regular cervical cancer screening with Papanicolaou and HPV tests, as recommended. The organization also supports policies that ensure universal access to HPV vaccination and cervical cancer screening and treatment. In the revised and reaffirmed "HPV Vaccination for the Prevention of Cervical Cancer" Position Statement (November, 2009), AWHONN endorsed the establishment of adolescent health visits (to include health counseling, physical assessment, and vaccinations) and called for the establishment of programs specifically designed to educate young women and men, parents, and providers about HPV and the importance of HPV vaccination.

In an effort to increase public awareness of the need for vaccination, Merck (manufacturer of Gardasil) launched a multimedia campaign about HPV and cervical cancer prevention using their vaccine. Other organizations including the CDC and the National Federation of Planned Parenthood have created consumer education Web sites. And recently, the Society for Adolescent Medicine, the National Basketball Association, the Women's National Basketball Association, and Sanofi Pasteur (a vaccine manufacturer) have collaborated in launching a national program designed to heighten public awareness of the importance of vaccinations for teens.

 Collaboration in Caring— *A team approach to a teen-targeted immunization campaign*

The NBA and the WNBA have collaborated with the Society for Adolescent Medicine and Sanofi Pasteur (a vaccine manufacturer) to create "Vaccines for Teens," a national program designed to educate parents and their teens about the need to get vaccinated. The campaign Web site (www.vaccinesforteens.net/) is one component of the larger effort to make parents and teens aware of the dangers of four serious diseases (meningococcal disease/meningococcal meningitis, pertussis, influenza, and HPV) that can easily be spread from person to person. The Web site, which includes a brief athlete-narrated video, describes each disease and provides links for additional resources.

HPV EDUCATION AND COUNSELING FOR TEENS AND THEIR PARENTS

An essential area for nurses in HPV awareness and prevention centers on education and counseling for adolescents and teens and their parents. Because both males and females may be at risk for acquiring HPV, educational efforts should target both genders (Pollack, Balkin, Edouard, Cutts, & Broutet, 2007). It is important that

reproductive health counseling provide developmentally appropriate information. Preteens tend to be concrete thinkers, and teenagers are more likely to engage in risky health behaviors. Understanding the tasks associated with normal adolescent development is an essential element that guides the nurse in establishing and directing a therapeutic dialogue. Communicating with young patients about HPV, the HPV vaccine, and other health issues may be enhanced by listening attentively, using terms the adolescent understands, remaining focused, and avoiding lectures and writing during the course of the conversation (Neinstein, 2008).

 Nursing Insight— *Understanding normal adolescent development*

The period of adolescence is characterized by rapid physical, emotional, and intellectual changes and development. Developmental tasks of adolescence center on establishing autonomy and identity, integrating physical changes into a new body image, and operating within the peer group. Adolescents experience feelings of invulnerability that may lead to an increased willingness to expose them to risk. Adolescents often tend to underestimate the personal risk of health hazards and unhealthful behaviors (Kahn, 2008; Woodson, 2008).

During the course of the conversation, it is helpful to focus on strategies to minimize HPV risk (e.g., minimizing sexual partners, using condoms, avoiding smoking) and discuss the HPV vaccination in terms of its value for the prevention of genital warts and cervical dysplasia. The nurse should emphasize the importance of completing the HPV vaccine series, once initiated. The nurse can encourage the teen to take responsibility for her health by discussing how a healthy lifestyle can contribute to disease prevention. Teens should also be reminded of the importance of cervical cancer screening beginning at age 21 (Taylor & Smith, 2009; Woodson, 2008).

 Optimizing Outcomes— **NASPAG: A resource for health professionals who provide gynecologic care for adolescents**

The North American Society for Pediatric and Adolescent Gynecology (NASPAG) is a nonprofit organization dedicated to educating health-care professionals in pediatric and adolescent gynecology. NASPAG's mission is to provide a forum for education, research and communication among health professionals who provide gynecological care to children and adolescents. The Web address for NASPAG is www.naspag.org.

Nurses can also teach parents about strategies to enhance effective HPV communication with their daughters. Some parents may believe that giving their daughters the HPV vaccine somehow implies that they are encouraging sexual activity. In this situation, it may be beneficial to use a seat belt analogy: Just as the seat belt does not give someone permission to drive recklessly, the HPV vaccination does not imply that it is okay to have sex (Woodson, 2008). Nurses should encourage frequent, age-appropriate dialogue between parents and their children. For younger girls, ongoing parent–adolescent communication about issues such as personal sexual risk and partner relationship dynamics is an important strategy in STD prevention (Teitelman et al., 2009). The nurse can model for parents how to have honest, open communications about HPV information and use discussion about HPV and the vaccine as a basis for future discussions about sexuality and reproductive health as their daughters grow older (Woodson, 2008). Parent–daughter communication about partner sexual pressure has been associated with increased condom use (Teitelman, Ratcliffe, & Cederbaum, 2008).

TREATMENT FOR HPV

The risk of developing genital warts after sexual intercourse with someone who has warts is greater than 65%. Once exposed to genital warts, most individuals will develop them within 4 weeks to 8 months. Genital warts are usually not painful, but they can interfere with normal bodily functions, such as urination and defecation, making these actions painful and uncomfortable. Although no treatment has been developed for latent HPV infection, several therapies are available to manage external genital warts and clearly identifiable subclinical HPV lesions on the vulva, cervix, and vagina. The goal of all therapies is to destroy the visible lesions and reduce patient symptoms. In the majority of patients, treatment produces wart-free periods. Treatment, however, does not eliminate HPV infection. Eradication of the virus is not considered to be conclusive even after there is no visible evidence of wart tissue because of the high incidence of recurrence (Woodson, 2008).

 Optimizing Outcomes— With treatment for HPV

Treatment options for HPV include the provider-administered medications podophyllin resin, trichloroacetic acid (TCA), or bichloracetic acid (BCA), which are carefully applied to each wart and allowed to air-dry. Patient-applied medications include podofilox solution or gel (Condylox) and imiquimod cream (Aldara). Podophyllin, podofilox, and imiquimod should not be used during pregnancy. No one treatment is ideal for all warts. Surgical therapies used to eliminate the lesions include cryosurgery, manual excision, electrosurgical excision, and laser vaporization. Injection of interferon is another treatment but one that is usually reserved for recurrent lesions unresponsive to standard treatments such as cryosurgery with liquid nitrogen or cryoprobe, electrocautery, and laser vaporization. Interferon is a naturally occurring substance that boosts the immune system and interferes with the ability of viruses to reproduce (CDC, 2006).

One's degree of contagiousness following treatment depends on how successful the treatment was in destroying the HPV lesions (where potentially infectious HPV particles are known to be present) and how successful the individual's immunity is in suppressing any HPV that might still be present in apparently normal skin. Most people treated for external warts do not experience a complete resolution even after several treatments. This is because most treatments destroy the HPV lesions but cannot eliminate any HPV in surrounding apparently normal skin. Until the individual's immune system responds and suppresses the remaining HPV, new lesions may appear (ASCCP, 2010).

Once no further HPV lesions are detectable by clinical exam, and no new lesions have appeared over several subsequent months, the chance of shedding enough HPV to be contagious dramatically falls. Although it is impossible to advise anyone exactly when they have little to no chance of passing HPV to a partner, as months pass with no new lesions found by a clinician, the possibility of being contagious becomes increasingly remote (ASCCP, 2010).

 Now Can You— Discuss HPV education, vaccination, and treatment?

1. Develop HPV educational programs specifically suited for adolescents, parents of adolescents, reproductive-age women, and older women?
2. Identify six risk factors associated with HPV infection and HPV-related cervical disease?
3. Discuss HPV vaccination: identify who should receive the vaccines, how and when the vaccines should be given, nursing implications for administration, and patient education concerning vaccination?
4. Identify medical and surgical treatment modalities for HPV-related genital warts?

Cervical Cancer

Cervical cancer is a malignant neoplasm that forms in the tissues of the cervix. Worldwide, cervical cancer is the second most common type of cancer in women. It is much less common in the United States because of the routine use of cervical cytological screening. Cervical cancers originate in the cells on the surface of the cervix, which are composed of squamous and columnar epithelium.

Nursing Insight— The uterine cervix and cervical cancers

Approximately 80% to 90% of cervical cancers are squamous cell carcinomas—neoplasms that originate in the squamous cells that cover the surface of the exocervix. Most of the remaining cervical cancers are adenocarcinomas, which are becoming increasingly more common in women born in the last 20 to 30 years. Cervical adenocarcinoma develops from the mucus-producing gland cells of the endocervix. Less commonly, cervical cancers have features of both squamous cell carcinomas and adenocarcinomas and are called adenosquamous carcinomas or mixed carcinomas (ACS, 2009).

The development of cervical cancer, which is typically a very slow process, begins as dysplasia, a precancerous condition. Dysplasia, which can be detected by a Pap test, is 100% treatable. Most women who are diagnosed with cervical cancer today have not had regular Pap tests or they have not followed up on abnormal results. Undetected, precancerous changes can develop into cervical cancer and spread to the bladder, intestines, lungs, and liver (ACS, 2009).

 Collaboration in Caring— *The Pearl of Wisdom Campaign to Prevent Cervical Cancer*

The Pearl of Wisdom Campaign to Prevent Cervical Cancer is a united, global effort to raise awareness of the opportunities now available to prevent cervical cancer. The campaign reaches women, health-care providers, policy makers, health advocates, and the media in an effort to increase awareness of the new means of preventing cervical cancer, encourage women to take full advantage of these methods, and advocate for the implementation of these tools for girls and women everywhere. The Pearl of Wisdom Campaign was started by the European Cervical Cancer Association, which includes 100 organizations from across Europe, including cancer charities, cancer treatment centers, medical associations, university teaching hospitals, and health education organizations. The campaign promotes the "Pearl of Wisdom" as the global symbol for cervical cancer prevention in the same way as the pink ribbon serves the breast cancer campaign. Launched in the United States in 2009, the campaign is led by the national nonprofit organization Tamika and Friends, Inc. All profits from purchases of the Pearl of Wisdom pin go to the U.S. Pearl of Wisdom Campaign Fund to support cervical cancer prevention activities. Campaign partners, which include more than 24 national as well as local women's health and advocacy organizations, distribute simple, consistent key messages about cervical cancer to ensure that their collective voices effectively reach women. Additional information about the Pearl of Wisdom Campaign to Prevent Cervical Cancer may be found at the organization Web site: www.pearlofwisdom.us/about_us.

RISK FACTORS

Although the exact mechanism for the progression of cervical cancer is unknown, several key contributing factors have been identified (Box 6-5). Nurses must remain up-to-date about cancer risk factors so that they can appropriately identify and screen individuals at risk and provide accurate, culturally centered patient counseling and education. As is true in other areas of health promotion, it is useful to focus teaching efforts on risk factors such as lifestyle choices (e.g., tobacco and alcohol use, diet, sexual practices, HPV exposure) over which the woman has some control.

 Ethnocultural Considerations— **Cervical cancer**

Cervical cancer disproportionately affects low-income women and women of color. The CDC (2008) estimates that cervical cancer treatment costs $160 million each year. In this country, cervical cancer occurs most often in Hispanic women, at a rate that is more than twice what is seen in non-Hispanic Caucasian women. African American women develop this cancer about 50% more often than non-Hispanic Caucasian women and have the highest mortality (ACS, 2010). In Caucasian women in the United States, the rate of new-onset cer-

---

Box 6-5 **Cervical Cancer Risk Factors**

- HPV infection (the most important risk factor)
- Cigarette smoking (doubles the risk for cervical cancer)
- Immunosuppression (HIV increases the likelihood for infection with HPV, which increases the risk for cervical cancer. Also, the immune system normally destroys/slows the growth of cancer cells)
- Co-infection with other STDs (e.g., Chlamydia, herpes simplex virus)
- Diet (low in fruits and vegetables increases the risk; obesity increases the risk of cervical adenocarcinoma)
- Early onset of sexual activity (before age 16)
- Inadequate cervical screening
- Male sexual partner who has had other partners, especially if a previous partner had cervical cancer
- Multiple sexual partners (three or more in a lifetime)
- An uncircumcised sexual partner
- Oral contraceptives (long-term use increases the risk; however, the risk returns to normal after discontinuation)
- Multiple full-term pregnancies (three or more full-term pregnancies are associated with an increased risk; reasons unknown)
- Young age at first full-term pregnancy (women younger than 17 years with first full-term pregnancy are almost two times more likely to get cervical cancer later in life than those who postpone pregnancy until 25 years or older)
- Poverty (most likely related to lack of cervical cancer screening)
- In utero exposure to diethylstilbestrol (DES) (increased risk for clear-cell adenocarcinoma of the vagina or cervix; risk is greatest if DES exposure occurred during the first 16 weeks of pregnancy; there may also be an increased risk of squamous cell cancers and precancers of the cervix linked to HPV)
- Family history of cervical cancer (if the mother or a sister had cervical cancer, the woman's chances of developing the condition are two to three times higher)
- Alcoholism

Sources: ACS (2009); Moore & Seybold (2007); Wysocki et al. (2007).

---

vical cancer peaks in the middle of the fifth decade of life and then decreases. The peak incidence in Hispanics is in the early 70s, and for women of Asian or Pacific Island ethnicity, the incidence peaks in the late 70s. The incidence of cervical cancer continues to increase throughout life in African American women in the United States (Ries et al., 2009). Factors that may influence cervical screening behaviors for these populations of women include a lack of a health promotion/disease prevention perspective, a lack of knowledge about Pap tests, financial barriers, and failure of health-care providers to recommend screening (Giarratano, Bustamante-Forest, & Carter; Wysocki et al., 2007).

SYMPTOMS

Most of the time, early cervical cancer produces no symptoms. In fact, patients with cervical cancer usually do not experience any problems until the cancer is advanced and has spread. An important nursing role in cervical cancer education centers on emphasizing the importance of routine cervical cancer screening and teaching women about symptoms that may be associated with cancer of the cervix.

Optimizing Outcomes— Teaching about symptoms of cervical cancer

Nurses should emphasize that although early cervical cancer usually produces no symptoms, patients should remain alert to the following signs and symptoms that may be associated with the disease:

* Continuous vaginal discharge, which may be pale, watery, pink, brown, bloody, or foul smelling
* Abnormal vaginal bleeding between menstrual periods, after intercourse, or after menopause
* Menstrual periods that become heavier and last longer than usual
* Any vaginal bleeding after menopause

Signs and symptoms that may be associated with *advanced* cervical cancer include:

* Loss of appetite
* Weight loss
* Fatigue
* Pelvic pain
* Back pain
* Leg pain
* Single swollen leg
* Heavy vaginal bleeding
* Leaking of urine or feces from the vagina
* Bone fractures

 Optimizing Outcomes— With a new tool to predict cervical cancer risk

A new tool for assessing cervical cancer risk may offer health-care professionals a simpler method for making treatment decisions. Katki and colleagues (2009) at the National Cancer Institute are developing a tool that uses cervical precancer (i.e., CIN Grade 3 or higher) as a common treatment threshold. The tool, which is based on the established predictability of cervical precancer, will allow clinicians to use their personal digital assistants or computers to accurately calculate a patient's current, 1-year, 3-year, and 5-year risk of developing cervical precancer based on the woman's age, current test results, and available past test results. This information can then be used to guide development of an appropriate plan of care.

DIAGNOSTIC WORKUP AND TREATMENT OF CERVICAL CANCER

Once a diagnosis of cervical cancer has been made, the physician orders additional tests to determine if the cancer is confined to the local area or has spread to distant organs. This process is termed *staging*. Tests that may be appropriate include x-ray computed tomography (CT scan), magnetic resonance imaging (MRI), positron emission tomography (PET scan), cystoscopy, chest x-ray, and intravenous pyelogram (IVP). The cancer stage is based on where the cancer is found (Box 6-6).

Treatment for cervical cancer depends on the stage of the cancer—whether it is localized or has spread to surrounding tissues or distant organs. A high-grade, preinvasive lesion (i.e., carcinoma in situ [CIS]) is removed to

---

Box 6-6 Stages of Invasive Cervical Cancer

STAGE I
The tumor has invaded the cervix beneath the top layer of cells. Cancer cells are located only in the cervix.

STAGE II
The tumor extends to the upper part of the vagina. It may extend beyond the cervix into nearby tissues toward the pelvic wall. The tumor does not invade the lower third of the vagina or the pelvic wall.

STAGE III
The tumor extends to the lower part of the vagina. It may also have invaded the pelvic wall. If the tumor blocks the flow of urine, one or both kidneys may not be working well.

STAGE IV
The tumor invades the bladder or rectum, or the cancer has spread to other parts of the body.

RECURRENT CANCER
The cancer was treated but has returned after a time during which it could not be detected. The cancer may show up again in the cervix or in other parts of the body.

Source: NCI (2009).

---

prevent progression to invasive disease. A conization procedure is usually recommended, although hysterectomy may be advised, depending on the individual situation (ACOG, 2009a).

 Nursing Insight— Factors that influence cervical cancer prognosis

A number of factors influence the prognosis for a woman who has received a diagnosis of cervical cancer. These factors include the type of cancer, the stage of the disease, and the woman's age and general physical condition. Precancerous conditions are completely curable when followed up and treated properly. The 5-year survival rate for cancer that has not spread beyond the cervical area is 92%. However, the 5-year survival rate falls steadily as the cancer extends to other areas in the body (NCI, 2009).

 Collaboration in Caring— *Using a team approach to facilitate treatment of cervical cancer*

Depending on the cervical cancer stage, the health-care provider may wish to refer the woman to the care of a gynecological oncologist, a surgeon who specializes in treating gynecological cancers. Other members of the health-care team who may be involved in the patient's treatment plan include medical oncologists, radiation oncologists, oncology nurses, mental health professionals, and registered dieticians.

Surgery

For invasive cancer, radiation can be used alone or in combination with some form of surgery. Surgery options range from cervical conization to radical hysterectomy. A radical trachelectomy involves removal of the cervix, part of the vagina, and the lymph nodes in the pelvis. This surgery is reserved for a small number of women with small tumors who desire pregnancy in the future. Total hysterectomy involves removal of the cervix and the uterus. Radical hysterectomy involves removal of the uterus, cervix, parametrium (tissue surrounding the uterus), ovaries, fallopian tubes, upper vagina, and some or all of the local lymph nodes (NCI, 2009).

 Nursing Insight— *Understanding pelvic exenteration*

Pelvic exenteration is a rare, extreme procedure that is used to treat recurrent cervical cancer that has spread to surrounding organs. This surgery, which involves removal of the same organs and tissues as radical hysterectomy, may also include removal of the bladder, rectum, part of the colon, and/or the vagina.

Radiation Therapy

Radiation therapy (RT) uses high-energy x-rays to destroy cancer cells. Cancers that extend beyond the cervix into the pelvis, lower vagina, and urinary tract typically receive radiation. RT may be combined with surgery or chemotherapy to treat early cervical cancers and more invasive stages of the disease; it can also be used to relieve symptoms caused by advanced cancer. Radiation may be delivered by external beam, by radioactive implants placed directly at the cancerous site ("internal therapy"), or by a combination of these two therapies.

External Therapy

External beam radiation, administered the same way as a diagnostic x-ray, is usually given five times a week for 5 or 6 weeks, with an extra boost of radiation at the end of that time. With this treatment modality, the entire pelvic area is irradiated, including the rectum, large intestine, small intestine, bone, and skin. Providing education and emotional support are key components of nursing care for women receiving external beam radiation. The nurse can encourage the patient to remain as active as possible throughout the course of therapy. Patients should be counseled that they might experience certain side effects in the treatment target area, such as hair loss, dry or irritated skin, or permanent darkening of the skin. While undergoing external RT, patients are cautioned not to remove any skin markings made by the radiologist (NCI, 2009).

 Optimizing Outcomes— **With strategies to promote comfort during external radiation therapy**

Nurses can teach women who are undergoing external beam RT about strategies to promote comfort and healing. For example, the nurse can suggest that the patient:

- Practice good personal hygiene
- Use lotions or creams only with the physician's approval, and remain vigilant about skin care and the condition of the treatment area
- Wear loose clothing over the treatment area
- Wear cotton underwear

- Expose the treatment area to air whenever possible
- Avoid exposing the treatment area to temperature extremes
- Avoid the use of adhesive tape in the treatment area

After completion of the external RT, patients are taught about self-care strategies to promote comfort and healing, and they are advised that side effects from the therapy may persist for weeks after the therapy has ended.

"What to say" — *Teaching about self-care strategies after external radiation therapy*

Nurses can empower women with self-care strategies to promote comfort and healing after the completion of external RT. For example, the nurse may tell the patient to:

- Be sure to consume a nutritious diet
- Drink plenty of fluids
- Obtain adequate rest, and take naps as needed
- Take medications as prescribed; check with your health-care provider before taking any non-prescribed medications
- Maintain good oral and skin care
- Anticipate that the effects from the radiation may persist for 10 days to 2 weeks after the last treatment
- Anticipate that signs of healing will occur in about 3 weeks after the last treatment
- Avoid infection; report any symptoms of infection to your health-care provider
- Promptly report symptoms of complications, such as gastrointestinal symptoms (e.g., continued nausea, vomiting, anorexia, diarrhea) or skin symptoms (e.g., redness, swelling, pain, pruritus at the radiation site) to your health-care provider.

Internal Therapy

Implant radiation, also known as brachytherapy ("slow therapy"), involves placement of the radioactive material as close to the tumor as possible while sparing the adjacent healthy tissue. The radioactive material is either placed in a capsule and inserted into the cervix or placed in thin needles that are inserted directly into the tumor. This method of treatment takes place in the hospital setting. The patient stays in the hospital for 1 to 3 days while the implants remain in place; during this time, the patient is considered radioactive. The device is removed before discharge. Brachytherapy is then repeated several times over a period of 1 to 2 weeks. Once the radioactive material has been removed, no radioactivity remains in the body. In some situations, the internal radiation therapy is delivered during a brief treatment session, and the patient is able to go home afterward. In premenopausal women, sterility and cessation of menstruation usually occur after brachytherapy. Patients should be advised to promptly report signs of infection (i.e., vaginal or rectal bleeding, hematuria, foul-smelling vaginal discharge, fever, abdominal distention or pain) to their health-care provider (NCI, 2009).

Be sure to— Monitor and limit personal radiation exposure

Nurses and other health-care providers who come in direct contact with patients receiving internal radiation therapy should monitor their personal radiation exposure by wearing a film badge or other device to determine the amount of exposure received. When providing direct patient care, isolation techniques (i.e., good hand-washing technique, wearing gloves when handling bodily fluids) are observed, and time spent in close proximity to the patient is limited to 30 minutes or less per 8 hours to avoid exposure to gamma rays. It is important to use the principles of time, distance, and shielding to protect from personal radiation exposure and to explain to the patient and her family why nursing care is focused on providing only essential care during the course of internal radiation therapy. Also, the nurse explains that pregnant women and children younger than 16 should not visit the patient. If the radiation source becomes dislodged, a radiation specialist uses special long-handled tongs to remove the device and place it in a lead container. All linens and dressings are considered contaminated (Venes, 2009).

Along with physical care, education and emotional support remain central in the nursing care for all patients undergoing radiation therapy. Understandably, patients experience considerable emotional distress related to their diagnosis, fear of the anticipated treatment (e.g., pain, perceived personal radioactivity, adverse effects on bodily functions), and concerns about the impact of their treatment on family members. Potential nursing diagnoses for patients undergoing radiation therapy for the treatment of cervical cancer are presented in Box 6-7.

Nurses can advise patients undergoing external RT that although the affected area may look and feel sunburned, the treated tissues usually regain their normal appearance within 6 to 12 months. It is also important that all patients be counseled about common RT side effects, such as fatigue, diarrhea, frequent or uncomfortable urination, loss of hair in the genital area, and vaginal dryness, itching, and burning. Patients should also be advised to abstain from intercourse until a few weeks following completion of the RT. In general, patients who are treated with internal RT may resume intercourse in 7 to 10 days. Altered patterns of sexuality related to RT side effects are not unusual. Patients may experience a decrease in vaginal secretions and sensation, as well as vaginal stenosis (narrowing). These aftereffects can cause coital pain and discomfort and can contribute to diminished sexual desire. Depending on the specific problem, the nurse may offer suggestions such as applying water-based lubricants for vaginal dryness and/or the regular use of a vaginal dilator for vaginal stenosis; patient/partner referral to other resources may be appropriate (NCI, 2009). Other complications of external beam radiation and brachytherapy are listed in Box 6-8.

Chemotherapy

Chemotherapy may be used for cervical cancer that has either metastasized too far from its origin to be treated by surgery or radiation or that has recurred. It may also be used to relieve pain associated with advanced cervical cancer or to shrink cancer to an operable size before surgery is performed. This treatment modality is termed *neoadjuvant chemotherapy*, and it can help to prevent cervical cancer from spreading. Chemotherapeutic agents most often used to treat advanced or recurrent cervical cancer include cisplatin (Cisplatinum, Platinol), ifosfamide (Ifex), paclitaxel (Taxol), cyclophosphamide (Cytoxan), and 5-fluorouracil (5-FU). The medications are either administered by mouth or via IV infusion. Chemotherapy treatments are usually alternated with "recovery periods" that allow the patient a rest time before beginning a new cycle of therapy (NCI, 2009).

Combination chemotherapy, which involves the combination of two or more chemotherapy medications, may be more effective than any single agent. When used in association with surgery or radiation, chemotherapy can help to prevent the spread or recurrence of cervical cancer. Nurses

---

Box 6-7 Potential Nursing Diagnoses for Patients Undergoing Radiation Therapy for Cervical Cancer

Knowledge Deficit related to planned treatment procedures

Fear and Anxiety related to
- diagnosis
- pain
- interference with sexual functioning
- concerns about personal radioactivity
- responses of family members and significant others

Disturbed Sensory Perception related to
- internal radiation therapy
- restricted contact with visitors and health-care professionals

Risk for Skin Integrity Impairment related to
- external radiation exposure
- immobility and bedrest (with internal radiation therapy)

Risk for Physical Injury related to dislodgment of the radiation source (with internal RT)

Acute Pain related to internal radiation applicators

Box 6-8 Complications of External Beam Radiation and Brachytherapy

Proctitis (inflammation of the rectum)

Cystitis (inflammation of the bladder)

Vaginal scarring and stenosis

Anemia and/or bruising

Thrombophlebitis, pulmonary embolism, pneumonia (related to immobility associated with internal radiation therapy)

Increased risk of infection

Skin rash, inflammation, pruritus

Sexual difficulties

Premature menopause

Vesicovaginal fistula (development of an abnormal connection between the vagina and the bladder or rectum)

Source: NCI (2009).

can counsel patients undergoing chemotherapy about common side effects associated with these medications, which include nausea and vomiting, change in appetite, oral lesions, vaginal sores, temporary hair loss, fatigue, bruising and bleeding, skin rash, joint pain, swelling in the legs and feet, susceptibility to infection, anemia, menstrual cycle changes, onset of early menopause, and infertility. In most situations, women who undergo chemotherapy for cervical cancer are already infertile as a result of surgery or RT. Physicians may prescribe hormones to help offset the symptoms associated with premature menopause (NCI, 2009).

 Optimizing Outcomes— **Biological therapy to boost cervical cancer treatment**

Biological therapy may be used to treat cancer that has metastasized to other body organs. Interferon, a cell protein that provides immunity to viral infections, is the type of biological therapy most often used. Biological therapy is usually administered on an outpatient basis and is sometimes combined with chemotherapy. Nurses can counsel women about possible side effects associated this treatment modality, including:

- Flulike symptoms: fever and/or chills; muscle aches; weakness; diarrhea, nausea, or vomiting
- Rash
- Loss of appetite
- Easy bleeding or bruising (NCI, 2009)

 Optimizing Outcomes— **Supportive care for cancer patients**

Nurses can inform women who have received a diagnosis of cancer about supportive care that is available at any stage of the disease. Patients may find information about relief from the side effects of treatment, tips to help to control pain and other symptoms, and emotional support to help them cope with the feelings associated with a diagnosis of cancer. Resources for coping are available on the NCI Web site at www.cancer.gov/cancertopics/coping and from NCI's Cancer Information Service at 1-800-4-CANCER or LiveHelp (www.cancer.gov/help).

Nurses are perfectly situated to provide women with factual information about cervical cancer screening, HPV, and cervical cancer. For example, nurses can explain that while HPV is the cause of cervical cancer, most HPV infections resolve without treatment and do not progress to cervical cancer, especially when regular screening is performed. Most new HPV infections occur in women in their 20s, but the most common decades of life for cervical cancer to be diagnosed is in the 40s and 50s, and 25% of new diagnoses occur in women over age 60. Sharing this information empowers patients with the essential knowledge they need to make informed choices about seeking continued screening at the recommended intervals (Ruhl, 2008; Saslow, 2008).

Teaching women about risk factors for cervical cancer may motivate them to stop smoking or seek regular cervical cancer screening, if they have not done so in the past.

Sharing information about strategies to reduce exposure to HPV (e.g., using condoms, limiting sexual partners, practicing monogamy) may assist in making decisions about intimate relationships. Women of all ages should be educated about the HPV vaccine—although the upper age limit for the vaccine is 26, they may be mothers, grandmothers, aunts, or sisters of preteen or teen girls. Because one concern about the HPV vaccine centers on a potential for patient and care provider complacency about cervical cancer screening, it is imperative that nurses continue to emphasize the importance of routine screening according to current early-detection guidelines (Ruhl, 2008; Saslow, 2008).

Nurses who care for pregnant women can use prenatal visits as an opportunity to counsel patients about the HPV vaccine and cervical cancer prevention and encourage them to begin the series during the postpartum visit. Nurses can support funding for programs that increase access to Pap testing and HPV vaccination for economically disadvantaged women. Finally, through age-appropriate, culturally sensitive educational efforts, nurses can empower patients to make informed choices about the HPV vaccine and, if they do choose to initiate the vaccine, encourage completion of the series (Teitelman et al., 2009).

 Now Can You— **Discuss aspects of cervical cancer?**

1. Identify at least 15 risk factors for cervical cancer?
2. Teach a woman how to recognize symptoms of cervical cancer?
3. Describe the various treatment modalities for cervical cancer?
4. Discuss the nursing role in caring for patients undergoing treatment for cervical cancer?

summary points

- Cervical cancers originate in the cells on the surface of the cervix, which are composed of squamous and columnar epithelium.

- Cytological screening for cervical cancer should begin at age 21 years, regardless of the woman's sexual history.

- An important nursing role in cervical cancer education centers on emphasizing the importance of routine cervical cancer screening and teaching women about symptoms that may be associated with cancer of the cervix.

- Infection with human papillomavirus (HPV) is known to be the primary cause of cervical cancer.

- An essential area for nurses in HPV awareness and prevention centers on education and counseling for adolescents and teens and their parents.

- The HPV vaccines are indicated for the prevention of cervical cancer, genital warts, and dysplastic or precancerous cervical lesions caused by several of the HPV viruses types.

- Routine Pap test screening is recommended for women regardless of whether they have received the HPV vaccine.

◆ Nurses are perfectly situated to provide women with factual information about cervical cancer screening, HPV, and cervical cancer.

review questions

Multiple Choice

1. The squamocolumnar junction of the cervix:
A. Is shed during menstruation
B. Is devoid of cellular growth and replacement
C. Is the area where the squamous epithelium and the columnar epithelium come together
D. Surrounds the vaginal introitus

2. The nurse teaches the patient that she can enhance the accuracy of her Pap test screening by:
A. Avoiding intercourse for 48 hours before the test
B. Douching 24 hours before the test
C. Scheduling the appointment to occur during menstruation
D. Using lubricants with intercourse 24 hours before the test

3. The liquid-based process for cervical cytology screening can also be used to test for:
A. HIV
B. Syphilis
C. Bacterial vaginosis
D. Chlamydia trachomatis

4. If an abnormal Pap test result requires further evaluation, a procedure that allows for a close-up visualization of the vagina and cervix is:
A. Colposcopy
B. Cryosurgery
C. Endocervical curettage
D. Conization

5. The nurse teaches about risk factors for cervical cancer, which include:
A. Initiation of sexual activity after age 26
B. A history of three or more sexual partners
C. A history of infection with the varicella virus
D. Nulliparity

REFERENCES

American Cancer Society (ACS). (2009). *Cervical cancer: Prevention and early detection.* Retrieved April 10, 2010, from http://www.cancer.org/docroot/CRI/content/CRI_2_6x_cervical_cancer_prevention_and_early_detection_8.asp?sitearea=PED

American Cancer Society (ACS). (2010). *Detailed guide: Cervical cancer.* Retrieved April 10, 2010, from http://www.cancer.org/docroot/CRI/content/CRI_2_4_2X_What_are_the_risk_factors_for_cervical_cancer_8.asp

American College of Obstetricians and Gynecologists (ACOG). (2007). *Guidelines for women's health care: A resource manual.* Washington, DC: Author.

American College of Obstetricians and Gynecologists (ACOG). (2008, December). *ACOG Practice Bulletin No. 99, Management of abnormal cervical cytology and histology* (pp. 402–427). Washington, DC: Author.

American College of Obstetricians and Gynecologists (ACOG). (2009a, December). *ACOG Practice Bulletin No. 109, Cervical cytology screening* (pp. 1409–1420). Washington, DC: Author.

American College of Obstetricians and Gynecologists (ACOG). (2009b, June). ACOG Committee Opinion No. 436, Evaluation and management of abnormal cervical cytology and histology in adolescents. *Obstetrics and Gynecology, 113*(6), 1422–1425.

American Society for Colposcopy and Cervical Pathology. (2010). *Human papillomavirus (HPV).* Retrieved April 13, 2010, from http://www.asccp.org/hpv_history.shtml

Association of Women's Health, Obstetric, and Neonatal Nurses. (2009). AWHONN Position Statement: HPV vaccination for the prevention of cervical cancer. *Journal of Obstetric, Gynecologic, & Neonatal Nursing, 39*(11), 129–130.

Association of Women's Health, Obstetric, and Neonatal Nurses. (2010). *Nursing association launches HPV awareness & education campaign.* Retrieved April 20, 2010, from https://www.awhonn.org/awhonn/content.do?name=07_PressRoom/7B7_Jan06_HPVBeConfident.htm

Bickley, L. S., & Szilagyi, P. G. (2007). *Bates' guide to physical examination and history taking* (9th ed.). Philadelphia: Lippincott Williams and Wilkins.

Brewer, N. T., & Fazekas, K. I. (2007). Predictors of HPV vaccine acceptability: A theory-informed, systematic review. *Preventive Medicine, 45*(2-3), 107–114.

Burchell, A. N., Tellier, P. P., Hanley, J., Coutlee, F., & Franco, E. L. (2010). Human Papillomavirus infections among couples in new sexual relationships. *Epidemiology, 21*(1), 31–37.

Burkman, R. T. (2010). New screening recommendations: Benefits and harms are in the eye of the beholder. *Female Patient, 35*(3), 12–13.

Burns, J. L., Walsh, L. J., & Popovich, J. M. (2010). Practical pediatric and adolescent immunization update. *Journal for Nurse Practitioners, 6*(4), 254–266.

Cates, J. R., Brewer, N. T., Fazekas, K. I., Mitchell, C. E., & Smith, J. S. (2009). Racial differences in HPV knowledge, HPV vaccine acceptability, and related beliefs among rural Southern women. *Journal of Rural Health, 25*(1), 93–97.

Centers for Disease Control and Prevention (CDC). (2006). *Sexually transmitted diseases treatment guidelines 2006.* Retrieved April 20, 2010, from http://www.cdc.gov/std/treatment/2006/genital-warts.htm

Centers for Disease Control and Prevention (CDC). (2009a). *Genital HPV infection—CDC fact sheet.* Retrieved April 20, 2010, from http://www.cdc.gov/STD/HPV/STDFact-HPV.htm

Centers for Disease Control and Prevention (CDC). (2009b). *HPV vaccine—questions & answers.* Retrieved April 20, 2010, from http://www.cdc.gov/vaccines/vpd-vac/hpv/vac-faqs.htm

Centers for Disease Control and Prevention, Advisory Committee on Immunization Practices (CDC ACIP). (2009). *Provisional recommendations for HPV vaccine.* Retrieved April 18, 2010, from http://www.cdc.gov/vaccines/recs/provisional/downloads/hpv-vac-dec2009-508.pdf

Chase, D. M., & Tewari, K. S. (2010). Update on cervical cancer screening. *Female Patient, 35*(1), 16–21.

Coker, A. L. (2007). Does physical intimate partner violence affect sexual health? A systematic review. *Trauma Violence and Abuse, 8*(2), 149–77.

Dillon, P. M. (2007). *Nursing health assessment: A critical thinking, case studies approach* (2nd ed.). Philadelphia: F. A. Davis.

Duffy, P. J. (2009). Cervical cancer risk management: A legal perspective. *Female Patient (Suppl.), 34*(1), S1–12.

Dunne, E. F., & Markowitz, L. E. (2006). Genital human papillomavirus infection. Emerging Infections. *Clinical Infectious Diseases, 43*(1), 624–629.

Escobar, P. F., & Orr, J. W. (2008). The human papillomavirus vaccine: Current status. *Female Patient, 33*(11), 18–22.

English, A., Shaw, F. E., McCauley, M. M., & Fishbein, D. B. (2008). Legal basis of consent for health care and vaccination for adolescents. *Pediatrics, 121*, S85–87.

Fazekas, K., Brewer, N., & Smith, J. (2008). HPV acceptability in a rural Southern area. *Journal of Women's Health, 17*(6), 539–547.

Frazer, I. H., Cox, J. T., Mayeaux, E. J., Jr., Franco, E. L., Moscicki, A. B., & Palefsky, J. M., et al. (2006). Advances in prevention of cervical cancer and other human papillomavirus-related diseases. *Pediatric Infectious Disease Journal, 25*(2 Suppl.), S65–S81.

Garfield, S., Gavaghan, M., Poret, A., & Ilika, K. (2010). HPV DNA co-testing adoption and its effect on patient annual visits. *Female Patient, 35*(4), 53–56.

Giarratano, G., Bustamante-Forest, R., & Carter, C. (2005). A multicultural and multilingual outreach program for cervical and breast cancer screening. *Journal of Obstetric, Gynecologic, and Neonatal Nursing, 34*(4), 395–402.

Gottlieb, S. L., & Brewer, N. T. (2009). Disparities in how parents are learning about the human papillomavirus vaccine. *Cancer Epidemiology, Biomarkers & Prevention, 18*(2), 363–372.

Gupton, N. E. (2007). Are Pap tests in danger of being phased out? *Clinical Advisor, 10*(4), 89–92.

Hachey, K. J., Allen, R. H., Nothnagle, M., & Boardman, L.A. (2009). Requiring human papillomavirus vaccine for immigrant women. *Obstetrics & Gynecology, 114*(5), 1135–1138.

Hellwig, J. P. (2006). HPV linked to common skin cancer. *AWHONN Lifelines, 10*(4), 289–294.

Howley, P. M., Yang, Y. C., Spalholz, B. A., & Rabson, M. S. (1986). Papillomavirus transforming functions. *Ciba Foundation Symposium, 120*, 39–52.

Hutchinson, M. K., Thompson, A. C., & Cederbaum, J. A. (2006). Multisystem factors contributing to disparities in preventive health care among lesbian women. *Journal of Obstetric, Gynecologic & Neonatal Nursing, 35*(3), 393–402.

Kahn, J. A. (2008). Human papillomavirus infections and anogenital warts. In L. Neinstein, C. M. Gordon, D. K. Katzman, D. S. Rosen, & E. R. Woods (Eds.), *Adolescent health care* (5th ed., pp. 842–849). Philadelphia: Lippincott Williams & Wilkins.

Kahn, J., Rosenthal, S., Jin, Y., Huang, B., Namakydoust, A., & Zimet, G. (2008). Rates of Human papillomavirus vaccination, attitudes about vaccination, and human papilloma-virus prevalence in young women. *Obstetrics and Gynecology, 111*(4), 1103–1110.

Katki, H. A., Wacholder, S., Solomon, D., Castle, P. E., & Schiffman, M. (2009). Risk estimation for the next generation of prevention programmes for cervical cancer. *Lancet Oncology, 10*(11), 1022–1023.

Kiviat, N. B., Hawes, S. E., & Feng, Q. (2008). Screening for cervical cancer in the era of the HPV vaccine: The urgent need for both new screening guidelines and new biomarkers. *Journal of the National Cancer Institute, 100*(5), 290–291.

Lara-Torre, E., & Murchison, A. B. (2009). Case management of cervical cytology and histology in the adolescent patient. *Female Patient, 34*(11), 34–37.

Lindstrom, A. K., Ekman, K., Stendahl, U., Tot, T., Henriksson, R., Hedman, H., & Hellberg, D. (2008). LRIG1 and squamous epithelial uterine cervical cancer: Correlation to prognosis, other tumor markers, sex steroid hormones, and smoking. *International Journal of Gynecological Cancer, 18*(2), 312–317.

Markowitz, L. E., Dunne, E. F., Saraiya, M., Lawson, H. W., Chesson, H., & Unger, E. R. (2007). Quadrivalent human papillomavirus vaccine: Recommendations of the advisory committee on immunization practices (ACIP). *Morbidity and Mortality Weekly Report, Recommendations and Reports, 56*(RR-2), 1–24.

Marrazzo, J. M., Koutsky, L. A., Kiviat, N. B., Kuypers, J. M., & Stine, K. (2001). Papanicolaou test screening and prevalence of genital human papillomavirus among women who have sex with women. *American Journal of Public Health, 91*(6), 947–952.

Marshall, H., Phillip, R., Don, R., & Peter, B. (2007). A cross-sectional survey to assess community attitudes to introduction of human papillomavirus vaccine. *Australian and New Zealand Journal of Public Health, 31*(3), 235–242.

Moore, S. L., & Seybold, V. K. (2007). HPV vaccine. *Clinician Reviews, 17*(1), 36–42.

National Association of Nurse Practitioners in Women's Health. (2007). Guidelines for screening and management of cervical disease. *Women's Health Care: A Practical Journal for Nurse Practitioners, 6*(1), 24–32.

National Cancer Institute (NCI). (2009). *Cervical cancer treatment.* Retrieved April 27, 2010, from http://www.cancer.gov/cancertopics/pdq/treatment/cervical/healthprofessional

Neinstein, L. S. (2008). Office visit and interviewing. In L. Neinstein, C. M. Gordon, D. K. Katzman, D. S. Rosen, & E. R. Woods (Eds.), *Adolescent health care* (5th ed., pp. 25–41). Philadelphia: Lippincott Williams & Wilkins.

Oh, J. K., Ju, Y. H., Franceschi, S., Quint, W., & Shin, H. R. (2008). Acquisition of new infection and clearance of type-specific human papillomavirus infection in female students in Busan, South Korea: A follow-up study [Electronic version]. *BMC Infection Diseases,* 8(13). Retrieved April 30, 2010, from http://www.biomedcentral.com/content/pdf/1471-2334-8-13.pdf

Olbrys, K. (2010). Cervical screening: Assessment and referral. *Journal for Nurse Practitioners, 6*(2), 151–152.

Policar, M. S. (2008). Female genital tract cancer screening. In R. A. Hatcher, J. Trussell, A. Nelson, F. Cates, F. Stewart, & D. Kowal. (Eds.). *Contraceptive technology* (19th ed., pp. 559–581). New York: Ardent Media.

Pollack, A. E., Balkin, M., Edouard, L., Cutts, F., & Broutet, N. (2007). Ensuring access to HPV vaccines through integrated services: A reproductive health perspective. *Bulletin of the World Health Organization, 85*(1), 57–63.

Ries, L. A., Melbert, D., Krapcho, M., Stinchcomb, D. G., Howlader, N., Horner, M. J., et al. (Eds.). (2009). *SEER cancer statistics review, 1975-2006.* Bethesda, MD: National Cancer Institute. Retrieved April 22, 2010, from http://seer.cancer.gov/csr/1975_2006/

Rome, E. S., & Hicks, C. W. (2009). Human papillomavirus vaccine: The current picture. *Female Patient, 34*(10), 34–39.

Ruhl, C. (2008). The future of the Pap: Where is cervical cancer screening headed? *Nursing for Women's Health, 12*(5), 427–431.

Saslow, D. (2009). Current issues in cervical cancer screening. *Female Patient, 33*(7), 20–23.

Schmidt, J. V. (2007). HPV vaccine: Implications for nurses and patients. *Nursing for Women's Health, 11*(1), 83–87.

Shanbhag, S., Clark, H., Timmaraju, V., Bhattacharya, S., & Cruickshank, M. (2009). Pregnancy outcome after treatment for cervical intraepithelial neoplasia. *Obstetrics & Gynecology, 114*(4), 727–735.

Taylor, J. S., & Smith, J. (2009). Concurrent STIs in adolescents with abnormal cervical cytologic findings. *Women's Health Care: A Practical Journal for Nurse Practitioners, 8*(12), 17–23.

Teitelman, A. M., Ratcliffe, S. J., & Cederbaum, J. A. (2008). Parent–adolescent communication about sexual pressure, maternal gender norms about relationship power and HIV protective behaviors of minority urban girls. *Journal of the American Psychiatric Nurses Association, 14,* 50–60.

Teitelman, A.M., Stringer, M., Averbuch, T., & Witkoski, A. (2009). Human papillomavirus, current vaccines, and cervical cancer prevention. *Journal of Obstetric, Gynecologic, and Neonatal Nursing, 38*(1), 69–80.

Theroux, R. (2008). The HPV vaccine: Rates, attitudes and acceptability. *Nursing for Women's Health, 12*(5), 423–426.

U.S. Preventive Services Task Force. (2007). *Guide to clinical preventive services 2007: Recommendations of the U.S. Preventive Services Task Force* (AHRQ Publication No. 07-05100). Available at http://www.ahrq.gov

Venes, D. (2009). *Taber's cyclopedic medical dictionary* (21st ed.). Philadelphia: F. A. Davis.

Watts, L. A., Joseph, N., Wallace, M., Rauh-Hain, J. A., Muzikansky, A., Growdon, W. B., & del Carmen, M. G. (2009). HPV vaccine: a comparison of attitudes and behavioralperspectives between Latino and non-Latino women. *Gynecologic Oncology, 112*(3), 577–582.

Woodson, S.A. (2008). *HPV counseling: A clinician resource.* Washington, DC: Association of Women's Health, Obstetric and Neonatal Nurses (AWHONN).

Wright, T. C., Massad, L. S., Dunton, C. J., Spitzer, M., Wilkinson, E. J., & Solomon, D. (2007). 2006 consensus guidelines for the management of women with abnormal cervical cancer screening tests. *American Journal of Obstetrics and Gynecology, 197*(4), 346–355.

Wysocki, S., Reiter, S., & Berman, N.R. (2007). Strategies for preventing cervical cancer and HPV-related disease: The role of vaccination. *Women's Health Care, 6*(1), 6–22.

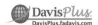 **For more information, go to http://davisplus.fadavis.com/**

Promoting Menopausal Health

Shelton M. Hisley, PhD, RNC, WHNP-BC

You can't turn back the clock.
But you can wind it up again.

—Bonnie Pruden

LEARNING TARGETS *At the completion of this chapter, the student will be able to:*

◆ Identify physiological changes that occur during the menopausal period.

◆ Identify self-care strategies to promote health during midlife and the later years.

◆ Recognize various risk factors for cardiovascular disease and osteoporosis.

◆ Develop an educational program for perimenopausal women that focuses on potential health threats and empowers women with strategies to optimize physical and emotional well-being.

Introduction

This chapter explores the years surrounding the menopausal transition. By 2025, 1.1 billion women worldwide will be postmenopausal. In 1900, the average age of menopause was 46 years and the average life expectancy was 51 years, although many women lived well beyond this age. In contemporary times, American women, on average, can expect to live to be 80 years old and spend close to one-third of their lives as postmenopausal women. For the modern woman, menopause does not mark the end of life. Instead, it represents a transition into another phase, with a potential life span of another 30 to 50 years (Burdette, Moore, Speroff, & Wysocki, 2009; Edelman, 2010).

A healthy lifestyle that balances optimal nutrition and regular exercise with mental and social stimulation helps women to lead productive, enriched lives well into the ninth decade. The period surrounding the menopause offers a unique time for women to evaluate their physical and emotional health, make plans for the future, and prepare for many, many healthy years ahead. With evidence-based information about menopause and the normal aging process, as well as various health issues such as cardiovascular disease and osteoporosis, nurses can empower women with the tools they need to prepare for and embrace the coming years with energy, enthusiasm, and strategies for optimizing their health and well-being. Armed with factual information, women can actively partner with their health-care provider in the decision-making process. Nurses are perfectly positioned to provide ongoing menopausal education and counseling to assist women in making fully informed choices.

While menopause is a natural, inevitable process, women do have control over how they pass through this special time of life. They can engage in strategies to ease uncomfortable symptoms and minimize their risks of chronic disease. For example, refraining from smoking, maintaining appropriate weight through exercise and diet, limiting alcohol intake, reducing stress, remaining socially active, and recognizing that happiness and long-term health come about through a personalized approach are tools that help women to enjoy good health during the later years of life. As a noted author observed, "the wise woman achieves menopause, it does not overcome her" (Weed, 2002). During this special time in their lives, many women describe an enhanced sense of well-being, hard-won individuality, and a positive attitude for living life to its fullest.

The Climacteric, Premenopause, Menopause, Perimenopause, and Postmenopause

The *climacteric* is a transitional time in a woman's life marked by declining ovarian function and decreased hormone production. The climacteric begins at the onset of ovarian decline and ends with the cessation of postmenopausal symptoms. *Menopause*, a term derived from Latin *mensis* for "month" and Greek *pausis*, meaning "to cease," refers to the last menstrual period and can be dated with certainty only 1 year after menstruation ceases. Menopause is defined as the permanent cessation of menses resulting from reduced ovarian hormone secretion that occurs naturally or is induced by surgery, chemotherapy, or radiation. The average age at menopause in the United States is 51.4 years; the normal age at menopause ranges from 40 to 58 years (Nelson, Haney, Humphrey, Miller, Nedrow, Nicolaidis, Vesco, Walker, Bougatsos, & Nygren, 2005).

Premenopause is the time up to the beginning of perimenopause, but the term is also used to define the time up to the last menstrual period. *Perimenopause* is the period of time preceding menopause, usually between 2 and 8 years before menopause. The age at onset of perimenopause ranges from 39 to 51 years. Although perimenopause may last as few as 2 or as many as 10 years; on average, it lasts 4 years. During this time of transition, levels of estrogen and progesterone increase and decrease at uneven intervals, causing the menstrual cycle to become longer, shorter, and eventually absent. Ovulation is sporadic. Symptoms of perimenopause, including irregular menses, hot flashes, vaginal dryness, dyspareunia, and mood changes are associated with the fluctuation and decline in hormone levels. *Postmenopause* begins when ovarian estrogen terminates, ovulation ceases, and menstrual periods have stopped for 12 consecutive months. During postmenopause, estrogen is produced solely by the adrenal glands. Women typically enter postmenopause between the ages of 40 and 58; the average age is 51 (Edelman, 2010; Nelson et al., 2005).

 Nursing Insight— **Perspectives on the perimenopausal period**

Every woman travels her own unique course through perimenopause. Interestingly, the term *perimenopause* is a relatively new concept—the word was not even listed in a medical dictionary until after 1989. The term *menopausal transition* describes the years from the onset of the loss of ovarian cycling to the last menstrual period. Menopause occurs regardless of a woman's age when the number of remaining ovarian follicles falls below a critical level of about 1000. The health habits established during the perimenopausal and early postmenopausal years can determine the woman's health status and quality of life for her critical elderly years after age 75, when serious health problems are greatest (Nelson & Stewart, 2008).

Throughout the menopausal transition, changes take place in both the physiological and emotional domains. Hormone levels shift, readjust, and reach new balances, and the tissues and organs whose function is influenced by these hormones also change structurally and functionally. At the same time, mental and emotional alterations occur as well. While some of the changes are physiological in nature, others involve various dimensions of self-perception and self-concept as women are challenged to deal with this natural passage into a new phase of life.

 Ethnocultural Considerations— **Views on menopause**

Cross-cultural studies have revealed that the menopausal experience is greatly influenced by the attitudes of the culture and community in which women reside. In the United States, owing in part to the present-day graying of the baby-boom generation, attitudes toward menopause and aging are undergoing change. For many traditional cultures throughout the world, menopause represents a time for women to assume leadership roles in the community and a time for honor and recognition as one of the tribal members with an accumulation of wisdom. American women are embracing this broad cultural perspective as an opportunity to shift self-perception and create a positive cultural image of women during this stage of life. Today, the majority of American women do not believe that menopause interferes with their quality of life (National Institutes of Health [NIH], 2005).

Signs and Symptoms of Menopause

A number of signs and symptoms typically herald the physical changes that take place during the menopausal transition. During this time, nurses can empower women with various strategies to promote mental and physical well-being. Potential nursing diagnoses for women experiencing the perimenopausal period are presented in Box 7-1.

 Nursing Insight— **Body systems affected by the natural decline in estrogen**

Estrogen secretion naturally declines as women age. Estrogen receptors are plentiful throughout the female body. During the childbearing years, estrogen is a dominant hormone that regulates the menstrual cycle and exerts important effects on the reproductive and urinary tracts, the heart and blood vessels, bones, breasts, skin, hair follicles, mucous membranes, pelvic muscles, and the brain. Loss of estrogen is associated with a multitude of acute symptoms, including hot flashes, sleep disruptions, and mood changes. For many women, menopause-related estrogen depletion is also associated with longer-term manifestations such as urogenital symptoms (Allmen & Moore, 2010).

MENSTRUAL CYCLE CHANGES

It is rare for a woman to cease menstruation all at once. Most often, the menstrual periods become progressively more irregular. The volume of blood flow is variable as well and may be accompanied by midcycle spotting. Changes in bleeding patterns largely result from a lack of ovulation. The absence of ovulation interrupts the production of progesterone, the hormone that stabilizes the endometrium, or uterine lining. Under the influence of prolonged, continuous estrogen, the endometrium continues to proliferate and may only be irregularly sloughed off. When bleeding does occur, it may be heavier or more prolonged. The endometrial lining may also develop irregular or thickened areas; it may not slough off evenly or in its entirety, and these events cause the menses to stop and start again.

Box 7-1 Potential Nursing Diagnoses for Perimenopausal Women

- Knowledge deficit related to menopause and its management
- Risk for injury related to osteoporosis and coronary heart disease
- Sexual dysfunction related to physiological changes associated with declining estrogen levels
- Readiness for enhanced family coping related to the menopausal transition
- Risk for situational low self-esteem related to the physical and emotional changes during the menopausal transition

Although irregular menses is usually a normal part of the perimenopausal process, any heavy bleeding should be investigated. Uterine fibroids, a frequent cause of increased bleeding, are common in perimenopausal women. Cervical or uterine cancer should also be considered as a possible cause of this symptom. If heavy bleeding is an ongoing problem and cancer has been ruled out, hormonal intervention in the form of low-dose oral contraceptives, progesterone alone, or another form of hormone therapy (HT) may be suggested. If fibroids are the cause of heavy bleeding, medical or surgical intervention may be advised. (See Bonus Chapter 4 for a discussion of uterine cancer and fibroid tumors and Bonus Chapter 6 for a discussion of cervical cancer.) It is important to remember that although fertility declines during this transitional period, it does not disappear until menopause is complete. Menopause is signaled by the passage of one full year without menstruation. For most women, birth control remains an important consideration during the perimenopausal period (Alexander, 2007; Nelson & Stewart, 2008; Secor & Simon, 2006).

HORMONAL CHANGES

During the perimenopausal period, hormone levels are frequently erratic, with highs and lows occurring without the usual synchronicity. A common hormonal pattern that occurs when ovulation becomes unpredictable is an elevated estrogen level throughout the cycle with low progesterone levels during the second half of the cycle, when progesterone is normally at its peak. Some women develop very low levels of estrogen as well. At this time, ovarian function declines and the ovaries lose their ability to manufacture large amounts of sex hormones. The physiological feedback loops between the ovaries, the hypothalamus, and the pituitary glands also lose their synchronized pattern. Progesterone undergoes the most dramatic drop during menopause because its production depends upon ovulation and the development of the corpus luteum.

Small amounts of estrogen continue to be produced by the ovaries for up to 10 years following cessation of menses. The body has other means of estrogen production, however. The woman's fat cells convert androgens produced by the adrenal glands to estrogens. Androgens are female forms of "male-type" hormones that are produced by the ovaries and the adrenal glands. Androgens are responsible for the maintenance of muscle strength and the sex drive. As estrogen and progesterone levels fall, the effects of the androgens often become relatively more pronounced. For example, these hormones can produce an increase in facial hair often noted after menopause. For some women, androgen levels (including testosterone) fall as well, producing symptoms of low libido or decrease in muscle mass with a relative increase in the amount of adipose (fat) tissue (Wysocki, 2009a).

SKIN AND HAIR CHANGES

Declining levels of estrogen affect many tissues throughout the body. The skin and mucous membranes become dry. The fatty layer beneath the skin tends to shrink, and this change is associated with an overall decrease in elasticity and moisture. The skin feels rougher to the touch, and the outer skin may be looser than the deeper layers, which results in wrinkling. The skin produces less melanin, and it can burn more easily. The increasing predominance of androgens often causes a darker, thicker, more wiry hair to appear on the symphysis pubis, underarm area, chest, lower abdomen, and back. Some women experience an increase in facial hair, and the hair on the head may become dry. Pubic and axillary hair often thins. Genetically susceptible women may experience female pattern (scalp) hair loss, a condition most likely related to the altered estrogen-to-androgen ratio that accompanies menopause (Bergfeld & Harrison, 2009; Freeman, 2009).

BREAST CHANGES

Glandular tissues in the breasts shrink during the menopausal period. The breasts may lose their fullness and flatten and drop. The nipples may become smaller and flatter.

UROGENITAL CHANGES

Vaginal changes may accompany the perimenopausal period, or they may not occur for several years after menopause. The mucous membranes, previously supported by estrogen stimulation, become thin, dry, and fragile. The vagina loses its rough texture and dark pink coloration and becomes smooth and pale. The vagina also shortens and narrows. Women may experience vaginal itching, burning, bleeding, or soreness. The vagina lubricates more slowly, and there is a diminished amount of cervical mucus produced. Owing to these changes, intercourse often becomes painful. Bleeding and/or pain may occur following minimal trauma, such as that occurring during intercourse or a pelvic examination. Vulvar changes may also make activities such as riding a bicycle uncomfortable. There is also an alteration in the normal vaginal flora, which results in a decrease in the normal protective mechanisms of the vagina. Declining estrogen secretion is accompanied by a corresponding reduction in the lactobacilli needed to maintain a healthy acidic vaginal environment. With these changes in pH, normally harmless pathogens may colonize the more alkaline vagina, potentially leading to infection. When the vaginal mucosa becomes inflamed, the condition is termed "atrophic vaginitis," a condition characterized by burning, leukorrhea and malodorous yellow discharge (Greenblum, Greenblum, & Neff, 2009; Mehta & Bachmann, 2008; North American Menopause Society [NAMS], 2007; Wysocki, 2009a).

A & P review **Estrogen Deficiency and Urogenital Atrophy**

Estrogen plays a critical role in maintaining the structure and function of the vagina. The layers of the vaginal mucosa, which is estrogen sensitive, are composed of *parabasal* (the least mature), *intermediate* or *basal* (larger and polygon-shaped), and *superficial* squamous cells (the most mature). Prior to menopause, the matured vaginal epithelium has more superficial cells than parabasal cells, indicating the presence of estrogenic stimulation. In menopausal women, systemic declines in estrogen levels correspond to decreased cellular maturation. The proportion of superficial cells present on cytological examination is expressed as the *vaginal maturation index* (VMI). The VMI is a ratio of parabasal, intermediate, and superficial squamous cells found on a cytological smear of cells taken from the upper one-third of the vagina. Although infrequently used in clinical practice today, the maturation index of vaginal cells is useful in evaluating the qualitative response of the vaginal tissue to estrogen. Under the influence of estrogen, mature superficial cells predominate; when estrogen levels are low, parabasal cell numbers fall, leading to gradual atrophic changes in the tissues of the vagina, vulva, urethra, and trigone area of the bladder. Some menopausal women experience urinary problems, including increased urinary tract infections (Allmen & Moore, 2010; Greenblum, Greenblum, & Neff, 2009; Mehta & Bachmann, 2008; NAMS, 2007; Wysocki, 2008, 2009a). ◆

Menopause-induced changes in the genitourinary tract can produce symptoms that include urinary urgency, increased frequency, stress or urge incontinence, and recurrent urinary tract infections. Unlike other symptoms associated with menopause, such as hot flashes, those of urogenital atrophy often worsen with advancing age. Vulvovaginal or urinary atrophic symptoms in postmenopausal women can cause significant reductions in quality of life, avoidance of sexual intercourse, and emotional distress (Burdette, 2009; Goldstein & Alexander, 2005). More than one-third of women over the age of 60 in the United States have some form of urinary incontinence (Alexander, 2007). The prevalence of incontinence appears to increase gradually during young adult life, peak around middle age, and then steadily increase during the later years. The estimated annual direct cost of urinary incontinence in women in this country is around $12.43 billion (ACOG, 2007).

A & P review **Estrogen Deficiency and Urogenital Changes**

In the urinary tract, estrogen deficiency causes urethral and bladder mucosal thinning, urethral shortening, weakening of the sphincter, decreased bladder capacity, increased postvoid residual urine volume, and uninhibited detrusor muscle contractions. After menopause, the urethral mucosa atrophies, and the collagen content in the connective tissue surrounding the urethra decreases; blood flow in the urethra is also reduced. These changes may cause dysuria, urinary frequency, and stress incontinence; estrogen-deficient women may also be susceptible to recurrent urinary tract infections. Owing to a decrease in collagen and elastin, declining estrogen levels also contribute to loss of mechanical support of the pelvic diaphragm (Goldstein & Alexander, 2005; Palacios, 2009; Wysocki, 2008). ◆

Nursing Insight— *Menopause and pelvic floor dysfunction*

Pelvic organ support is provided by the physiologically complex interactions between the vagina, the levator ani muscles and their fascial coverings, the connective tissue attachments to the bony pelvis (including the uterosacral ligaments), the arcus tendineus fascia pelvis, and the perineal body and perineal membrane. The pelvic floor muscles atrophy after menopause, becoming weak and unable to adequately support the pelvic structures and organs. As the pelvic organs shift position, they begin to press against the vagina, resulting in prolapse, usually of the vagina or bladder. A prolapse can result in pain during intercourse and urinary incontinence. Exercises can strengthen the muscles; however,

muscle damage cannot be reversed. Surgery is the primary treatment for pelvic prolapse; the timing of the surgery depends on the woman's symptoms and their effect on her daily activities. Some symptoms can be medically managed until surgery is appropriate. Many treatment options are available for urinary incontinence, especially if it is not accompanied by a cystocele, which results when the bladder herniates into the vagina (Jones, Bryson, & Harmanli, 2010).

Urinary incontinence has been shown to affect women's social, clinical, and psychological well-being. It is estimated that fewer than one-half of all incontinent women seek medical assistance for this problem, even though urinary incontinence can often be treated (ACOG, 2007). Loss of estrogen supply to the estrogen-dependent tissues of the genitourinary tract results in a decrease in muscle tone and control in the bladder and urethra. Stress urinary incontinence (SUI) is a disturbance in urinary control (e.g., loss of urine) due to sudden increases in intra-abdominal pressure that often occurs during sneezing, coughing, or laughing. SUI is more likely to occur in women who have given birth. For most women, pelvic muscle exercises, known as Kegel exercises, can be very effective in strengthening the pelvic floor and in improving symptoms associated with SUI. Some practitioners provide patients with "Kegel beads" to encourage and remind them to perform the exercises. Patients are instructed to slide the beads from one side of the chain to the other until all sets (10) are performed for the day (Jones, Bryson, & Harmanli, 2010).

"What to say" — *Teaching patients how to perform Kegel exercises*

To teach patients about Kegel exercises, the nurse may provide the following information:

Kegel exercises strengthen the pelvic floor and should help decrease your urinary symptoms. To perform the Kegel exercise:

- First, contract the vaginal opening as if you are trying to stop the flow of urine.
- Now hold to a count of 6.
- Relax to a count of 10, then repeat these steps 10 more times.
- Perform 5 to 10 sets of Kegel exercises each day.

For patients who are unable to isolate the levator ani, electrical stimulation and/or muscle biofeedback may be helpful. Electrical stimulation during Kegel exercises stimulates and contracts the pelvic muscles in a manner similar to the Kegels. This approach, conducted in the health-care practitioner's office, may be helpful for women who have difficulty contracting the pelvic muscles voluntarily. It involves the use of a device that delivers current to the pudendal nerve through a vaginally placed probe (Jones, Bryson, & Harmanli, 2010).

Biofeedback therapy has been used to assist the re-education of patients with pelvic floor spasms and has been shown to result in significant symptomatic improvement after several months of therapy. Biofeedback utilizes a vaginal sensor that measures the level of muscle activity generated by voluntary pelvic floor contraction. With biofeedback, the patient is taught to voluntarily control the pelvic muscles and bladder. With an electrode attached to the skin, biofeedback machines measure the electrical signals elicited when the pelvic muscles and urinary sphincter are contracted. Through the visual cues from the graph shown on the monitor, patients can learn to control these muscles voluntarily (Jones, Bryson, & Harmanli, 2010).

Vaginal cones, which may also be vaginal weights, can be used to strengthen the vaginal muscles as well. The woman is instructed to insert the tampon-shaped cone into the vagina while in a standing position, beginning with the lightest weight. Once inserted, the patient should contract the levator ani muscles in an effort to keep the cone in place for 15 to 20 minutes. As the muscles strengthen, the patient then transitions, one at a time, to the next heaviest cone. It is helpful to use the cone while doing Kegel exercises as well. As the pelvic muscles strengthen, patients can use the cones while engaging in exercise (Jones, Bryson, & Harmanli, 2010).

Some women choose to use a pessary, which is a device inserted into the vagina to support the prolapsed bladder or uterus. This device must be fitted by a health-care practitioner and needs to be removed and cleaned regularly with soap and water to reduce the risk of infection. Surgical intervention for a prolapsed bladder usually involves an anterior repair (colporrhaphy). This procedure involves shortening of the pelvic muscles to provide better support for the bladder.

Urinary urgency and/or frequency combined with an involuntary loss of urine are common signs of an overactive bladder. Pharmacologic management of incontinence is aimed at relaxing the involuntary contractions that occur at the bladder. For overactive bladder, common medications include tolterodine (Detrol), oxybutynin (Ditropan), and imipramine (Tofranil). Common side effects associated with these medications include dry mouth, nausea, dizziness, drowsiness, and constipation. Low-dose vaginal estrogen creams, tablets, or rings may also be prescribed to provide relief of urinary symptoms (Alexander, 2007).

Promoting Sexual Health During the Menopausal Years

Years ago, researchers Masters and Johnson studied sexuality in menopausal women and found that there is a general reduction in the four phases of the sexual response cycle with increasing years after menopause. However, they also discovered that women who maintained regular sexual activity experienced vaginal lubrication similar to levels expected in women who were premenopausal, and these women continued to be capable of full sexual response and enjoyment. Sexual activity is also beneficial in improving tone and blood flow to the pelvic floor.

 Nursing Insight— *Sexual responsiveness in older women*

Sexual responsiveness reaches a peak for women in their late 30s and can remain on a high plateau into the 60s. Some women report an increased sexual desire after menopause. The fear of unwanted pregnancy often frees women to be much more sexually expressive and responsive than they were in their premenopausal years.

The two most important influences on older women's sexual activity are the strength of the relationship and the health status of each partner. The lack of an available partner can have a negative effect on sexual intimacy for many midlife and older women. Older widowed, divorced, and lesbian women may have fewer opportunities to develop close relationships because they are less sought after. When discussing sexuality issues with older women, it is important for nurses to provide accurate information and offer support and nonjudgmental guidance. The nurse can reassure the woman that the desire for sex into old age is a natural one and the body continues to have the capacity for sexual satisfaction (ACOG, 2007).

Many women do, however, experience changes in libido (sex drive), reduction in vaginal lubrication, discomfort during intercourse, and changes in orgasmic response in the years after menopause. The use of various oils (e.g., vegetable, vitamin E, olive) or vaginal lubricants that are specifically formulated for menopausal vaginal discomfort allows many older women to continue to enjoy sexual intercourse. Lengthening the foreplay time may promote enhanced vaginal lubrication as well.

"What to say" — *Initiating dialogue about menopausal sexual difficulties*

When discussing menopause-related problems, it is important to use patient-friendly terms such as *vaginal dryness, discomfort,* or *irritation,* rather than *sexual dysfunction.* Owing to the fact that the patient may be reluctant to initiate dialogue about sexual or urinary problems, the nurse may enhance the woman's comfort level with questions such as

- "Many women come to our office with various complaints such as vaginal dryness, itching, and pain with sex. Have you experienced any of these problems?"

- "Have you had any problems with frequent urination, leaking urine, or burning during urination?"

- "Have you tried any vaginal lubricants or other products to enhance comfort during intercourse?" (Allmen & Moore, 2010; Reiter, 2009).

Nurses can empower perimenopausal women with strategies to help combat vaginal dryness. Depending on the situation, the nurse may offer the following suggestions:

- Remain sexually active—sexual activity increases blood flow to the vagina, increases elasticity and lubrication of the vaginal tissues, and maintains muscle tone. Orgasm, achieved by any means, helps to decrease vaginal atrophy.

- Consume phytoestrogen-containing foods and herbs.

- Consider vitamin E, which has an estrogenic effect— apply vitamin E oil to the vagina; take vitamin E supplements (contraindicated in women with hypertension) (Constantino & Guaraldi, 2008).

- Consider the use of vegetable or olive oil, which is more soothing to the genital tissue than the commercially available alcohol-based products, but be aware that the oils can degrade latex condoms (Allmen & Moore, 2010).

- Consider vitamin C and bioflavonoids, substances that increase estrogen levels.

If natural remedies and interventions do not alleviate the discomfort associated with vaginal dryness, a number of nonprescription, nonhormonal products are available. For example, Replens, Me Again, Astroglide, Good Clean Love, and KY Liquibeads assist with moisture, lubrication, coital comfort, and normalization of vaginal pH. The duration of effectiveness is generally 24 to 48 hours. However, nonhormonal lubricants and moisturizers do not restore the integrity of the vagina. Nurses should caution women to avoid the use of Vaseline and other petroleum-based products, which can increase the chance for infection. Also, some over-the-counter products have an alcohol base and can have an undesirable drying effect (Alexander, 2007; Allmen & Moore, 2010; Kellogg-Spadt, 2010).

For women who experience a significant decrease in sex drive along with intolerable vaginal symptoms, the use of estrogen therapy, delivered in the form of a vaginal cream, tablet, or a silastic device may be helpful (ACOG, 2007). Presently, U.S. Food and Drug Administration (FDA) guidelines recommend the use of a vaginal hormonal preparation for menopausal women whose only symptom is vaginal atrophy (Alexander, 2007; Nelson & Stewart, 2008; NAMS, 2007, 2010a).

⑤ **Optimizing Outcomes— With the therapeutic effects of vaginal estrogen therapy**

Vaginal estrogen therapy promotes a healthy vaginal ecology by restoring vaginal pH to premenopausal levels and normalizing vaginal cytology. Treatment also leads to substantial subjective relief and marked improvement of vulvovaginal atrophy manifestations. Restoration of the vaginal mucosa with subsequent improvement in symptoms associated with vaginal atrophy is likely to improve sexual function by facilitating intercourse. Vaginally delivered estrogen therapy may also reduce urinary urge incontinence and diminish the recurrence of urinary tract infections (Allmen & Moore, 2010).

Low-dose vaginal estrogen cream (e.g., Premarin, Estrace) has been shown to significantly improve symptoms associated with vaginal dryness and reduce the incidence of urinary tract infections. Because systemic absorption of estrogen is minimal, most experts do not recommend the concomitant use of progestins to prevent endometrial hyperplasia in women who have a uterus. Typically, the woman is instructed to insert the estrogen cream into her vagina every day for the first 3 weeks, and then twice a week or as needed. Nurses need to instruct patients to discontinue local estrogen therapy for several days before a Pap screening so as not to obscure the cytology slide. A tablet that contains a low dose of estradiol (i.e., Vagifem) is also available; it is inserted in the vagina twice a week. Nurses should counsel all women who use estrogen therapy to promptly report any vaginal bleeding

or breast pain (Alexander, 2007; Greenblum, Greenblum, & Neff, 2009; Secor & Simon, 2006; Wysocki, 2008).

Hormonal vaginal rings, which are silastic devices impregnated with estrogen (estradiol) offer another option. The vaginal rings Estring and Femring are designed to deliver a slow release of estrogen (estradiol) locally to the vagina. The vaginal ring is inserted for a period of 3 months and then replaced by the patient or physician. The Estring is formulated with an ultralow dose of estradiol (7.5 micrograms released per day) and is associated with minimal systemic absorption. No concomitant progestin therapy (to prevent endometrial hyperplasia in women who have a uterus) is necessary. The Femring is formulated with a higher dose of estradiol (available to deliver 0.05 mg per day or 0.1 mg per day) and women with an intact uterus who use this product should almost always receive a progestin to avoid endometrial hyperplasia. Some older women with limited dexterity may experience difficulty positioning the vaginal ring, and the ring may become dislodged with intercourse, douching, or defecation (Greenblum, Greenblum, & Neff, 2009; Secor & Simon, 2006; Wysocki, 2008).

⑤ **Be sure to— Consider Lichen sclerosus et atrophicus as another cause of vulvovaginal symptoms**

Lichen sclerosus et atrophicus (LS&A) is a rare, benign, chronic, and progressive skin condition that usually affects the vulva in postmenopausal women. Lesions of vulvar LS&A appear as thin, white, glistening scaly patches with diffuse borders affecting the labia majora and minora. Diagnosis is made by the histological examination of a vulvar punch biopsy. Hormonal factors, genetics, immunological abnormalities, and local factors such as infection have been suggested as possible causes, although the actual etiology of LS&A is unknown. Most patients complain of nonspecific vulvar irritation or discomfort of variable intensity. Interestingly, some women are completely asymptomatic; others with severe disease and related symptoms (e.g., intense pruritus, pain, ulceration) may develop dysuria, dyspareunia, and vaginal or meatal stenosis. Treatment usually consists of the nightly application of a topical corticosteroid such as clobetasol (Temovate, Clobex) or halobetasol propionate (Ultravate). Because patients with genital LS&A are at an increased risk for the development of squamous cell cancer, routine follow-up is essential (Patel & Nunley, 2010; Pugliese, Morey, & Peterson, 2007).

HOT FLUSHES, HOT FLASHES, NIGHT SWEATS, AND SLEEP DISTURBANCES

One of the hallmarks of menopause is the occurrence of the vasomotor symptoms hot flushes, hot flashes, and night sweats. A *hot flush* is a visible red flush of skin and perspiration. A *hot flash* is a sudden warm sensation in the neck, head, and chest; heat may be radiated from all parts of the body. During a hot flash, skin temperatures rise as a result of peripheral vasodilation and sweating begins primarily on the upper body. Most women describe a sudden sweeping wave of heat sensation that spreads over the body. An increase in the heart rate of about 7 to 15 beats per minute occurs at approximately the same time as the peripheral vasodilation and sweating. It may take up to 30 minutes or longer for skin temperatures to return to normal. Hot flashes can occur infrequently (e.g., monthly; weekly) or frequently (hourly), although there is usually an individual pattern. A circadian rhythm has been observed, with hot flash frequency peaking in the early evening hours—about 3 hours after the peak in core body temperature (NAMS, 2007).

Night sweats are characterized by profuse perspiration and heat radiating from the body during the night. The woman's sleep may be interrupted each night because her nightclothes and bed linens become soaked with perspiration. Hot flashes constitute the most common symptom reported by women experiencing menopause and are present in 68% to 90% of women. They can occur often throughout the day and create anxiety, distress, and a significantly decreased quality of life (Edelman, 2010; Nelson & Stewart, 2008).

 Nursing Insight— Vasomotor symptoms and NAMS terminology

The terms *vasomotor symptoms, hot flash,* and *hot flush* are often used to describe the same phenomenon. The North American Menopause Society (NAMS) defines vasomotor symptoms as a global term that encompasses both hot flashes and night sweats. NAMS prefers the term *hot flash* rather than *hot flush* (NAMS, 2007).

For some women, hot flashes are only a significant problem for 1 to 2 years; others experience vasomotor symptoms that can persist for up to 15 years. Approximately 10% to 15% of women characterize their hot flashes as "debilitating." In many non-Westernized cultures, hot flashes either do not occur or are so minimal they are barely noticed. In this country, hot flashes cause women to seek medical advice more than any other symptom of menopause (Alexander, 2007; Secor & Simon, 2006).

The cause of the alternating vasodilation and vasoconstriction associated with hot flashes is not well understood, but it is known that this symptom is related to hormonal changes that affect the temperature-regulating centers in the hypothalamus. Low levels of estrogen alone are not responsible. It is believed that the presence of estrogen, followed by its withdrawal, triggers an imbalance in the body's temperature control center, which subsequently decreases the core body temperature. The body then attempts to activate heat centers to readjust the body's thermostat (Alexander, 2007). Other problems that may be associated with vasomotor instability include dizziness, numbness, or tingling in the fingers and toes and headaches. Environmental and lifestyle factors such as being in a crowded or warm room, consuming hot drinks, alcohol, or spicy foods, and stress can precipitate or aggravate an episode of vasomotor symptoms.

 Be sure to— Consider alternate causes for various vasomotor symptoms

The nurse should be aware of other conditions that may cause vasomotor symptoms in women. These include thyroid disease, epilepsy, infection, pheochromocytoma (a rare tumor of the adrenal gland), leukemia, pancreatic tumors, autoimmune disorders, new-onset hypertension, and mast-cell disorders. Also, some medications, such as tamoxifen (Nolvadex) and raloxifene (Evista) can cause hot flashes. Night sweats may be associated with more serious diseases, such as tuberculosis and lymphoma (NAMS, 2007).

Sleep disturbance is a more prevalent complaint for women than men. It is associated with menopausal symptoms (e.g., hot flashes, night sweats) and most importantly, with comorbidities (e.g., obesity, diabetes, depression, esophageal reflux) and stress. Sleep disorders in midlife women should not be attributed solely to the menopausal symptom experience. Referral for clinical evaluation to assess for primary sleep disorders such as restless legs, insomnia, or sleep-disordered breathing may be appropriate (Minarik, 2009; Reeve & Bailes, 2010; Valerio, 2009).

 Now Can You— **Discuss certain aspects of menopause?**

1. Differentiate among the terms *climacteric, premenopause, perimenopause,* and *postmenopause*?
2. Identify menstrual cycle changes, hormonal changes, skin and hair changes, and urogenital changes that typically accompany menopause?
3. Describe four strategies for maintaining and promoting sexual health and enjoyment during the menopausal transition and later years?
4. Identify and describe various vasomotor symptoms that frequently accompany menopause?

Promoting Comfort During the Menopausal Transition

COMPLEMENTARY AND ALTERNATIVE MEDICINE

Complementary and alternative medicine (CAM) includes a broad base of healing philosophies, approaches, and therapies that conventional medicine has not commonly understood or used. In general, a therapy is termed "complementary" when it is used *in addition to* conventional treatment, and it is called "alternative" when it is used *instead of* conventional treatment (NAMS, 2007).

Many women use CAM approaches such as stress management, guided imagery, biofeedback, massage therapy, yoga, chiropractic care, acupuncture, and dietary supplements to relieve various menopausal symptoms. Other nonmedicinal interventions for the relief of mild vasomotor symptoms include engaging in regular exercise; consuming cool, refreshing foods such as cabbage, cucumbers, and pineapple; minimizing the intake of alcohol, fatty foods, sugar and caffeine; avoiding "triggers" such as hot drinks, alcohol, or spicy foods; and dressing in layers to keep cool. Wearing clothing made of cotton, washable linen, or fabrics that wick perspiration away from the skin and increase air movement can increase comfort. Synthetic fabrics such as polyester should be avoided, as they can trap body heat and trigger hot flashes. Nurses can also counsel women to drink 8 to 10 glasses of water each day and perform deep-breathing or paced-respiration exercises at the beginning of a hot flash to diminish its effects (Alexander, 2009; Burdette

---

Box 7-2 Alternative Medical Systems, Mind–Body Medicine, Manipulative and Body-Based Methods, and Energy Medicine

ALTERNATIVE MEDICAL SYSTEMS
Traditional Chinese Medicine (TCM)
Traditional Chinese medicine (TCHM) is a system of healing that in written form dates back to 200 BC. TCM emphasizes the proper balance of two opposing and inseparable forces: yin and yang. Yin represents the cold, slow, or passive principle, and yang represents the hot, excited, or active principle. An imbalance of these two forces is thought to lead to blockage in the flow of qi (pronounced "chee" and meaning vital energy) and of blood along pathways known as meridians. TCM consists of a group of techniques and methods, including acupuncture, herbal medicine, oriental massage, and qi gong, to bring the body back into harmony and balance (NAMS, 2007).

Ayurveda
Ayurveda is India's traditional system of medicine. Meaning "science of life," Ayurvedic medicine is a comprehensive system that places equal emphasis on body, mind, and spirit and strives to restore the innate harmony of the individual. Some of the primary Ayurvedic treatments include diet, exercise, meditation, herbs, massage, exposure to sunlight, and controlled breathing (NAMS, 2007).

Homeopathic Medicine
Homeopathy is an unconventional Western system that is based on the principle that "like cures like" (i.e., large doses of a particular substance may produce symptoms of an illness; very small doses will cure it). Very small doses of specially prepared plant extracts and minerals are used to stimulate the body's defense mechanisms and healing processes to treat illness. The homeopathic approach focuses on the links among an individual's physical, emotional, and mental symptoms (NAMS, 2007).

Naturopathic Medicine
In naturopathic medicine, disease is viewed as a manifestation of alterations in the processes by which the body naturally heals itself, and emphasis is placed on health restoration rather than on disease treatment. Practitioners of naturopathic medicine employ a variety of healing practices, including diet and clinical nutrition, homeopathy, acupuncture, herbal medicine, hydrotherapy, spinal and soft-tissue manipulation, physical therapies involving electric currents, ultrasound and light therapy, therapeutic counseling, and pharmacology (NAMS, 2007).

MIND–BODY MEDICINE
Mind–body medicine focuses on the interactions among the brain, mind, body, and behavior and the powerful ways in which emotional, mental, social, spiritual, and behavioral factors can directly affect health. Mind–body medicine is an approach that respects and enhances each person's capacity for self-knowledge and self-care and emphasizes techniques that are grounded in this approach. Hypnosis, dance, music, and art therapy, prayer and mental healing, relaxation and visual imagery, meditation, and yoga are typical techniques used with this approach (NAMS, 2007).

MANIPULATIVE AND BODY-BASED METHODS
These methods are based on manipulation and/or movement of structures and systems of the body, including bones and joints, the soft tissues, and the circulatory and lymphatic systems. While there is considerable variation in the training and approaches of manipulative and body-based providers, they all share certain principles, such as the belief that the human body is self-regulating and has the ability to heal itself. Practitioners of manipulative and body-based methods include osteopathic physicians (DOs), massage therapists, and reflexologists (NAMS, 2007).

ENERGY MEDICINE
Energy therapies focus on either energy fields originating within the body (putative energy fields [biofields], which cannot be measured) or those from other sources that involve the use of measurable wavelengths and frequencies, also called electromagnetic fields). Examples of putative energy medicine include qi gong, reiki, intercessory prayer, and healing touch (NAMS, 2007).

---

et al., 2009; Kupferer, Dormire, & Becker, 2009; Nachtigall et al., 2006; Nelson et al., 2006).

Daily aerobic exercise helps to reduce the frequency and severity of hot flashes by assisting in body temperature regulation. Exercise is also beneficial in reducing cardiovascular disease and osteoporosis risk and helps to maintain normal glucose levels and weight. Midlife women who engage in regular exercise report a higher quality of life, and routine exercise can help to improve depression, muscular soreness or stiffness, palpitations, memory, and sleep quality (Alexander, 2009).

In 1998, the U.S. Congress established The National Center for Complementary and Alternative Medicine (NCCAM) at the National Institutes of Health to stimulate, develop, and support research on CAM for the benefit of the public. NCCAM was charged with providing the American public with reliable information about the safety and effectiveness of CAM practices. NCCAM groups CAM therapies into the following five major domains: Alternative Medical Systems, Mind-body Medicine, Manipulative and Body-based Methods, Energy Medicine, and Biologically-based Treatment (NAMS, 2007).

Alternative Medical Systems

Alternative medical systems include complete systems of theory and practice that have evolved independently of and often prior to the conventional biomedical approach. Many are traditional systems of medicine practiced by individual cultures throughout the world. Alternative medical systems, mind–body medicine, manipulative and body-based methods, and energy medicine are briefly described in Box 7-2.

 Nursing Insight— *Traditional Chinese medicine and menopause*

Traditional Chinese medicine (TCM) includes menopause as part of a phenomenon that involves an imbalance of body energy. The TCM practitioner may use herbs, meditative or breathing exercises, massage, or diet to help a woman restore and balance the energy and therefore reduce menopausal symptoms. TCM practitioners may also use acupuncture for treating symptoms associated with menopause (NAMS, 2007).

Biologically Based Treatments

Biologically based complementary and alternative medicines include biologically based practices, interventions, and products, many of which overlap with conventional medicine's use of dietary supplements. Botanical therapies are complex mixtures of preparations made from the whole plant or plant part, such as root, leaves, gum, resin, or essential oil. Most botanical therapies are medicinal herbs. A medicinal herb is a plant or plant part that produces and contains chemical substances that act upon the body (NAMS, 2007).

 Complementary Care: *Herbal therapies: Modes of administration*

Herbal therapies intended for ingestion may be administered in a variety of ways, such as:
- Tea infusions (soft, aromatic parts of the plant are steeped, not boiled, in water)

- Tea decoctions (barks and roots, boiled in water)
- Essential oils (highly concentrated)
- Tinctures and fluid extracts (herbs macerated into water-alcohol mixtures)
- Dried standardized extract (these typically contain part of a plant but can contain the whole plant; extracts are standardized to one ingredient only)
- Homeopathic preparations (extremely diluted) (NAMS, 2007)

The most studied of the botanicals for menopause-related conditions are compounds often termed *phytoestrogens* (sometimes called "dietary estrogens"). Phytoestrogens are a diverse group of naturally occurring nonsteroidal plant compounds that have a structural similarity with estradiol and are able to exert estrogenic and/or antiestrogenic effects. There are three principal groups of phytoestrogens: isoflavones, coumestans, and lignans. Because herbal compounds containing phytoestrogens are not FDA regulated, there is no proof of the efficacy, safety, or overall quality of the products. Until such information becomes available, these remedies should be considered to have the same issues as traditional menopausal hormone therapy (discussed later in this chapter) (Alexander, 2006; Alexander, 2007; Lake, 2007; McKee & Warber, 2005; NAMS, 2007).

 Be sure to— Advise women to use isoflavones with caution

Isoflavones (e.g., red clover, soy) are the most widely used phytoestrogens for menopause. Isoflavones comprise a class of organic compounds, often naturally occurring, related to the isoflavonoids. Some isoflavones and isoflavone-rich foods possess activity against cancer, including certain types of breast and prostate cancer. Isoflavones are produced almost exclusively by members of the bean family, and soybeans are the most common source of isoflavones in human food. Soy and other isoflavone supplements are regulated in the United States as dietary supplements; their effectiveness has not been well established, and they are not monitored for purity, amount of active ingredient, or health claims (Alexander, 2009; Geller & Studee, 2008; NAMS, 2007).

Phytoestrogens interact with estrogen receptors in the body. Foods that contain phytoestrogens include wild yams, cashews, peanuts and almonds, dandelion greens, apples, cherries, alfalfa sprouts, sage, black beans, and soy products (e.g., beans, flour, milk, sauce). The use of soy-rich foods has also been investigated as an alternative to hormone therapy for menopausal symptoms. According to the Natural Standard database, there is good evidence for sage and soy for menopause symptom management (http://www.naturalstandard.com/). NAMS concedes that soy products may have small benefits in the treatment of vasomotor symptoms in the short term (12 weeks), but not for longer periods (6 to 12 months). According to NAMS (2007), there is strong evidence that soy is non beneficial in the prevention of postmenopausal bone loss, but may be useful in maintaining cognitive function; however, additional studies are needed (Albertazzi, 2005; NAMS, 2007).

An important role for nurses centers on counseling women to become informed about any herbal preparations they are considering and to consult with their health-care providers before using any of them. Nurses should explain that before using any substance, it is important to understand the mechanisms of action, contraindications, and potential adverse effects. Herbs may be beneficial in resolving physical symptoms as well as mood swings and depression. To obtain current information about various dietary supplements, health professionals and consumers may consult various Internet sites such as those offered by the U.S. National Library of Medicine and the National Institutes of Health (http://www.nlm.nih.gov/medlineplus/dietarysupplements.html and http://www.nlm.nih.gov/medlineplus/druginformation.html) and the U.S. Department of Agriculture National Agricultural Library (http://fnic.nal.usda.gov/nal_display/index.php?info_center=4&tax_level=2&tax_subject=274&topic_id=1331). Nurses may also inform patients who wish to use soy, herbs, or other dietary supplements about ConsumerLab (http://www.consumerlab.com), an independent company that tests and provides objective reviews of many over-the-counter consumer supplements; there is an annual subscription fee to access the information (Alexander, 2009).

Oriental herbal teas composed of licorice, ginseng, sage, coptis, red raspberry leaf, and Chinese rhubarb may provide some relief for hot flashes. Dong quai and black cohosh have been used for various menopausal discomforts. Dong quai, the most commonly prescribed Chinese herbal medicine for "female problems," purportedly regulates and balances the menstrual cycle and is said to "strengthen the uterus." It is also purported to exert estrogenic activity. However, Dong quai has not been found to be useful in reducing hot flashes and is not recommended for this symptom. Also, Dong quai can trigger heavy uterine bleeding and should never be used by women who have fibroids, hemophilia, or other blood-clotting problems; it is contraindicated for use with anticoagulants (ACOG, 2001; Alexander, 2009; NAMS, 2007).

Black cohosh (*Cimicifuga racemosa*) may be helpful in the short-term (less than 2 years) treatment of menopausal symptoms, including hot flashes, sleep disorders, anxiety, and depression. Black cohosh is not recommended for women with a history of liver problems or for those using hepatotoxic medications. Both Dong quai and black cohosh have been investigated for effectiveness, with varying results. According to NCCAM (http://nccam.nih.gov/), there is very little high-quality scientific evidence about the effectiveness and long-term safety of complementary and alternative medicine for menopausal symptoms (ACOG, 2001; Alexander, 2009; Geller & Studee, 2008; NAMS, 2007).

Complementary Care: *St. John's wort, valerian, chasteberry, and ginseng*

St. John's wort and valerian root have been used for mood disturbances during menopause. The flower *hypericum perforatum,* known as St. John's wort, has been used for centuries to treat mild to moderate depression. Commercial preparations typically contain the generally recommended doses and one capsule is taken three times a day. Side effects are similar to, but much less than, those associated with standard antidepressant medications and include fatigue, dry mouth, dizziness, and constipation. St. John's wort should not be used concomitantly with psychotropic medications. Valerian root (*Valeriana officinalis*), has traditionally been used as a tranquilizer and soporific. Valerian improves subjective experiences of sleep when taken nightly for 1 to 2 weeks. Although it has no demonstrable toxicity, there have been reports of adverse reactions and visual disturbances. Little is known about the actions, effects, or potential interactions of valerian with other medications (ACOG, 2001; NAMS, 2007).

Some practitioners have recommended chasteberry and ginseng for menopausal loss of libido. Chasteberry, or vitex, is also known as Chaste tree, Monk's pepper, agnus castus, Indian spice, sage tree hemp, and tree wild pepper. It has been used for vaginal dryness at menopause and also for depression and to enhance libido in menopausal women. Asian ginseng (*Panax ginseng*) is promoted as an "adaptogen" that helps one cope with stress and boost immunity. Ginseng is also reputed to be an aphrodisiac, although this claim has not been substantiated by medical evidence (ACOG, 2001; NAMS, 2007). According to the Natural Standard database, there is poor evidence for ginseng and chasteberry in the treatment of menopausal symptoms. However, there is good evidence for both sage and soy in menopause symptom management.

 Now Can You— **Discuss various CAM therapies for menopausal symptoms?**

1. Identify and briefly describe three alternative medical systems?
2. Describe the major focus of mind–body medicine and identify six examples of typical techniques used with this approach?
3. Briefly explain the techniques of *intercessory prayer* and *healing touch*?
4. Provide appropriate counseling to a woman who wishes to use herbal products?

HORMONAL THERAPIES

Estrogen is the only pharmacologic therapy that is government approved in the United States and Canada for treating menopause-related symptoms. Estrogen-containing drugs for menopausal use are divided into two categories: estrogen therapy (ET) and combined estrogen-progestogen therapy (EPT) (NAMS, 2010a).

 Nursing Insight— NAMS menopausal hormone therapy terminology

Estrogen therapy (ET)—unopposed estrogen prescribed for postmenopausal women who have had a hysterectomy.
Estrogen plus progestogen (EPT)—a combination of estrogen and progestogen (either progesterone or progestin, synthetic forms of progesterone). Although the available data suggest that the benefits of EPT are almost exclusively due to the estrogen, progestogen reduces the risk of endometrial adenocarcinoma in women with a uterus—and this risk is significantly increased in women who use unopposed estrogen.

Hormone therapy (HT)—encompasses both ET and EPT. The FDA refers to EPT as HT.
Local therapy—vaginal ET administration that does not result in clinically significant systemic absorption.
Progestogen—encompasses both progesterone and progestin.
Systemic therapy—HT administration that results in absorption in the blood high enough to provide clinically significant results.
Timing of HT initiation—length of time after menopause when HT is initiated. (NAMS, 2010a)

Previously, the terms *estrogen replacement therapy* and *hormone replacement therapy* were used. However, according to NAMS, the term *replacement* is a misnomer because postmenopausal levels of HT provide only a small fraction of the estrogen the ovaries once produced. The FDA declared that "replacement" can no longer be used by marketers of products available in the United States. The FDA uses "ET" to describe unopposed estrogen therapy and "HT" to describe EPT. NAMS, however, prefers using "HT" to encompass all hormone therapy used for menopause and "EPT" to more clearly describe combined therapy (Bachmann, 2009; NAMS, 2007; Theroux, 2008).

Menopause hormone therapy (HT) is a controversial issue. A brief review of the historical background, recent research, and current guidelines for use of HT can assist women and their health-care providers in making the appropriate decisions concerning this treatment option.

Historical Background

The widespread practice of prescribing estrogen began in the 1960s. Estrogen was touted as a wonder drug that offered women the opportunity to age more slowly. By 1975, conjugated equine estrogen, marketed under the name of Premarin, was one of the most frequently prescribed drugs in the United States. Premarin is derived from the urine of pregnant mares. For many years, animal rights activists have promoted public awareness of cruelty to these animals and their offspring involved in the production of Premarin (National Women's Health Network, 2000).

In 1975, two studies were published that showed a 2- to 8-fold increase in the rate of uterine cancer among non-hysterectomized women receiving estrogen therapy. The risk was linked to estrogen dosage and the duration of treatment. In response to this finding, a number of women's organizations sought to heighten public awareness of the risks associated with estrogen use, claiming that women were not given adequate information to make informed choices. As this information became more widespread, use of estrogen in this country declined. Later studies were conducted to investigate combinations of estrogen and a progestin (a synthetic form of progesterone). Results of these studies revealed that the estrogen-progestin combination protected against precancerous changes of the uterine lining. Based on these findings, there was a shift to the use of estrogen-progestin combinations (National Women's Health Network, 2000).

By the late 1980s, results of several studies had shown that women who received estrogen were less likely to suffer heart attacks than those who did not receive estrogen. Although the FDA refused to grant the manufacturer approval for promoting estrogen as a heart disease preventive, many clinicians were recommending estrogen for this purpose. The combination of estrogen along with a progestin also began to be prescribed for this same purpose, even though the combination had not been in use long enough to evaluate its effect on heart disease. The Postmenopausal Estrogen/Progestin Interventions (PEPI) study, published in 1995, showed that the most commonly used progestin, medroxyprogesterone acetate (Provera), greatly interfered with the positive effect of estrogen alone on high-density lipoprotein (HDL) levels. Natural progesterone (i.e., oral micronized progesterone), also used in the study, did not negate the positive effects of estrogen on HDL levels (National Women's Health Network, 2000). Major findings from more recent studies, including the Heart and Estrogen/Progestin Replacement Study (HERS I and II), the Nurse's Health Study, and the Women's Health Initiative (WHI) are summarized in Box 7-3.

Menopausal Hormone Therapy: Considerations and Choices

Owing to the findings from large-scale prospective clinical trials such as the WHI, which demonstrated that hormone therapy is not without risks, the FDA and several professional organizations recommend prescribing the lowest effective dose for the shortest duration of time consistent with treatment goals for the individual patient. Growing evidence indicates that the benefits and risks vary with the type of estrogen and progestogen prescribed, as well as the route of administration, timing of therapy, baseline risk of disease, chronological age, age at menopause, cause of menopause, time since menopause, and previous use of

---

Box 7-3 **Major Findings From The HERS and WHI Studies**

THE HEART AND ESTROGEN/PROGESTIN REPLACEMENT STUDY (HERS), THE HEART AND ESTROGEN/PROGESTIN REPLACEMENT STUDY FOLLOW-UP (HERS II), AND THE NURSE'S HEALTH STUDY

- Designed to assess the relationship between hormone therapy (HT) and coronary artery disease events among postmenopausal women.
- Although findings from the HERS II study showed that HT did not provide cardiac protection in women who had previously been diagnosed with heart disease, re-analysis of data indicated that certain women (e.g., women on statin medications to lower cholesterol) experienced fewer problems associated with thromboembolic events (Alexander, 2007).

THE WOMEN'S HEALTH INITIATIVE (WHI)

- A long-term primary prevention trial conducted with 25,000 healthy postmenopausal women.
- Purpose: To evaluate the safety and effectiveness of estrogen as well as an estrogen/progestin combination given to healthy women over a 9-year period beginning in 1993, with final analysis planned for 2005.
- Designed to assess the major benefits and risks of hormone therapy with regard to coronary heart disease, venous thrombotic events, breast cancer, colon cancer, and fractures.
- Quality of life issues, such as a reduction in hot flashes and vaginal dryness, were not included (Secor & Simon, 2006).
- In July, 2002, after approximately 5 years of follow-up, the estrogen and progestin arm of the WHI trial was halted because the predetermined boundary for invasive breast cancer was exceeded. At this time, it was concluded that the risks outweighed the benefits for the indicators that were being studied.
- The risk of cardiovascular disease, coronary heart disease, stroke, and venous thromboembolism was increased as well (Theroux, 2008; Writing Group for the Women's Health Initiative Investigators, 2002).
- There was a 37% and a 24% decrease in colorectal cancer and total fractures, respectively.
- Of importance, there was no difference in rates of mortality between the two groups (i.e., those who did receive HT and those who did not receive HT).
- In 2004, the estrogen-only trial was also halted because the risk with the conjugated equine estrogen (Premarin) for stroke was elevated and the other endpoints were unlikely to change with continuation of the trial (Burdette et al., 2009; Hsia et al., 2006; Secor & Simon, 2006).
- Later analysis of the findings suggested that timing of hormone therapy use has an effect: In the age 50 to 59 cohort, coronary heart disease was decreased. Based on this information, it is believed to be safest to begin hormone therapy within 10 years of menopause.
- Another follow-up study of the WHI participants demonstrated that women ages 50 to 59 who were on estrogen therapy had lower amounts of calcium deposits in their coronary arteries.

Sources: Alexander, 2007; Dranov, 2007; Secor & Simon, 2006; Williams & Brownlee, 2010; Writing Group for the Women's Health Initiative Investigators, 2002.

---

where research and practice meet:
Considerations of the WHI Research Results

Findings from the WHI research may be used to guide patient education and counseling. Nurses should consider the following points (ACOG, 2007; Burdette et al., 2009; Secor & Simon, 2006; Theroux, 2008; Utian, 2008):

The HT arm of the WHI trial was stopped because the rate of breast cancer crossed a predetermined boundary set at the initiation of the trial. However, breast cancer rates had not reached statistical significance when the trial was halted.

The fact that that the slight increase in invasive breast cancer was noted during the fourth year of the study, along with the trend toward a later decrease in the total number of breast cancer cases, suggests that HT promotes the growth of existing breast cancer, rather than causes breast cancer. No increased risk in breast cancer was seen among women on estrogen therapy for an average of 7.1 years. Estrogen-progestin therapy, and to a lesser extent, estrogen therapy, increases breast cell proliferation, breast pain, and mammographic density. Hormone therapy may impede the diagnostic interpretation of mammograms. Women with risk factors for breast cancer (e.g., positive family history, early puberty, late parity) should be individually assessed before initiating HT for the relief of moderate to severe vasomotor symptoms.

For the first time in terms of any therapy, findings from the WHI study indicated that HT reduces hip fractures and colon cancer.

---

any hormone (Altman, 2008, 2009; Bachmann, 2009; Berga, 2009; Sherman, 2009a; Gersh, 2009; Nachtigall, 2009). A summary of NAMS (2010a) recommendations concerning HT for the treatment of various menopausal symptoms is presented in Box 7-4.

Today, clinicians have a wide variety of estrogen products from which to choose, including oral tablets; transdermal patches; and topical sprays, gels, and lotions, as well

Box 7-4　Summary of NAMS 2010 Recommendations for HT Use

Vasomotor symptoms: Moderate to severe vasomotor symptoms (e.g., hot flashes, night sweats) remain the primary indication for HT; it is also the best treatment for moderate to severe vulvar and vaginal atrophy; local vaginal ET is recommended for treating urogenital atrophy alone; systemic or local ET can relieve dyspareunia.

Osteoporosis: Extended HT is an option for women with decreased bone mass; benefits decrease quickly once therapy has ended.

Coronary heart disease (CHD): HT is not recommended as a sole or primary indication for coronary protection at any age; starting ET alone soon after menopause may slow development of calcified atherosclerotic plaque and lower CHD risk.

Stroke: HT is not recommended for primary or secondary prevention of stroke.

Venous thromboembolism (VTE): Most likely an increased risk of VTE with oral HT, especially in women with a history of VTE or factor V Leiden (a hypercoagulability disorder).

Diabetes mellitus: Inadequate evidence to recommend HT as the sole or primary indication for preventing diabetes in perimenopausal or post-menopausal women.

Endometrial cancer: Women with an intact uterus taking systemic ET should take concomitant progestogen to counteract the risk of endometrial cancer; HT is not recommended for women with a history of endometrial cancer.

Breast cancer: Diagnosis of breast cancer increases with EPT use longer than 3 to 5 years; women who start EPT shortly after menopause may have a greater risk than women who start more than 5 years afterward; ET use in breast cancer survivors has not been proven to be safe and may be associated with an increased risk of recurrence.

Ovarian cancer: Data on HT and ovarian cancer conflict; the association between ovarian cancer and HT beyond 5 years is rare.

Cognitive aging and dementia: HT is not recommended for the sole or primary indication of preventing cognitive aging or dementia or to enhance cognitive function in younger postmenopausal patients with intact ovaries.

Mood and depression: Although HT might have a positive effect on mood and behavior, HT is not an antidepressant and should not be considered as such; evidence is insufficient to support HT use for the treatment of depression.

Sources: Altman, 2009; Bachmann, 2009; Burdette, Moore, Speroff, & Wysocki, 2009; Freeman, 2009; Helmrich, 2010; Hess, London, Moore, & Simon, 2009; Henderson, 2009; Margolis, 2010; NAMS, 2010a; Utian, 2008.

Box 7-5　Examples of Estrogen and Progestogen Products for Menopause-Related Symptoms

ESTROGEN ONLY
Estrace (oral tablet, vaginal cream)
Femtrace (oral tablet)
Ogen (oral tablet)
Premarin (oral tablet, vaginal cream)
Estraderm, Vivelle, Climara (transdermal patch)
Divigel, EstroGel (transdermal gel)
Femring, Estring (vaginal ring)
Vagifem (vaginal tablet)
Evamist (topical spray)

PROGESTOGEN ONLY
Provera (oral tablet)
Prometrium (oral tablet)

ESTROGEN-PROGESTOGEN COMBINATIONS
CombiPatch (transdermal patch)
Climara Pro (transdermal patch)
Femhrt (oral tablet)
Prempro (oral tablet)

protection, osteoporosis prevention, short- and long-term hormone use, and alternatives to HT. Women who are taking or considering HT only for the prevention of cardiovascular disease should be counseled about other strategies to lower their risks of heart disease.

 Nursing Insight— **Hormone therapy and heart disease**

According to the American College of Obstetricians and Gynecologists (ACOG) (2008) and the North American Menopause Society (NAMS) (2010a), menopausal HT should not at present be used for the primary or secondary prevention of coronary heart disease. Recent analyses suggest that HT may not increase CHD (coronary heart disease) risk for select populations of women who have experienced menopause recently. Hormone therapy should be limited to the treatment of menopausal symptoms at the lowest effective dosage over the shortest duration possible and continued use should be reevaluated on a periodic basis.

as vaginal creams, tablets, and rings. The choice of therapy is often based on patient preference. Examples of estrogen and progestogen products for menopause-related symptoms are presented in Box 7-5; NAMS has prepared charts for health-care providers that include information about all estrogen and progestogen products that are currently available in the United States and Canada. The charts may be viewed at http://www.menopause.org/edumaterials/hormoneprimer.aspx (Bachmann, 2009; Margolis, 2010; NAMS, 2010a; Theroux, 2008; Utian, 2008; Utian, Archer, Bachmann, et al., 2008).

The Nursing Role in Menopausal Hormone Therapy Counseling

When counseling women about HT benefits and risks, it is helpful to consider a number of factors, such as cardiac

Women who are taking HT only for the prevention of osteoporosis should be assessed for their personal osteoporosis risk and should be advised to consult with their health-care provider about continuing HT for this purpose. There are many alternatives (i.e., bisphosphonates, calcitonin) that should be considered for women whose only need for HT is the prevention of osteoporosis (ACOG, 2004; Alexander, 2007; Bachmann, 2009; Dranov, 2007; National Osteoporosis Foundation [NOF], 2008; Secor & Simon, 2006). (See discussion of osteoporosis later in this chapter.)

For women who seek short-term (1 to 4 years) relief of menopausal symptoms, the benefits of HT most likely outweigh the risks. Although certain symptoms such as hot flashes and night sweats tend to be of short duration for most women, other menopausal symptoms such as vaginal dryness generally continue throughout the post-menopausal period. Also, many women believe that estrogen helps them to feel, think, and sleep better. These women may conclude that for them, the added benefits of fracture prevention and colon cancer reduction associated with HT outweigh the risks. Nurses may share information about alternatives to HT, such as the use of vaginal lubricants, and strategies for relief from sleep disturbances (Ruhl, 2010). However, the decision to continue with long-term HT is one that must be made on an individual basis following consideration of each woman's benefits and risks, including those benefits and risks that were not addressed in the WHI study.

Large randomized controlled trials, including the WHI, have suggested that hormone therapy reduces the incidence of diabetes among postmenopausal women. The reason for this benefit is unknown, although it may be related to lower weight gain or reduced insulin resistance among women using HT. However, there is inadequate evidence to recommend hormone therapy solely for diabetes prevention in perimenopausal women. Also, it is important to bear in mind that the WHI studied only one preparation of HT. Hence, data generated from the WHI study cannot be applied to all HT therapies. An important role for nurses who care for midlife women involves providing them with current evidence-based information about HT along with culturally appropriate resources for promoting menopausal health (Alexander, 2007; Dranov, 2007; NAMS, 2010a; Secor & Simon, 2006).

Estrogens do not cause endometrial cancer, as long as an appropriate dosage of progestogen (either as progestin or progesterone) is added to the hormonal regimen. Individual regimens and formulations differ and include both synthetic and natural formulations, and each route and type of progestogen carries different effects, risks, and benefits. Evidence shows that women who use combined HT are no more likely than those who have never used HT to develop overgrowth (hyperplasia) of the endometrium or endometrial cancer (LaCroix, 2005; Liu, 2007; NAMS, 2010a; Secor & Simon, 2006).

❝What to say❞ — *Counseling patients about bleeding symptoms when systemic HT is first initiated*

Nurses should educate women who plan to initiate HT about certain symptoms, such as vaginal spotting and unscheduled bleeding, that often occur as the body adapts to a new hormonal milieu. Nurses may offer the following information:

- Vaginal bleeding and spotting are most likely to occur in the first 3 months after initiation of therapy.

- Follow-up visits should be scheduled at 1 and 3 months—and improvement in symptoms should be noted at that time.

- It is important to promptly report the following symptoms: persistent bleeding, bleeding that stops but then starts again, or the presence of blood clots in the vaginal discharge (Liu, 2007).

Evidence that the risk of depression is higher in early menopause is mixed. Although two small randomly controlled trials found that short-term estrogen therapy is effective for the treatment of affected perimenopausal women, another trial found no such benefit for depressed older postmenopausal women. Presently, there is insufficient evidence for using hormone therapy to treat depression in general (Dranov, 2007). Also, despite earlier findings, no evidence has been generated to support the use of hormone therapy to prevent dementia or cognitive decline. Beginning estrogen-progestogen therapy after age 65 for these reasons may actually increase the risk of dementia within the subsequent 5 years. Studies that investigated whether dementia can be prevented in women who begin hormone therapy during the menopause transition or early postmenopause period provided insufficient evidence of help or harm. Estrogen therapy does not appear to have any effect on Alzheimer's disease (Gies & Lessick, 2009; Dranov, 2007). The U.S. Preventive Services Task Force (USPSTF) and ACOG advise against the use of HT to improve cognition or to prevent or treat dementia (ACOG, 2004b; Alexander, 2007; USPSTF, 2009).

Educating Patients About Hormone Therapy Options

In general, transdermal estrogen (estradiol) provides the same relief of menopausal symptoms as do the oral preparations but without the side effects of breast tenderness or fluid retention. Transdermal estradiol delivery systems have been shown to be safer than oral administration in reducing certain markers of cardiovascular risk. Since the hormones bypass the liver and are directly absorbed into the bloodstream, transdermal administration is more effective in maintaining stable blood levels of estrogen. Also, because the transdermal estradiol is absorbed directly into the body, first-pass metabolism by the gastrointestinal tract and liver is avoided. When given orally, larger doses of estrogen are required to achieve therapeutic levels and to offset metabolism by the liver and inactivation by the gut wall. In addition, when compared with the transdermal formulations, oral estrogen therapy has been shown to increase the risk of venous thromboembolic disease (Altman, 2009; Dranov, 2007; Secor & Simon, 2006; Shulman, 2008).

No large studies have compared the advantages and disadvantages of the different transdermal formulations. The patch, applied one or two times a week to a hairless area of the skin, is considerably more irritating to the skin than either the gel or emulsion. Also, the gel and the emulsion are more discrete than the patch. To use the gel or emulsion, the patient applies the product to clean, dry, intact skin at the same time each day. The emulsion is applied to the complete surface of both legs once a day; the gel is applied to one upper arm and shoulder once a day. An estradiol transdermal spray, now available, is applied to a small area on the inner forearm once daily; the dose can be increased to two or three sprays as needed for symptom control. The application site should be allowed to dry for 2 minutes before it is covered with clothing and the site should not be washed for 30 minutes after application. When applying two or three sprays, the applicator cone should be placed adjacent to, but not overlapping, the area of the previous administration. All of these products should be used for the shortest possible period of time and require 4 to 12 weeks before relief of symptoms is obtained (Altman, 2009; Minkin, 2010; Secor & Simon, 2006; Shulman, 2008).

Nurses can empower women with current evidence-based information about contraindications, risks, and side effects of various hormone therapies. Providing this information helps guide patients to make appropriate, informed decisions. The risks and side effects of estrogen and progestogen are presented in Box 7-6.

 Be sure to— Be knowledgeable of the contraindications to estrogen

Nurses who care for patients who use estrogen therapy must be knowledgeable of the absolute contraindications to estrogen. These include the following:

- Known or suspected estrogen-dependent cancer
- Known, suspected, or history of breast cancer except in appropriately selected patients being treated for metastatic disease
- Undiagnosed abnormal genital bleeding
- Active or history of deep venous thrombosis, pulmonary embolism
- Active or recent (within the past year) arterial thrombo-embolic disease (e.g., stroke, myocardial infarction)
- Liver dysfunction or disease
- Known or suspected pregnancy
- Known hypersensitivity to ET/EPT
(NAMS, 2007; Reiter, 2009)

 Optimizing Outcomes— Using the NAMS 2010 position statement to guide care

The North American Menopause Society's evidenced-based 2010 Position Statement emphasizes recent data on breast cancer, cognitive aging/decline and dementia, coronary heart disease, stroke, and discontinuation of therapy. It also includes new sections on ovarian and lung cancer. The full text is available on the NAMS Web site at http://www.menopause.org/PSHT10.pdf.

Bioidentical Compounds

The term *bioidentical hormones* was introduced by Jonathan Wright, MD, a practitioner who used the term to communicate his still unsubstantiated claim that plant-derived hormones are "identical" in molecular structure to human hormones. When used to describe hormones, "bioidentical" simply means chemically indistinguishable from the hormones produced in a woman's body (e.g., estradiol-17β and progesterone) during her reproductive years. Numerous FDA-approved drugs contain these hormones and therefore are also "bioidentical" (Box 7-7) (ACOG, 2005; Alexander, 2006, 2007; Altman, 2008, 2009; Burkman, 2009; Dranov, 2007; NAMS, 2010a; Rosenthal, 2008, 2009; Secor & Simon, 2006).

Compounded bioidentical hormones are plant-derived hormones (e.g., from wild yam or soy) that are prepared by a pharmacist and can be custom-made for a patient according to a physician's specifications. Bioidentical compounds have been promoted as a natural approach; the claim is that

---

Box 7-6 Risks and Side Effects of Estrogen and Progestogen

RISKS OF ESTROGEN

Breast cancer

Endometrial cancer

Increased risk of stroke

Small increase in the risk of venous thromboembolism

Possible small increase in the risk of coronary events

Worsening of hypertriglyceridemia

Possible worsening of gallbladder disease

Deterioration of liver function in women with severe liver disease

Worsening of edema in women with severe cardiac disease

Worsening of pain from benign breast disease

Increased risk of gallbladder disease

SIDE EFFECTS OF ESTROGEN

Worsening of estrogen-dependent conditions, such as uterine fibroids and endometriosis

Increase in fibrocystic breast problems

Vaginal bleeding

Hypertension

Nausea and vomiting

Headaches, jaundice, and fluid retention

Impaired glucose tolerance

Changes in the shape of the cornea (sometimes leading to contact lens intolerance)

SIDE EFFECTS OF PROGESTOGEN

Fluid retention

Breast tenderness

Jaundice

Nausea

Insomnia

Depression

Menstrual bleeding

Sources: Altman, 2009; NAMS, 2007; Reiter, 2009.

Box 7-7 FDA-Approved Pharmaceutical Bioidentical Hormone Preparations

- Oral estradiol (Estrace, Femtrace)
- Estradiol transdermal patches (Alora, Climara, Esclim, Estraderm, Menostar, Vivelle, Vivelle-dot)
- Estradiol transdermal gel (Divigel, Elestrin, EstroGel)
- Estradiol spray (Evamist)
- Estradiol topical emulsion (Estrasorb)
- Vaginal estradiol cream (Estrace) and ring (Estring, Femring)
- Progesterone as oral micronized progesterone (Prometrium) and vaginal gel (Crinone)
- Estradiol patches are available in combination with a synthetically produced progestin; no combination bioidentical preparations are on the market.

Sources: Minkin, 2010; Moore, 2010; Weil, 2009.

they replace specific hormones that are naturally present in a woman's body. Because the only truly natural source of human estradiol is the human ovary, all plant sources must be processed to synthesize estradiol. Therefore, all bioidentical products are, in actuality, synthetic (ACOG, 2005; Alexander, 2006, 2007; Altman, 2008, 2009; Burkman, 2009; Dranov, 2007; Moore, 2010; NAMS, 2010a; Secor & Simon, 2006; Weil, 2009).

Many bioidentical replacement hormones are compounded in private laboratories or pharmacies as individualized made-to-order products. The hormones prepared by a compounding pharmacist are not regulated and FDA approved. Women need to be made aware of the limitations and poor results that may be associated with this therapy (ACOG, 2005; Alexander, 2006, 2007; Altman, 2008, 2009; Dranov, 2007; Minkin, 2010; NAMS, 2010a; Secor & Simon, 2006). However, certain bioidentical preparations of estrogen or progestin are approved by the FDA for oral, intravaginal, transdermal, or percutaneous applications. These particular medications have undergone strenuous testing for safety, efficacy, and quality control. *Compounded* bioidentical formulations are not FDA-regulated in the same way. These products are not subject to rigorous testing or quality control standards. Also, the compounded products do not include a package insert that lists important contraindications, warnings, and precautions—which may make them appear to be safer than traditional therapy medications. These products lack standardization and in many cases, the specific active ingredients and minimally effective dosages are not known (ACOG, 2005; Alexander, 2006, 2007; Altman, 2008, 2009; Altman, Moore, Speroff, & Wysocki, 2009; Moore, 2010; NAMS, 2010a).

 Nursing Insight— *Being wary of compounded bioidentical hormone formulations is warranted*

Custom-made HT formulations, called *bioidentical hormone therapy,* or BHT, are compounded for an individual according to a health-care provider's prescription. Often touted as "natural," in actuality, bioidentical hormones are all synthesized, making terms such as *natural* and *nonsynthetic* inaccurate and meaningless. The American College of Obstetricians and Gynecologists (ACOG) and the North American Menopause Society (NAMS) consider the bioidentical hormone preparations to have the same safety risks as traditional hormone therapy and assert that they may carry additional risks associated with the compounding process. In addition, evidence-based data supporting the efficacy of bioidentical compounded preparations are lacking. The risks, benefits, and quality of these products have not been evaluated through rigorous testing, a standard requirement for traditional hormone therapy medications (ACOG, 2005; Alexander, 2007; Altman, 2008, 2009; NAMS, 2010a; Secor & Simon, 2006).

These products are custom compounded to "normalize" a woman's hormone levels. However, natural levels of estrone, estradiol, and other hormones are in constant flux, so they are impossible to normalize. Procedures such as having personal hormone levels measured via blood tests or saliva tests as a basis for compounding "individualized" HT products are expensive and useless; no scientific data exist to indicate what these levels should be (Altman, 2008, 2009; Altman, Moore, Speroff, & Wysocki, 2009; NAMS, 2010a).

 Across Care Settings: ETIQ, an estrogen therapy awareness campaign

In late 2010, the National Association of Nurse Practitioners in Women's Health (NPWH) launched ETIQ, a Web site, http://www.ETIQ.info, created to empower women with credible information about menopause and advances in estrogen therapy. The campaign was inspired by findings from a recent (2010) survey that revealed women were unaware of the differences between FDA-approved estrogen therapies and those that are compounded at the pharmacy level. The goal of the ETIQ campaign is to heighten awareness of bioidentical estrogen options that are FDA approved so that women can make more informed choices about how best to manage the symptoms of menopause. NPWH hopes to enhance awareness of the advances in new delivery methods of estrogen, such as transdermals, in the form of gels, sprays, and creams, which may be preferred options for some women. The organization also hopes to help women become aware that FDA-approved estrogen therapies are tightly monitored for safety and efficacy whereas compounded estrogen formulations are not.

NONHORMONAL PRESCRIPTION MEDICATIONS

Women who experience debilitating vasomotor symptoms and wish to avoid traditional hormone therapy (HT) may be willing to try certain prescription medications, including antidepressants, belladonna alkaloid preparations, anticonvulsants, or antihypertensive agents.

 Nursing Insight— *Nonhormonal medications for vasomotor symptoms*

Various nonhormonal medications have been prescribed for the relief of severe vasomotor symptoms. Antidepressant agents known as selective serotonin reuptake inhibitors (SSRIs), including fluoxetine (Prozac), paroxetine (Paxil), citalopram (Celexa), escitalopram (Lexapro), and sertraline (Zoloft), and serotonin/norepinephrine reuptake inhibitors (SNRIs), including venlafaxine (Effexor), and desvenlafaxine (Pristiq), may reduce hot flashes (Kupferer, Dormire, & Becker, 2009). However, studies that compared the efficacy of venlafaxine with that of medroxyprogesterone acetate (MPA, a progestational agent) found that a single dose of MPA alleviated hot flashes more effectively than did daily use of the antidepressant (Alexander, 2007; Hess, London, Moore, & Simon, 2009; Loprinzi et al., 2006).

Belladona alkaloid preparation is a combination of phenobarbital, caffeine, and belladonna. This medication may be useful for certain women with sleep-related vasomotor symptoms. However, this agent is contraindicated with a number of other medications and may interact with many other substances, including acetaminophen, alcohol, antacids, certain antibiotics, digoxin, metronidazole, and warfarin (Alexander, 2007).

In some women, clonidine (Catapres), an antihypertensive medication, and gabapentin (Neurontin), an anticonvulsant, have been useful in controlling hot flashes (Hess, London, Moore, & Simon, 2009; Minarik, 2010).

Now Can You— Discuss certain aspects of menopausal hormone therapy?

1. Identify the NAMS recommendations for HT use for the following conditions: vasomotor symptoms, osteoporosis, coronary heart disease, diabetes mellitus, and cognitive functioning?
2. Explain why a progestogen may be appropriate for a patient who wishes to use HT?
3. Counsel a patient about the proper use of various transdermal formulations?
4. Explain what is meant by the term *bioidentical hormones?*

Cardiovascular Disease

Cardiovascular disease (CVD) is the number-one killer of older American women; the diagnosis of heart disease presents a greater challenge in women than in men. This disease includes coronary heart disease (CHD), stroke, congestive heart failure (CHF), hypertension, and other diseases of the heart and vascular system. Over the past few decades, improved prevention and treatment have reduced the annual number of CVD deaths in men, but not in women. Cardiovascular disease is a particularly important problem among minority women. The death rate due to CVD is substantially higher in African American women than in Caucasian women. Despite the heightened public awareness of cardiovascular disease in women, the majority of women in this country continue to underestimate their risk of dying as a result of CVD (American Heart Association [AHA], 2010).

 Nursing Insight— Women and cardiovascular disease

Compared to men, many women before the age of menopause appear to be partly protected from coronary heart disease, heart attack, and stroke. As women age, their risk of heart disease and stroke begins to rise and keeps rising. The reasons for the lower incidence of coronary heart disease and stroke in younger women are not clear. Results from clinical trials have shown that estrogen therapy alone or in combination with progestin does not protect from heart disease or stroke. The American Heart Association does not advise women to undertake postmenopausal hormone therapy to reduce the risk of coronary heart disease or stroke (AHA, 2010).

Cardiovascular disease is a chronic, degenerative disease. While the exact mechanisms are not well understood, it is known that there is deterioration in arterial wall elasticity due to the deposition of plaque containing cholesterol and other compounds. The plaque formation may result from attempts by the body to repair damage to the lining of blood vessels. Blood flow is slowed through the narrowed areas, and clots tend to form around the deposits, causing further occlusion of the vessels (AHA, 2010).

According to the American Heart Association, the risk of heart disease and stroke increases with age. CVD ranks first among all disease categories in hospital discharges for women, and nearly 38% of all female deaths in this country occur from coronary heart disease, hypertension, stroke, congestive heart failure, and other cardiovascular diseases.

The risk of heart disease and stroke increases with age, and in the year 2006, more than 36 million American women were 55 and older. More women than men die of stroke. Interestingly, low blood levels of "good" cholesterol (high density lipoprotein or HDL) appear to be a stronger predictor of heart disease death in women than in men in the over-65 age group. High blood levels of triglycerides (another type of fat) may be a particularly important risk factor in women and the elderly (AHA, 2010).

THE AMERICAN HEART ASSOCIATION GUIDELINES FOR WOMEN

The AHA 2007 Guidelines for Preventing Cardiovascular Disease in Women emphasize that health-care professionals should focus on women's lifetime heart disease risk, rather than just the short-term risk. This approach underscores the importance of healthy lifestyles in women of all ages to reduce the long-term risk of heart and blood vessel diseases. The new guidelines for risk assessment include personal risk factors and family history, as well as the Framingham Risk Score, which estimates the risk of developing CHD within 10 years. The guidelines include expanded recommendations on lifestyle factors such as physical activity, nutrition, and smoking cessation, as well as specific recommendations on drug treatments for blood pressure and cholesterol control (AHA, 2010; McNeal & Birchem, 2009a; Mosca et al., 2007; Wenger, 2007).

 Nursing Insight— The Framingham Risk Score (FRS) and the Reynolds Risk Score (RRS)

Some experts have expressed concerns about the utility of the Framingham Risk Score (FRS) for women, pointing out that it does not reflect the risk of developing "soft" endpoints that are more common in women, such as stroke, angina, or need for coronary revascularization. Furthermore, the 10-year risk projection in the FRS may underestimate a woman's risk for developing CHD because women tend to live longer than men, resulting in an increased lifetime risk even if one risk factor is left untreated. To address these concerns, the Reynolds Risk Score (RRS) has recently been introduced, and it may be a superior indicator of CVD risk, especially in postmenopausal women. The Reynolds Score measures the same risk factors as the FRS but also includes family history, glycosylated hemoglobin value, and high sensitivity C-Reactive Protein (hs-CRP) levels (a biomarker associated with subclinical inflammation). Patients and health-care providers may learn more about the RRS by visiting http://www.reyoldsriskscore.org/ or http://www.hearthealthywomen.org/index.php?view=article&id=90&Itemid=1&option=com_content (Blumenthal, Michos, & Nasir, 2007; McNeal & Birchem, 2009a; Ridker, Buring, Rifai, & Cook, 2007).

The new guidelines state that the use of unregulated dietary supplements is not a proven method of preventing heart disease. Research that has become available since the last guidelines were developed suggests that health-care providers should consider recommending aspirin to women over age 65 to prevent stroke. For women younger than age 65, routine use of aspirin is not recommended to prevent myocardial infarction (MI), owing to an increased risk of cerebral and gastrointestinal bleeding. In addition, health-care providers should avoid the use of menopausal therapies such as hormone therapy or selective estrogen receptor modulators (SERMs) (e.g., raloxifene, tamoxifen) to prevent heart disease because they have been shown to be ineffective in protecting the heart and may, in fact, increase the risk of a stroke. Estrogen plus progestin can increase the risk of MI, breast cancer, venous thromboembolism, stroke, dementia, and ovarian cancer. In women who have undergone hysterectomy, estrogen alone confers a risk of stroke and dementia/memory loss. Likewise, no cardiovascular benefit has been shown for SERMs (AHA, 2010; Flores & Taylor, 2010; McNeal & Birchem, 2009b; Manson, 2009; Mosca et al., 2007; Wenger, 2007).

 Optimizing Outcomes— **With AHA Guidelines for women's heart health**

The AHA Guidelines for women include the following:

* Recommended lifestyle changes to help manage blood pressure include weight control; increased physical activity; alcohol moderation; sodium restriction; and an emphasis on eating fresh fruits, vegetables, and low-fat dairy products.
* Besides advising women to stop smoking, the 2007 guidelines recommend counseling, nicotine replacement, or other forms of smoking cessation therapy.
* Physical activity recommendations for women who need to lose weight or sustain weight loss include a minimum of 60 to 90 minutes of moderate-intensity activity (e.g., brisk walking) on most, and preferably all, days of the week.
* All women should be encouraged to reduce the intake of saturated fats to less than 7% of calories.
* All women should be encouraged to consume oily fish at least twice a week, and women with heart disease should consider taking a capsule supplement of 850 to 1000 mg of EPA (eicosapentaenoic acid) and DHA (docosahexaenoic acid) (2 to 4 grams for women with high triglycerides).
* Women at high risk for CVD should consider taking 325 mg of aspirin per day.
* Antioxidant supplements such as vitamins E, C, and beta-carotene should not be used for primary or secondary prevention of CVD.
* Folic acid should not be used to prevent CVD.
(AHA, 2010; Manson, 2009)

 where research and practice meet: **Women's Awareness of Heart Disease and Stroke**

Christian, Rosamond, White, and Mosca (2007) conducted a study to evaluate trends in women's awareness, knowledge, and perceptions related to cardiovascular disease since 1997, when the American Heart Association initiated a national campaign for women. An interviewer-assisted questionnaire was used to assess CVD awareness, knowledge, and perceptions among a nationally representative sample of 1005 women. Their findings indicated that while CVD awareness has increased significantly among women since 1997, the racial/ethnic gap in awareness has not narrowed. Based on their research, the investigators call for educational efforts to increase heart disease and stroke awareness that target racial/ethnic minorities, especially Hispanics.

 Across Care Settings: **The AHA Go Red For Women movement**

In 2004, the American Heart Association launched its multitiered marketing campaign, the "Go Red for Women" movement, to raise women's awareness of their risk for heart disease and empower them to take charge of their heart health. In 2010, the AHA set a strategic goal of reducing death and disability from cardiovascular disease and strokes by 20% while improving the cardiovascular health of all Americans by 20% by the year 2020. Nurses and patients can obtain accurate, up-to-date information about heart disease and stroke and the "Go Red for Women" movement by calling 1-888-MY-HEART or by visiting http://www.goredforwomen.org/.

 Be sure to— **Teach women about heart attack warning signs**

As with men, women's most common heart attack symptom is chest pain or discomfort. But women are somewhat more likely than men to experience some of the other common symptoms, particularly shortness of breath, nausea and vomiting, and back, neck, tooth, or jaw pain. Atypical symptoms that have been reported include fatigue, weakness of the arms or shoulders, dizziness, gaslike pain, indigestion, pain between the shoulder blades, restlessness, and a feeling of impending doom (AHA, 2010; Vassar, 2009).

RISK FACTORS FOR CVD

Women are considered to be at high risk for cardiovascular disease if they have established CVD or CHD, peripheral artery disease, cerebrovascular disease, chronic renal disease, or diabetes mellitus. Other risk factors for coronary disease are listed in Box 7-8.

Fortunately, many of the major CVD risk factors can be significantly modified through therapeutic lifestyle changes

Box 7-8 Risk Factors for Cardiovascular Disease

Increasing age (about 83% of people who die of CHD are 65 or older)

Heredity (including race). Children of parents with heart disease are more likely to develop it themselves. African Americans have more severe high blood pressure than do Caucasians and a higher risk of heart disease. Heart disease is also higher among Mexican Americans, Native Americans, native Hawaiians and some Asian Americans—and this is partly due to higher rates of obesity and diabetes in these populations.

Cigarette smoking

Obesity

Elevated serum cholesterol levels

Metabolic syndrome

Hypertension (often related to the use of alcohol, cigarettes, excessive sodium, and obesity)

Other modifiable factors such as a high-fat diet, sedentary lifestyle, stressful lifestyle

Sources: Mosca et al., 2007; Ruhl, 2009; Vassar, 2009.

and pharmacotherapy. Modifiable risk factors include smoking, hyperlipidemia, diabetes mellitus (DM), hypertension (HTN), and obesity. Educating women about strategies to control these five risk factors can empower them to make the changes that can greatly reduce their lifetime risk for CVD.

Smoking has been associated with early CVD events and doubles the risk of developing CVD by age 70. Nurses can encourage women to avoid both cigarette smoking and secondhand exposure to environmental tobacco smoke. When discussing smoking cessation strategies, it may be useful to identify and address barriers to smoking cessation, such as a fear of weight gain, a lack of support, a lack of interest, and a long-standing use of smoking as a stress reliever (Vassar, 2009).

 Optimizing Outcomes— **Medications to treat tobacco dependence**

Patients may benefit from medications to treat tobacco dependence. These include bupropion (Wellbutrin, Zyban), supplemental nicotine (Nicoderm CQ, Nicorette), varenicline (Chantix), clonidine (Catapres), and nortriptyline (Sensoval, Aventyl). All of these agents significantly increase the rate of long-term smoking abstinence, especially varenicline and nicotine nasal spray (Nicotrol NS) (McNeal & Birchem, 2009b).

Abnormal lipid levels—including elevated low-density lipoprotein cholesterol (LDL-C), low high-density lipoprotein cholesterol (HDL-C), elevated total cholesterol, and elevated triglycerides (TG)—are associated with an increased long-term likelihood of CVD. A fasting lipid profile should be obtained for women beginning at age 20 and then every 5 years thereafter. If a dyslipidemia is identified, secondary causes such as diabetes mellitus (DM), hypothyroidism, obstructive liver disease, chronic renal failure, and medication-induced changes should be considered (McNeal & Birchem, 2009b; Vassar, 2009).

DM is a significant risk factor for CVD. In women, having DM confers a myocardial infarction (MI) risk equal to that in someone who has established coronary artery disease (CAD). Women with DM have a 57.3% risk for CVD by age 75, compared with a 16.3% risk in women without DM (Vassar, 2009).

Hypertension (HTN) is also a significant risk factor for CVD, although the relative risk is closely correlated to how well women can control their blood pressure. Among U.S. women age 20 years and older, 15.5% have been diagnosed with HTN. Sadly, most of these women remain unaware that HTN constitutes a major risk factor for CVD (Vassar, 2009).

As of 2004, 61.9% of women in the United States were classified as overweight or obese. Obesity is more prevalent in women, especially minorities and those with a lower socioeconomic status. Overweight and obesity are independent and contributory risk factors to CVD. Body mass index (BMI) greater than 25 kg/m² is independently associated with an increased risk of CVD, with an even larger risk in persons with a BMI equal to or greater than 30. Those with a BMI of 40 kg/m² or greater tend to experience MI 12 years earlier than those with a normal

BMI (Madala, Franklin, & Chen et al., 2008). Moreover, overweight and obesity are known contributors to other risk factors, such as DM, HTN, and dyslipidemia (McNeal & Birchem, 2009b; Vassar, 2009).

 Nursing Insight— *Understanding the term cardiometabolic health*

The term *cardiometabolic health*, promoted by the American Diabetes Association (ADA) since 2006, describes an individual's level of risk for developing diabetes and CVD; it's based on an assessment of all the factors, called "cardiometabolic risk factors," that contribute to risk for these conditions. In 2006, the ADA launched its Cardiometabolic Risk Initiative, which is a national campaign to encourage health-care providers to focus on the prevention, recognition, and treatment of all risk factors (e.g., smoking, obesity, physical inactivity, psychological stress) for CVD and type 2 diabetes (ADA, 2006; Ruhl, 2009).

THE NURSING ROLE IN PROMOTING CARDIOVASCULAR HEALTH

Nurses have a central role in promoting cardiovascular health through education and counseling about heart disease. Nurses can empower women with strategies to make lifestyle modifications to address the five major risk factors (smoking, dyslipidemia, DM, HTN, and obesity) for cardiovascular disease. Diets high in saturated fat, trans-fatty acids, cholesterol, calories, alcohol, and salt and low in fiber, fruits, and vegetables have been shown to contribute to HTN, DM, dyslipidemia, and obesity. Dietary changes to reduce blood pressure may include incorporation of the Dietary Approaches to Stop Hypertension (DASH) diet. The DASH diet emphasizes low sodium intake (2.3 g/day or less) and the consumption of fruits, vegetables, low-fat/nonfat dairy foods, whole grains, lean meat, fish, poultry, nuts, and beans (McNeal & Birchem, 2009b; Vassar, 2009). Nurses and patients may learn more about the DASH Diet Eating Plan by visiting the Web site at http://www.dashdiet.org/.

Complementary Care: *Olive oil to promote cardiovascular health*

When counseling women about dietary modifications to promote CV health, nurses can encourage them to use olive oil in their cooking. In 2004, the U.S. Food and Drug Administration approved labeling olive oil as a nonpharmaceutical product that reduces the risk of coronary heart disease. Olive oil has been shown to reduce after-meal lipemia and to promote more rapid metabolism of the damaging, oxidative chylomicrons formed after eating fats (Covas, 2007; Ruano, Lopez-Miranda, & de la Torre et al., 2007; Sego, 2009). A botanical product, olive oil may produce allergic reactions in sensitive individuals, so skin patch testing for patients with significant sensitivity histories is advised. While there are no known drug interactions, highly antioxidant compounds can increase the potency of warfarin (Coumadin); nurses should advise patients who use this anticoagulant to proceed with caution. Most studies are conducted with extra virgin olive oil using a daily intake of 1 to 2 ounces (30 to 60 mL), the amount typically found in salad dressings, cooking, and spreads (Sego, 2009).

A lack of physical activity is also known to contribute to CVD. Exercise inhibits atherosclerosis (Fig. 7-1); reduces inflammatory responses; improves endothelial function; and reduces obesity, HTN, dyslipidemia, and insulin resistance (AHA, 2002; Lichtenstein, Appel, Brands, & Carnethon et al., 2006; Perry & Bennett, 2006; Slentz, Duscha, & Johnson et al., 2004; Vassar, 2009).

 Optimizing Outcomes— With exercise to decrease CHD and DM risk

Exercise has been documented to decrease the risk of CHD by 40%, stroke by 30%, and type 2 diabetes mellitus by 30%. Nurses can encourage patients to exercise for a total of at least 30 minutes over the course of a day; 60 minutes is optimal, and 90 minutes is recommended for weight loss (AHA, 2002; McNeal & Birchem, 2009b). Evidence indicates that community-based physical activity programs are effective in reducing new cases of cancer (i.e., breast, colon), type 2 diabetes, and heart disease. Community-based interventions may include mass communication efforts, social support networks, individualized physical activity goal-setting and monitoring, and enhanced access to services such as fitness centers, bike paths, and walking trails (Hellwig, 2009; Kapustin, 2010). "Choose To Move," offered by the AHA, is a free 12-week physical activity program for women that provides step-by-step instructions for simple exercises, motivational tips, and information about nutrition, heart disease and stroke. Women may register by visiting the Web site at http://www.choosetomove.org/.

Nurses can also explore and address barriers to prevention and treatment of CVD. Barriers may be perceived or actual; mental or physical; or economic, geographic, or cultural. Exploring these barriers in a nonthreatening, culturally sensitive, therapeutic environment empowers women to identify and overcome them so that they may take action to improve their cardiovascular health (Ruhl, 2009; Vassar, 2009). It is well established that women who have limited access to health care have more adverse health outcomes, including CVD (Ruhl, 2009; Zhang, Geiss, Cheng, Beckles, Gregg, & Kahn, 2008).

 Nursing Insight— Barriers to CVD prevention and treatment

Nurses can help women identify barriers to actions that promote their cardiovascular health. Barriers may include:

- Confusion concerning information in the media
- The belief that a supreme being ultimately determines one's health
- The perception that one is not at risk for CVD
- A reluctance to make a change in lifestyle
- The belief that nothing can be done to prevent CVD
- A lack of time, energy, support, willpower
- An overwhelming feeling of stress that prevents participation in CVD prevention or treatment activities
- A lack of resources (financial, access to healthy foods, access to exercise space, family obligations) (Christian, Rosamond, White, & Mosca, 2007; Mosca, Mochari, & Christian et al., 2006; Mosca, Ferris, Fabunmi, & Robertson, 2004; Thanavaro, 2005; Vassar, 2009).

When counseling women about personal risk for CVD, nurses can inform them about the Reynolds Risk Score, developed by experts at Brigham and Women's Hospital in Boston. The interactive tool calculates the risk of having a heart attack, stroke, or other form of heart disease in the next 10 years. Nurses can also inform women about HeartHub (http://www.hearthub.org/), the AHA's patient portal for information, tools, and resources about CVD and stroke. This Internet resource offers a wealth of current information about various cardiovascular-related topics, such as warning signs for heart attack, stroke, and cardiac arrest, and provides self-assessment activities for personal risk of diabetes, heart attack, and high blood pressure. The HeartHub Internet site offers information in Spanish, Vietnamese, and simplified and traditional Chinese.

Across Care Settings: **The National Coalition for Women with Heart Disease**

For more than a decade, WomenHeart Champions have been educating, supporting, and advocating in communities nationwide for prevention, early detection, timely and accurate diagnosis and treatment, and effective health-care policy to help women better understand about heart

Figure 7-1 A. Cross-section of normal coronary artery. **B.** Coronary artery with atherosclerosis narrowing the lumen. (Scanlon V.C., & Sanders T.: *Essentials of anatomy and physiology*, 5th ed., Philadelphia, F. A. Davis Company, 2007, p. 280.)

Normal artery

Atherosclerotic artery

A

B

disease. Often misdiagnosed and undertreated, more than 41 million American women are living with or at risk for developing heart disease. WomenHeart, the National Coalition for Women with Heart Disease, is the only national organization dedicated to promoting women's heart health. To learn more about this organization, women may visit the organization's Web site at http://www.womenheart.org.

Remaining up-to-date about current, evidence-based CVD information empowers nurses to offer care that promotes and optimizes women's cardiovascular health. Nurses can appropriately counsel patients about interventions that have been found harmful or are ineffective in preventing CVD in women. For example, both folic acid and antioxidant supplementation have been found ineffective in the primary and secondary prevention of CVD. Also, women younger than age 65 should not routinely use aspirin to prevent myocardial infarction. Finally, hormone therapy and estrogen-receptor modulators are no longer recommended for primary or secondary prevention of CVD in women (Manson, 2009; Mosca, Banka, & Benjamin et al., 2007; Smith, Allen, & Blair et al., 2006; Vassar, 2009).

 Optimizing Outcomes— **Resources for health-care providers**

The American Heart Association (AHA) and American College of Cardiology (ACC) have published guidelines to assist practitioners in the prevention of CVD. The AHA has published *Evidence-Based Guidelines for Cardiovascular Disease Prevention in Women: 2007 Update*, and the AHA and ACC have jointly published AHA/ACC *Guidelines for Secondary Prevention for Patients With Coronary and Other Atherosclerotic Vascular Disease: 2006 Update: Endorsed by the National Heart, Lung, and Blood Institute*. This publication summarizes the highlights of these guidelines and is a rich resource for health-care professionals. Both sets of guidelines focus on major CVD risk factor reduction and the use of pharmacotherapy in patients with established CVD (Mosca, Banka, Benjamin, & Berra et al., 2007; Smith, Allen, & Blair et al., 2006; Vassar, 2009).

 Now Can You— **Discuss certain aspects of cardiovascular disease?**

1. Discuss the utility of two tools specifically developed to determine risk for cardiovascular disease?
2. Identify at least five AHA guidelines for promoting heart health in women?
3. Develop a patient teaching program that focuses on five modifiable risk factors for cardiovascular disease?

Osteoporosis

As individuals age, their bone density progressively decreases. Osteoporosis is a generalized, metabolic disease characterized by decreased bone mass and an increased incidence of bone fractures (Fig. 7-2). Osteopenia is a condition where bone mineral density is lower than normal, and many clinicians consider it to be a precursor to osteoporosis. Osteoporosis is a largely preventable complication of menopause. Screening strategies and pharmacological interventions are available to prevent and treat osteoporosis.

 Nursing Insight— Appreciating the full impact of osteoporosis-related fractures

Hip fractures, which occur on average at age 82, elicit a particularly devastating toll, resulting in higher cost, disability, and mortality than all other osteoporotic fracture types combined. Hip fractures cause up to a 25% increase in mortality within 1 year of the incident. Approximately 25% of women require long-term care after a hip fracture, and 50% will experience some long-term loss of mobility. Vertebral fractures may cause substantial pain as well as loss of height and exaggerated thoracic kyphosis (abnormal curvature of the thoracic spine). Spinal pain and deformity can greatly restrict normal movement, including bending and reaching. Thoracic fractures may restrict lung function and cause digestive problems. Osteoporotic fractures exert a psychological toll as well. Pain, loss of mobility, change in body image, and loss of independence can exert a strong negative impact on self-esteem and mood (NAMS, 2010b).

Normal Bone

Osteoporosis

A

B

Figure 7-2 A. Normal spongy bone, as in the body of a vertebra. **B.** Spongy bone thinned by osteopososis. (Scanlon V.C., & Sanders T.: *Essentials of anatomy and physiology,* 5th ed., Philadephia, F. A. Davis Company, 2007, p. 113.)

NORMAL BONE PHYSIOLOGY

Bone is a living tissue. It is involved in a wide range of biochemical processes, which result in the constant breakdown and reformation of new bone replacing weakened areas with new, well-formed tissue. Bone is composed of two types of cells, osteoblasts and osteoclasts (Fig. 7-3), as well as an intercellular matrix. The intercellular matrix is composed of organic compounds, such as collagen and other proteins, and inorganic components responsible for bone rigidity, including minerals such as calcium phosphate, calcium carbonate, magnesium, fluoride, sulfate, and other trace elements that form crystalline structures called *hydroxyapatites* (NAMS, 2010b).

A & P review **The Bone Remodeling Unit**

The bone-remodeling unit is the site on the surface of the bone where osteoblasts and osteoclasts act to form and resorb bone. Bone is constantly being remodeled to provide optimal support and to repair damage occurring from daily activities. An osteoblast (from the Greek words for "bone" and "germ," or embryonic) is a mononucleate cell that is responsible for bone formation. Osteoblasts produce osteoid, which is composed mainly of collagen. Osteoblasts are also responsible for mineralization of the osteoid matrix. Bone is a dynamic tissue that is constantly being reshaped by osteoblasts, which build bone, and osteoclasts, which resorb bone. An osteoclast (from the Greek words for "bone" and "broken") is a type of bone cell that removes bone tissue by removing its mineralized matrix and breaking up the organic bone, a process termed *bone resorption*. Osteoclasts and osteoblasts are instrumental in controlling the amount of bone tissue: osteoblasts form bone; osteoclasts resorb bone. Osteoblast cells tend to decrease as individuals age, thus decreasing the natural renovation of bone tissue (Fig. 7-4) (ACOG, 2004; NAMS, 2010b). ◆

 Nursing Insight— *Gonadal hormones and bone metabolism*

Estrogen inhibits bone resorption by binding to estrogen receptors in bone tissue and also by blocking the production of cytokines, substances that increase the number of osteoclasts. Estrogen, however, is not the only hormone that has an important influence on the health of bone. Two other hormones produced by the ovaries, progesterone and dehydroepiandrosterone (DHEA), influence bone metabolism as well. Testosterone (one of the male hormones also produced by women) may also play a role in bone health (ACOG, 2008, NOF, 2008).

There are two major types of bone: cortical and trabecular. Cortical bone forms the outer shell of all bones and accounts for 75% of total bone mass. Trabecular bone is the spongy, interlacing network of struts that forms the internal support within the cortical bone. Trabecular bone is concentrated in the vertebral bodies and pelvis and at the ends of the long bones. Trabecular bone accounts for only 25% of total bone mass, but because of its spongy, open architectural structure, it accounts for most of the bone volume. Bone remodeling units are limited to the bone surface. Because trabecular bone has a larger surface area, it has a higher turnover rate than cortical bone. Trabecular bone is most likely to show early bone loss, but it also is the first bone type to show response to therapy (ACOG, 2004).

Bone formation and resorption are ongoing processes that are usually "in balance" in young adults who have adequate nutrition and exercise and experience normal puberty. Bone mass peaks at approximately 30 years in both men and women. After reaching peak bone mass, approximately 0.4% of bone is lost per year in both genders. Bone strength is determined by the total bone mass and the integrity of its protein and crystal matrix. Bone strength is also related to the efficiency of bone repair in response to mild trauma, which produces microfractures. Remodeling tends to occur along lines of stress, increasing the strength in those weakened areas (NOF, 2008).

 Nursing Insight— *The menopause–bone loss link*

In addition to the bone loss with aging that naturally occurs in both genders, women lose approximately 2% of cortical bone and 5% of trabecular bone per year for the first 5 to 8 years after menopause. With menopause and aging, the coordinated "balance" between osteoclasts and osteoblasts may be disturbed, resulting in excessive bone resorption and loss of both bone density and structure. In women who are recently menopausal, excess bone loss commonly is caused by excessive osteoclast-mediated resorption. In later postmenopausal years, suppressed osteoblast activity and inadequate formation of bone may play a major role in the progression of osteoporosis, providing an opportunity for new therapeutic approaches, such as stimulating bone formation. Osteoporosis is more common in women than in men in part because of the accelerated loss of bone that occurs after menopause (ACOG, 2004).

Bone health promotion typically centers on methods of ensuring adequate intake of calcium. However, bone health maintenance and the prevention of fractures should encompass other strategies, such as preventing the loss of calcium and other minerals from the bone, maintaining the soft tissue components around the bone, and promoting the efficiency of bone repair (NOF, 2008; Speroff & Fritz, 2005).

Figure 7-3 Osteoclast. (Venes, D.: *Taber's cyclopedic medical dictionary*, 21st ed., Philadelphia, F. A. Davis Company, 2009, p 1655.)

B Epiphyseal disc

Chondrocytes producing cartilage

Osteoblasts producing bone

Bone

Epiphyseal disc

Cartilage

Medullary cavity containing marrow

Compact bone

Secondary ossification center

Compact bone

Cartilaginous model

Bone collar and calcifying cartilage in ossification center

Medullary cavity and development of secondary ossification centers

Spongy bone

Articular cartilage

A

Figure 7-4 The ossification process in a long bone. **A.** Progression of ossification from the cartilage model of the embryo to the bone of a young adult. **B.** Microscopic view of an epiphyseal disc showing cartilage production and bone replacement. (Scanlon V.C., & Sanders T.: *Essentials of anatomy and physiology*, 5th ed., Philadelphia, F. A. Davis Company, 2007, p. 110.)

Nursing Insight*— *Fractures commonly associated with osteoporosis

Three major types of fractures may occur as a result of osteoporosis:

Spontaneous vertebral crush fracture—the vertebrae become so weak that one vertebra collapses under the minimal stress of lifting or due to the weight of the woman's body. This action causes a loss of height and kyphosis, or dowager's hump, the curvature of the upper back often present in older people.

Colle's fracture—a transverse fracture of the distal radial metaphysis with displacement of the hand posteriorly and outward. This fracture occurs when a person breaks a fall by landing on a hand, causing fracture of the radius (Venes, 2009).

Osteoporotic hip fracture—The hip fracture related to the osteoporotic process is the most severe form of these three types of fractures.

Tooth loss and periodontal disease represent other aspects of osteoporosis.

In the United States, it is estimated that 10 million individuals have osteoporosis and almost 34 million more are estimated to have osteopenia, or low bone mass, placing them at increased risk for osteoporosis. Of the 10 million Americans estimated to have osteoporosis, 8 million are women and 2 million are men. Although osteoporosis is often considered to be an older person's disease, it can strike at any age. Both osteopenia and osteoporosis increase the risk of fracture (ACOG, 2007; NOF, 2008b).

Ethnocultural Considerations*— Osteoporosis

Osteoporosis varies among ethnic groups. Asian Americans and Caucasians are more often affected by osteopenia/osteoporosis than are African Americans. African American women have approximately a 6% higher bone mineral density than Caucasian women. Among non-Hispanic African American women who are older than age 50, 5% have osteoporosis and 35% have osteopenia. Among Hispanic women over age 50, 10% have osteoporosis and 49% have osteopenia. When compared with other ethnic/racial groups, the risk of osteoporosis is increasing most rapidly among Hispanic women. And among non-Hispanic Caucasian women and Asian American women who are 50 and older, approximately 20% have osteoporosis, while 52% have osteopenia. (ACOG, 2004; NOF, 2008b; Speroff & Fritz, 2005)

Osteoporosis constitutes a major health threat for women. In this country, the incidence of osteoporosis-related fractures has increased over the past 20 years. Most fractures occur at the femoral neck, the vertebrae, and the distal radius. Postmenopausal women who experience a hip or symptomatic vertebral fracture have a 6- to 8-fold increased risk of death in the year following their fracture. On an annual basis, the associated costs of osteoporosis-related fractures exceed $14 billion, and this figure is expected to increase as life expectancy increases and the population ages (Alexander, 2007; Nelson & Stewart, 2008).

Nursing Insight*— *Heredity and bone mass

The single largest factor that influences a woman's peak bone mass (i.e., the maximal bone mineral density [BMD] gained during the skeletal development and maturation phase) is genetics. Up to 80% of the variability in peak bone mass is attributable to genetic factors alone. Female children of women with osteoporotic fractures have lower bone mass than would be expected for their age when compared with unrelated individuals. First-degree relatives of women with osteoporosis have lower bone mass than those with no family history of osteoporosis. (ACOG, 2004; NAMS, 2007; NAMS, 2010b)

CAUSES

Stated in simple terms, osteoporosis occurs when the normal balance of bone formation and bone resorption is disrupted. In women and young adults, bone growth and calcium deposition take place continuously throughout young adulthood. Bone mass generally reaches a peak around age 30. As women grow older, net bone loss gradually occurs due to an imbalance in bone tissue and metabolism. A deficiency of estrogen worsens the situation, as does the inefficiency in calcium and vitamin D assimilation that naturally occur as women age (Nelson & Stewart, 2008; NOF, 2008; Speroff & Fritz, 2005).

During the first five to six years following menopause, women lose bone density six times more rapidly than men. By the age of 65, one-third of women have experienced a vertebral fracture; by the age of 80, women have lost approximately 47% of the trabecular bone, which is concentrated in the vertebrae, pelvis, and other flat bones, and the epiphyses. The most well-defined risk factor for the development of osteoporosis is the loss of the protective effects of estrogen, which occurs with declining ovarian function during perimenopause (NOF, 2008).

Osteoporosis may result from other causes, including rheumatoid arthritis, chronic lung disease, anorexia nervosa, and endocrine diseases such as diabetes, hypogonadism, overactive thyroid, and hyperparathyroidism. Also, certain prescription drugs, including glucocorticoids (e.g., prednisone), anticoagulants (e.g., heparin), chemotherapeutic agents, anticonvulsants (e.g., phenytoin), and some diuretics (e.g., furosemide), as well as some over-the-counter aluminum-containing antacids (e.g., Maalox), can contribute to bone loss. An excessive caffeine intake increases calcium excretion, and excessive alcohol use (i.e., three or more drinks per day) interferes with calcium absorption and depresses bone formation (NOF, 2008).

Optimizing Outcomes— **With routine postmenopausal osteoporosis risk assessment**

All postmenopausal women should be assessed for risk factors associated with osteoporosis and fracture. This assessment requires a history, physical examination, and any necessary diagnostic tests. The goals of this evaluation are to evaluate fracture risk, to rule out secondary causes of osteoporosis, to identify modifiable risk factors, and to determine appropriate candidates for pharmacologic therapy (NAMS, 2010b).

RISK FACTORS

There are a number of risk factors for osteoporosis. Non-modifiable factors include genetic background and medical conditions (presented in Box 7-9). Modifiable risk factors related to lifestyle include smoking (active or passive); alcohol use; low dietary calcium; vitamin D insufficiency; high dietary intake of sodium, protein, caffeine, phosphates, sugar, and refined flour products; lack of sun exposure or a deficiency of vitamin D; and lack of exercise (NOF, 2008).

 Nursing Insight— Tobacco use and osteoporosis risk

Compared with nonsmokers, women smokers tend to lose bone more rapidly, have lower bone mass, and reach menopause 2 years earlier, on average. The mechanisms by which smoking might adversely affect bone mass are not known, although some experts suggest that cigarette smokers may have impaired calcium absorption and lower estradiol levels (NAMS, 2010b).

DIAGNOSING OSTEOPOROSIS

A *clinical* diagnosis of osteoporosis is made when a postmenopausal woman suffers a nontraumatic, nonpathological fracture of the spine. A *radiological* diagnosis is based on the T score, which is obtained from bone densitometry

analysis. The first-line technique for assessing BMD (bone densitometry) is the central dual-energy x-ray absorptiometry, or C-DEXA (or DEXA). This test assesses BMD in the spine, hip, and waist.

 diagnostic tools Bone Density Scan (DEXA)

Bone density scanning, also called dual-energy x-ray absorptiometry (DEXA) or bone densitometry, is an enhanced form of x-ray technology that is used to measure bone loss. Central DEXA is today's established standard for measuring BMD and is most often performed on the lower spine and hips. Central DXA devices, consisting of a large, flat table and an "arm" suspended overhead, are usually located in hospitals and medical offices. Peripheral devices (pDEXA) that use x-ray or ultrasound are sometimes used to screen for low bone mass. Peripheral devices measure bone density in the wrist, heel, or finger and are often available in drugstores and mobile health vans in the community. The pDEXA device, much smaller than the central DEXA device, is a portable box-like structure with a space for the foot or forearm to be placed for imaging. Although bone tests at peripheral sites can identify women at risk of fracture, they are not useful for the diagnosis of osteoporosis and have limited or no value in the follow-up of patients. In some communities, a computed tomography (CT) scan with special software can also be used to diagnose or monitor low bone mass. This is accurate but less commonly used than DEXA scanning. DEXA is effective in tracking the effects of treatment for osteoporosis and other conditions that cause bone loss; the DEXA test can also assess an individual's risk for developing fractures (NAMS, 2010b).

DEXA works by measuring a specific bone or bones (e.g., spine, hip, waist). The density of these bones is then compared with an average index based on age, sex, and size to determine risk for fractures and the stage of an individual's osteoporosis. Results are generally scored by two measures, the T-score and the Z-score. The T-score refers to the extent of bone loss and is reflective of the number of standard deviations by which a patient's BMD falls below the expected BMD score for healthy young women. Every decrease of 1 standard deviation represents approximately a 12% reduction in BMD, which translates into a 1.5- to 3.0-fold increase in fracture risk (NOF, 2008).

 Nursing Insight— Understanding the BMD Z-score and T-score

The Z-score is the number of standard deviations above or below the mean for the patient's age, sex, and ethnicity. The Z-score is used in premenopausal women, men under the age of 50, and in children. The T-score, which is also the number of standard deviations above or below the mean, is a comparison of a patient's BMD to that of a healthy 30-year-old of the same sex and ethnicity. This value is used in postmenopausal women and men over age 50 because it better predicts risk of future fracture. The World Health Organization T-score criteria are as follows:

- Normal: a T-score of –1.0 or higher
- Osteopenia: a T-score less than –1.0 and greater than –2.5
- Osteoporosis: a T-score equal to or less than –2.5 (i.e., the bone density is 2.5 standard deviations below the mean of a 30-year-old healthy woman)

Scores indicate the amount one's bone mineral density varies from the mean. Negative scores indicate lower bone density; positive scores indicate higher bone density.

Box 7-9 Nonmodifiable Risk Factors for Osteoporosis

Gender: Eighty percent of the 10 million Americans who have osteoporosis are women.

Race: Caucasian, Asian, and Latina women are at the highest risk; African American women have a lower risk.

Advanced age

History of:
- Previous fractures that occurred without any major trauma, or fracture after the age of 50
- Poor absorption of calcium and other minerals or nutrients due to celiac disease, chronic diarrhea, low stomach acid (common in older individuals), surgical removal of part of the stomach or intestines

Family history of female osteoporosis or fractures or both

Body build: Women who are small-boned and slim and have small muscle mass are at greater risk than women with other body builds

Current osteopenia

Early menopause (before age 40 years, or if surgically induced); amenorrhea; never having gone through a pregnancy

Diabetes; liver disease; kidney disease with dialysis; daily use of thyroid replacement medication (greater than 2 grains); hyperthyroidism; hyperparathyroidism

Lactose intolerance: Present in 60% of women with osteoporosis and in only 15% of the general population

Use of phenytoin sodium (Dilantin), a medication that interferes with the body's ability to absorb calcium; aluminum-containing antacids; steroid medications

Sources: ACOG, 2004; NAMS, 2007; NAMS, 2010b; NOF, 2008.

"What to say" — *Preparing patients for a C-DXA examination*

The nurse can do much to allay the patient's anxiety about a scheduled bone densitometry test. The nurse explains why the test is performed, how the test is performed, and what information will be gained from the test results. The nurse may also counsel the patient about how to prepare for the test. For example, the nurse may say:

- The bone density test is a quick, noninvasive, painless procedure.
- The amount of radiation used is extremely small—less than one-tenth the dose of a standard chest x-ray and less than a day's exposure to natural radiation.
- DXA bone density testing is the most accurate method available for the diagnosis of osteoporosis and is also considered an accurate estimator of fracture risk.
- No radiation remains in your body after an x-ray examination.
- On the day of the exam, you may eat normally. You should not take calcium supplements for at least 24 hours before your exam.
- You should wear loose, comfortable clothing and avoid garments that have zippers, belts, or buttons made of metal. Objects such as keys or wallets that would be in the area being scanned should be removed.
- You may be asked to remove some or all of your clothes and to wear a gown during the exam. You may also be asked to remove jewelry, dentures, eyeglasses, and any metal objects or clothing that might interfere with the x-ray images.
- You will be positioned on a padded table and your legs will be supported on a padded box (to flatten the pelvis and lumbar spine).You must hold very still and you may be asked to hold your breath for a few seconds while the x-ray picture is being taken.
- The DEXA bone density test is usually completed within 10 to 30 minutes, depending on the equipment used and the parts of the body being examined.
- You should inform your health-care provider if you recently had a barium examination or have been injected with a contrast material for a CT scan or radioisotope scan. In this event, you may have to wait 10 to 14 days before undergoing the DEXA test.
- You should inform your health-care provider and the x-ray technologist if there is any possibility that you may be pregnant.

Optimizing Outcomes— **Routine height assessments to detect asymptomatic osteoporosis**

As women grow older, routine height assessments should become standard practice during annual examinations. Loss of height may indicate bone loss in asymptomatic women. Height loss in women who are in their 40s or early 50s should signal a need for further testing to determine the cause. After achieving maximal height, women can lose up to 1.0 to 1.5 inches (2.0 to 3.8 cm) of height as part of the normal aging process, primarily as a result of degenerative arthritis and shrinkage of intervertebral disks. Height loss greater than 1.5 inches increases the likelihood that a vertebral fracture is present. The nurse should measure height using an accurate method such as a wall-mounted ruler or a stadiometer (an instrument used to measure both sitting and standing height) (NAMS, 2010b; NOF, 2008).

According to recommendations established by the ACOG, the USPSTF, NAMS, and NOF, health-care providers should routinely screen all women older than 65 for osteoporosis, regardless of risk factors. Women with risk factors should be screened beginning at age 60.

Be sure to— **Teach women about osteoporosis early warning signs**

Teaching women about the early warning signs of osteoporosis constitutes an important nursing role in the promotion of bone health. Nurses should alert women to the following signs and symptoms that may signal bone loss and advise them to promptly contact their health-care provider if they experience them:

- Sudden onset of insomnia and restlessness
- Leg and foot cramps that occur frequently during the night
- Persistent low back pain
- Gradual loss of height
- Development of gum disease or loose teeth

In this country, women typically reach menopause around age 51, and most bone loss occurs during the first 5 to 7 years after cessation of menses. Thus, it may be prudent to begin screening at an earlier age. It is generally recommended that the BMD be reassessed every 3 to 5 years. For certain women, including those who are undergoing treatment for osteoporosis and those who are immobilized, the BMD may need to be measured beginning at an earlier age and more often, such as every 6 to 24 months (ACOG, 2008b; Goldstein, 2008; NAMS, 2010b; NOF, 2008, USPSTF, 2002).

 Nursing Insight— *ACOG recommendations for bone mineral density (BMD) testing*

ACOG (2008b) has published the following recommendations for BMD testing:

- Bone mineral density testing should be recommended to all postmenopausal women aged 65 years or older regardless of risk factors.
- Bone mineral density testing may be recommended for postmenopausal women younger than 65 years who have one or more risk factors for osteoporosis. According to current risk factors, all Caucasian postmenopausal women younger than 65 years would be candidates for BMD testing.
- Bone mineral density testing should be performed on all postmenopausal women with fractures to confirm the diagnosis of osteoporosis and determine disease severity.

Optimizing Outcomes— **With the FRAX Assessment Tool**

The launch of the World Health Organization (WHO) technical report *Assessment of Osteoporosis at the Primary Health Care Level* and the related Fracture Risk Assessment Tool (FRAX) are major milestones toward helping health professionals worldwide to improve identification of patients at high risk of fracture. The practical Web-based tool FRAX assesses the 10-year risk of osteoporosis fracture. An individual's risk factors such as age, sex, weight, height, and femoral neck BMD (if available) are entered into the tool, followed by clinical risk factors, which include a prior fragility fracture, parental history of hip fracture, tobacco smoking, long-term use of glucocorticoids, rheumatoid arthritis, other causes of secondary osteoporosis, and daily alcohol consumption. The FRAX tool then provides a figure indicating a 10-year fracture probability as a percentage, which, together with a clinical assessment, provides guidance for determining access to treatment in health-care systems. Estimates are available for U.S. Caucasian, African American, Hispanics, and Asian Americans. It is expected that the software needed to provide the FRAX model calculations will be loaded into most DEXA machines by 2011. The FRAX algorithm is intended for use with postmenopausal women and men age 50 and older and applies only to previously untreated patients. The FRAX model is available on the NOF Web site (http://www.nof.org) or at the FRAX Web site (http://www.shef.ac.uk/FRAX/) (Ettinger & Ettinger, 2009; Goldstein, 2008; Kessenich, 2009; Nelson, 2009; Watts, Ettinger, & LeBoff, 2009).

PROMOTING BONE HEALTH THROUGH OPTIMAL NUTRITION

Although it is impossible to determine the precise effect of diet on bone health, there is at least circumstantial evidence that the standard American diet, which frequently contains excessive sugar, refined grains, and caffeine, promotes the development of osteoporosis. Other dietary factors that adversely affect bone health include alcohol and protein, phosphorus, and sodium. The relationship between these substances and their impact on bone loss is presented in Box 7-10.

Nurses can empower women with information about the value of optimal nutrition in reducing osteoporosis risk. Consuming a diet that is composed primarily of plant-based, unprocessed whole foods is an important strategy in the promotion of bone health and the prevention of osteoporosis. Examples of plant-based nutritious substances include legumes, fresh fruits and vegetables, whole grains, nuts, and seeds. These foods provide a rich supply of nutrients in the right proportions to enhance their absorption and use. In addition to calcium, many vitamins, such as vitamins K, B₆, C, and D, and minerals, such as manganese, magnesium, boron, and zinc, play an important role in maintaining bone mass and in preventing bone loss (Box 7-11) (NAMS, 2010b; NOF, 2008c).

Calcium

Calcium deficiency is only one of the predisposing factors for the development of osteoporosis in women,

---

Box 7-10   Selected Dietary Substances and Their Association With Bone Loss

Sugar: The average American ingests 139 pounds of refined sugar each year. Sugar intake may be associated with large increases in urinary calcium excretion. Owing to the fact that 99% of the body's calcium is stored in bone, and the blood maintains a very narrow concentration range of calcium, when the body loses calcium, it is likely to be from bone.

Refined grains: The nutrient-rich portions of grains have been removed through refinement, including vitamin B complex, calcium, magnesium, and zinc.

Caffeine: Caffeine in coffee, tea, and soft drinks, as well as similar substances in chocolate and some drugs, causes calcium to be excreted in the urine. Increased calcium excretion causes a systemic acidosis that stimulates bone resorption.

Alcohol: Excessive alcohol intake interferes with calcium absorption and depresses bone formation.

Protein, phosphorus, and sodium: The typical American diet contains excessive amounts of protein, phosphorus, and sodium. Calcium is mobilized to neutralize the acidic by-products and is then excreted in the urine, causing a loss of calcium from the body. Phosphorus is an ingredient in many soft drinks, and excess protein results from the high consumption of meat and dairy products in the average American diet.

Oxalate and phytate sodium: Foods with high amounts of oxalate and phytate reduce the absorption of calcium contained in those foods. Examples of foods high in oxalate include spinach, rhubarb, and beet greens. Legumes (e.g., pinto beans, navy beans, peas) are high in phytate. To reduce the phytate level, soak the legumes in water for several hours; discard the water, then cook them in fresh water. Wheat bran is also high in phytate; take calcium supplements 2 or more hours before eating any foods with 100% wheat bran.

---

and not everyone with osteoporosis is deficient in calcium. Calcium balance and metabolism in the body are complex and involve a number of factors, including ingestion, absorption, use, and excretion. In addition, calcium balance is modulated by various hormonal systems. Adequate calcium intake for osteoporosis prevention should begin early in life when bone mass is reaching its peak. This important period for bone health occurs during the late teens to early 20s (Speroff & Fritz, 2005).

 Optimizing Outcomes— **With skeletal health promotion in children and adolescents**

An important role for nurses who work with men, women, and families centers on promoting bone health and preventing osteoporosis. Ideally, protection against osteoporosis should begin in childhood and adolescence, with efforts focused on building bone mass. Children should be encouraged to eat calcium-rich foods, and nurses should teach parents to encourage regular exercise, including participation in school gym classes and sports programs, to build strong bones and establish healthy lifestyle habits. Parents also should be informed about the negative effects that eating disorders, excessive dieting, excessive exercise, alcohol consumption, and smoking exert on bone density. From the mid-20s through age 35, focus should continue to be placed on building and maintaining bone mass

The National Institutes of Health Office of Dietary Supplements (2009) recommends the following calcium dietary allowances for women, which represent the amounts of calcium required to maintain adequate rates of calcium retention and bone health in healthy individuals:

- 9 to 13 years: 1300 mg/day
- 14 to 18 years: 1300 mg/day (same amount for pregnant and lactating individuals)
- 19 to 50 years: 1000 mg/day (same amount for pregnant and lactating individuals)
- 50+ years: 1200 mg/day

When considering dietary sources of calcium, most people are aware that dairy products are rich in calcium, but many do not realize that the animal protein in these products can interfere with the body's ability to absorb the calcium. Other substances that can inhibit calcium absorption are found in wheat bran, raw spinach, salt, caffeine, alcohol and tobacco, and fructose (present in many soft drinks). An important nursing role in promoting bone health centers on teaching women about good nutritional sources of calcium.

❝What to say❞ — *Educating women about dietary calcium*

Nurses can teach women about calcium-rich dietary sources. The nurse may offer the following information:

- Dietary sources are the preferred means of obtaining adequate calcium intake because there are other essential nutrients in high-calcium foods.

- Milk, yogurt, ice cream, and cheese are rich sources of calcium.

- Nondairy calcium sources include vegetables such as Chinese cabbage, kale, and broccoli.

- Most grains do not have high amounts of calcium unless they are fortified; however, they contribute calcium to the diet because they do have small amounts and people consume them frequently.

- Seafood, including sardines and salmon, are good sources of calcium.

- Puddings, instant breakfast drinks, cottage cheese, and sour cream are good sources of calcium.

- Many products, such as soy milk, rice, yogurt, cereals, and orange juice, are now available with extra calcium added.

- Reduced-fat or low-fat products contain at least as much calcium per serving as high-fat dairy products, and they offer an alternative for women concerned about body weight and lipid profiles.
  (Dawson-Hughes et al., 2008; NAMS, 2007)

through a calcium-rich diet. After age 35, bone resorption exceeds bone formation. At that time, emphasis should be placed on preventing bone loss through a healthy diet, use of calcium supplements, and engaging in weight-bearing exercises such as weight-lifting, walking, jogging, dancing, and climbing stairs (Venes, 2009).

Some individuals are lactose intolerant and have difficulty digesting dairy products because they lack the enzyme lactase, which is needed to break down the milk sugar lactose. Lactose intolerance is fairly common in adults, particularly African Americans, Asians, Native Americans, and Inuits (Alaska natives). Persons with lactose intolerance experience abdominal cramping, bloating, and diarrhea following milk consumption, although many can tolerate small amounts of milk without symptoms. Calcium sources such as yogurt, sweet acidophilus milk (fermented with certain bacteria), buttermilk, cheese, chocolate milk, and cocoa may be tolerated even when fresh milk is not. Lactase supplements such as Lactaid are available to consume with milk, and lactase-treated milk is also available in many markets. The lactase in these products digests the lactose in the milk so that lactose-intolerant persons can drink milk without experiencing unpleasant intestinal symptoms (NOF, 2008c).

 Optimizing Outcomes— **Teaching women about strategies to enhance calcium absorption**

The absorption of calcium depends upon adequate acidity in the stomach. Low stomach acid is a common problem that becomes more prevalent with increasing age. When counseling women about strategies to optimize the absorption of calcium, the nurse can offer the following advice:

* Eat slowly and chew well.
* Limit fluid intake with meals.
* Consider the use of digestive enzymes.

Most women will need an additional 600 to 900 mg of calcium per day over their usual daily dietary intake to reach recommended levels. Among the many calcium supplements are various formulations available in oral tablets, chewable tablets, dissolvable oral tablets, and liquids. Patients should be advised that the "best" supplement for them is the one that best meets their needs, based on tolerance, convenience, cost, and availability. Nurses can teach women that when choosing a calcium supplement, special consideration should be given to the product's purity, absorbability, tolerance, and possibility of interactions with other drugs. Although vitamin D is necessary for the absorption of calcium, it is not necessary that it be included in the calcium supplement. Calcium citrate tends to be better tolerated than calcium carbonate; however, it is a more expensive form of calcium supplement. Most individuals adequately absorb calcium carbonate, a less expensive calcium source, unless there is a problem with insufficient stomach acid. Antacids are not the best sources of calcium, as they can cause other problems, such as kidney stones, and they may aggravate other medical conditions as well. Furthermore, some antacids also contain aluminum, which can cause the body to lose calcium. Nurses can reassure women that total calcium intakes of up to 1500 mg/day do not appear to increase the risk of developing renal calculi and may actually reduce it. Also, women should not exceed the recommended daily requirement for calcium, as there appears to be no benefit to consumption of amounts in excess of 1500 mg/day (NAMS, 2007, 2010b; NOF, 2008c).

❝What to say❞ — *Providing guidance to assist women in choosing calcium supplements*

When discussing calcium supplements, the nurse may offer the following advice:

* *Purity:* Choose only those supplements that are known brand names that have proven reliability. The product label should include the term *purified* or have the USP (U.S. Pharmacopeia) symbol, although the USP label is voluntary and not all products display this symbol. Avoid calcium extracted from unrefined oyster shell, bone meal, or dolomite without the USP—these products historically have contained higher lead levels or other toxic materials (NOF, 2008).

* *Absorbability:* Most brand-name calcium products are readily absorbed by the body. If the product label does not state that it is absorbable, it is easy to determine absorbability by doing this: place the tablet in a small amount of warm water for 30 minutes and stir occasionally. If the tablet has not dissolved within this time period, it probably will not dissolve in the stomach. Calcium supplements in chewable and liquid form dissolve well because they are broken down before they enter the stomach. Calcium, whether in the diet or from supplements, is best absorbed when it is taken several times a day in amounts of 500 mg or less. Calcium carbonate is absorbed best when taken with food; calcium citrate can be taken any time (NOF, 2008).

* *Tolerance:* Although calcium supplements are well tolerated by most people, certain preparations can cause side effects such as gas or constipation in some individuals. If simple strategies such as increased fluids and fiber intake do not resolve the symptoms, try another calcium source. A combined calcium-magnesium product may be helpful if constipation is a problem. It is best to increase the intake of any calcium supplement gradually, beginning with 500 mg a day for several days, and add additional calcium slowly (NOF, 2008).

* *Interactions with other drugs:* Before taking any calcium supplement, it is important to talk with your health-care provider or pharmacist about possible interactions between prescription or over-the-counter medications and the calcium supplements. For example, calcium supplements may interfere with the absorption of the antibiotic tetracycline. Calcium also interferes with iron absorption and should not be taken at the same time as the iron supplement unless the iron supplement is taken with vitamin C or calcium citrate. Any medication that is to be taken on an empty stomach should not be taken with a calcium supplement (NOF, 2008c).

* *Dietary factors that limit calcium absorption:* Consumption of certain foods, including those that contain oxalic acid (found in spinach, rhubarb, and some other green vegetables), large amounts of grains that contain phytates (e.g., wheat bran, soy protein isolates), and, possibly, tannins (found in tea) are known to limit calcium absorption from the intestines (NAMS, 2007)

 Optimizing Outcomes— **With NOF resources for patients and health-care professionals**

Boning Up on Osteoporosis is a 100+ patient-care handbook that offers current information on the prevention, diagnosis, and treatment of osteoporosis. The handbook also includes detailed nutrition information and exercises for individuals with low bone density and osteoporosis. It may be purchased from the NOF online store at http://www.nofstore.org/.

The *Clinician's Guide to Prevention and Treatment of Osteoporosis* was published in 2008, and an online updated version became available in January 2010. This resource was developed to inform clinical decision making for the management of men and women at high fracture risk. It integrates the expression of a patient's fracture risk as a 10-year probability with current clinical recommendations for the management of osteoporosis. Health-care professionals may obtain a single print copy of the 2008 *Clinician's Guide* at no charge; additional quantities may be purchased from the NOF online store.

PROMOTING BONE HEALTH THROUGH PHYSICAL ACTIVITY

Immobilization and bedrest are associated with an increase in bone loss. During travel in space, astronauts have experienced accelerated rates of bone loss. It is known that overall bone mass is directly related to weight-bearing physical exercise. Women who regularly engage in exercise programs that include weight-bearing and muscle-strengthening elements can help prevent postmenopausal bone loss and reduce their risk of falling. The bone-building effect of exercise results mainly from the repetitive physical stress applied to the bones. With weight-bearing exercise, pressure is placed on the bones either by the weight of the body or by the force of muscular contractions. Effective exercises for menopausal women that are generally safe and contribute to cardiovascular health and bone mass are walking, stair climbing, gardening, weight lifting, and low-impact aerobics. An effective program involves regular exercise for at least 30 minutes, every day of the week. Also, the 30 minutes do not need to be done all at once—physical activity may be divided into 10-minute segments, if desired (NOF, 2008d).

 Optimizing Outcomes— With exercises to promote balance, posture, and function

Nonimpact exercises improve balance, posture, and movement and help to increase muscle strength and decrease the risk of falls and fractures. Balance exercises such as Tai Chi strengthen the legs and enhance the balance. Posture exercises that improve one's posture and help reduce rounded shoulders decrease the risk of fractures, especially in the spine. Functional exercises enhance the performance of daily activities and decrease the risk of falls and fractures. Yoga and Pilates can also improve strength, balance, and flexibility. Individuals with osteopenia or osteoporosis should avoid certain positions such as forward-bending exercises to prevent fractures (NOF, 2008d).

When counseling older women, it is helpful to include information about safety and prevention of falls. Many factors, such as frailty, altered balance, poor vision, and use of certain medications can contribute to falls (Box 7-12). Strategies to minimize falls include lowering the bed, removing throw rugs, illuminating dark areas with night lights, using safety treads and safety rails in the bathroom, ensuring ready access to a telephone, eliminating exposed electrical cords, ensuring stair safety (handrails, good condition, nonslip surfaces), and removing all clutter from the floors. Also, older women should be advised to avoid

---

Box 7-12 Medical Risk Factors for Falls

- Age
- Anxiety and agitation
- Arthritis of the lower extremities
- Arrhythmias
- Dehydration
- Depression
- Female gender
- Impaired transfer and mobility
- Malnutrition
- Medications that cause oversedation (e.g., narcotic analgesics, anticonvulsants, psychotropics)
- Orthostatic hypotension
- Poor vision and use of bifocals
- Previous fall
- Reduced problem solving or mental acuity and diminished cognitive skills
- Urgent urinary incontinence
- Vitamin D insufficiency
- Kyphosis
- Poor balance
- Reduced proprioception
- Muscle weakness

Sources: Dawson-Hughes et al., 2008; NAMS, 2010b.

---

wearing slippery-soled shoes or slippers, since they provide insufficient support, traction, and stability (Kaunitz, 2008; Nelson & Stewart, 2008).

 Optimizing Outcomes— Potential nursing diagnoses for women with osteoporosis

Nursing diagnoses for women with osteoporosis may focus on potential or real problems such as trauma, pain, or impaired mobility:

Risk for Trauma (related to loss of bone density/integrity; increasing risk of fracture with minimal or no stress)

Acute/Chronic Pain (related to vertebral compression on spinal nerves/muscles/ligaments, spontaneous fractures, possibly evidenced by verbal reports, guarding/distraction behaviors, self-focus, and changes in sleep pattern)

Impaired Physical Mobility (related to pain and musculoskeletal impairment, possibly evidenced by limited range of motion, reluctance to attempt movement/expressed fear of re-injury, and imposed restrictions/limitations) (Venes, 2009)

MEDICATIONS FOR THE PREVENTION AND/OR TREATMENT OF OSTEOPOROSIS

A number of medications are effective in preserving bone mineral density. FDA-approved osteoporosis treatments have been shown to decrease fracture risk in patients who have had fragility fractures and/or osteoporosis as diagnosed by DEXA. NOF treatment guidelines state that treatment should be recommended to anyone who faces at least a 3% risk of suffering hip fracture in the next 10 years and to anyone who has at least a 20% risk of sustaining any major bone fractures in that time frame; this is based on a cost-effectiveness model. Pharmacotherapy may also reduce fractures in patients with osteopenia without fractures. There is no consensus about when to initiate therapy to prevent fractures; the health-care provider should assess the potential benefits and risks of therapy in each patient on an individual basis (Cadarette, Katz, Brookhart, Levin, Stedman, Choudhry, & Solomon, 2008; Nelson, 2009; NOF, 2008a).

 Nursing Insight— *ACOG and NAMS recommendations for osteoporosis pharmacotherapy*

ACOG (2008b) recommends osteoporosis pharmacotherapy for the following women:

* Postmenopausal women who have experienced a fragility or low-impact fracture
* Postmenopausal women with no risk factors who have a BMD T-score determined by central dual energy x-ray absorptiometry (C-DEXA) of less than –2
* Postmenopausal women with risk factors for fracture who have a BMD T-score by C-DEXA of less than –1.5

NAMS (2010) recommends osteoporosis pharmacotherapy for:

* All postmenopausal women who have had an osteoporotic vertebral or hip fracture
* All postmenopausal women who have BMD values consistent with osteoporosis (i.e., T-scores equal to or worse than –2.5 at the lumbar spine, femoral neck, or total hip region)
* All postmenopausal women who have T-scores from –1.0 to –2.5 and a 10-year risk, based on the FRAX calculator, of major osteoporotic fracture (spine, hip, shoulder, or wrist) of at least 20% or hip fracture of at least 3%

The FDA has approved a number of medications for the prevention and/or treatment of postmenopausal osteoporosis. These include, in alphabetical order, bisphosphonates (alendronate, alendronate plus D, ibandronate, resedronate, risedronate with 500 mg of calcium carbonate and zoledronic acid), calcitonin, estrogens (estrogen and/or hormone therapy), estrogen agonist/antagonists (raloxifene), and parathyroid hormone (PTH). Certain medications are available in oral and intravenous forms; specific information about each medication is presented in Box 7-13. Combination therapy (usually a bisphosphonate with a nonbisphosphonate) can provide additional small increases in BMD when compared with monotherapy. However, the impact of combination therapy on fracture rates is unknown. Presently, combination therapy is reserved for treatment failures when compliance has been assured (Dawson-Hughes, Lindsay, Khosla, Melton, Tosteson, Favus, & Baim, 2008; NAMS, 2010b; Pinkerton & Dalkin, 2007).

 Nursing Insight— *Empowering women with information about medication options*

An intravenous bisphosphonate may be an appropriate choice when a patient prefers less frequent dosing. Because an IV formulation must be administered by a health-care professional (in an infusion center or infusion-equipped office setting), use of an IV bisphosphonate ensures adherence for the indicated treatment period. Prior to the initiation of any therapy, it is important to inform the patient of various medication dosing and delivery options so that she may participate in the decision-making process, when possible (Bachmann, 2008; Sunyecz & Derman, 2007).

 Nursing Insight— *FDA-approved expanded use of Forteo*

In late 2009, the FDA approved a new use for the osteoporosis medication Forteo (teriparatide) to treat osteoporosis associated with sustained, systemic glucocorticoid therapy in men and women who have a high risk of fracture. Glucocorticoid therapy is the most common cause of secondary osteoporosis—approximately 50% of individuals who are prescribed chronic glucocorticoid therapy will eventually have an osteoporotic fracture. Glucocorticoid medication can lead to a reduction in bone formation, and Forteo has been shown to counter this effect by stimulating bone formation (Scott, 2009).

The Nurse's Role in Fostering Safe Use of Osteoporosis Medications

Nurses have an essential education and counseling role in caring for women who take prescribed osteoporosis medications in terms of advising them about potential risks and side effects as well as the importance of adhering to specific dosing recommendations for the bisphosphonates. The oral bisphosphonates share a common risk profile in terms of their potential to cause gastrointestinal problems, including difficulty swallowing, gastroesophageal reflux, inflammation of the esophagus, and gastric ulcer. Oral bisphosphonates are contraindicated in individuals with reflux, gastroesophageal reflux disease, and other esophageal abnormalities. Neither IV ibandronate nor IV zoledronic acid has been associated with adverse upper gastrointestinal events. Side effects for all of the bisphosphonates may include abdominal, bone, joint, or muscle pain. The nurse should emphasize that deviating from the dosing instructions increases the likelihood of experiencing gastrointestinal symptoms (ACOG, 2004; Cole, 2009; Dawson-Hughes et al., 2008; Kaunitz, 2008; NAMS, 2010b; Pinkerton & Dalton, 2009; Wysowski, 2009).

It is essential that the oral bisphosphonates be taken on an empty stomach first thing in the morning with 8 ounces of plain water, with no additional food or drink consumption for at least 30 minutes, and that the patient remain upright during this time. Not following the instruction to take the medication with only plain water can substantially reduce bisphosphonate absorption; substituting coffee or juice for water can reduce drug absorption by as much as 60%. Oral bisphosphonates are contraindicated in women with uncorrected hypocalcemia, an inability to sit or stand for 30 to 60 minutes, esophageal stricture, or severe renal impairment. Side effects associated with the IV administration of bisphosphonates include flu-like symptoms: fever, pain in the muscles or joints, and headache. Eye inflammation (uveitis) is a rare side effect (ACOG, 2004; Cole, 2009; Dawson-Hughes et al., 2008; Gertz, Holland, Kline,

Box 7-13 **FDA-Approved Medications for the Prevention and/or Treatment of Postmenopausal Osteoporosis**

BISPHOSPHONATES

Bisphosphonates are synthetic forms of a class of compounds found in the body. These compounds bind to the crystals in the bone matrix and inhibit bone resorption. Women who cannot or who choose not to take estrogen are good candidates for bisphosphonate therapy. Bisphosphonates inhibit normal physiological bone resorption as well as abnormal bone resorption, thereby halting bone loss, increasing bone mineral density, and reducing the risk of fractures (Dawson-Hughes et al., 2008; Kagan, 2009; Miller, 2009).

Alendronate (Fosamax, Fosamax Plus D) is FDA approved for the prevention (5 mg PO daily or 35 mg PO weekly) and treatment (10 mg PO daily or 70 mg PO weekly) of postmenopausal osteoporosis. A liquid formulation is available, as well as a formulation that contains 5600 IU of vitamin D. This medication is now available as a generic preparation in the United States. Alendronate reduces the incidence of spine and hip fractures by about 50% over 3 years in patients with a prior vertebral fracture, and it reduces the incidence of vertebral fractures by about 48% over 3 years in patients without a prior vertebral fracture (Dawson-Hughes et al., 2008; Pinkerton & Dalkin, 2009).

Etidronate (Didrocal) is approved in Canada for osteoporosis prevention and treatment in postmenopausal women (400 mg/day for 14 days every 3 months, with calcium taken between cycles). In the United States, etidronate is approved only for treatment of Paget's disease, not for osteoporosis therapy (NAMS, 2010b).

Ibandronate (Boniva) is FDA approved for the treatment of postmenopausal osteoporosis (2.5 mg daily tablet, 150 mg monthly tablet, and 3 mg every 3 months by intravenous injection). The oral preparations are also approved for the prevention of postmenopausal osteoporosis. Ibandronate reduces the incidence of vertebral fractures by about 50% over 3 years (Dawson-Hughes et al., 2008; Pinkerton & Dalkin, 2009).

Risedronate (Actonel, Actonel with Calcium) is approved by the FDA for the prevention and treatment of postmenopausal osteoporosis (5 mg daily tablet or 35 mg weekly tablet, packaged with 5 tablets of 500 mg calcium carbonate or 75 mg tablets on 2 consecutive days every month, or 150 mg monthly tablet). This medication reduces the incidence of vertebral fractures by about 41% to 49% and nonvertebral fractures by about 36% over 3 years, with significant risk reduction occurring after 1 year of treatment in patients with a prior vertebral fracture (Dawson-Hughes et al., 2008; Pinkerton & Dalkin, 2009).

Zoledronic acid (Reclast—USA; Aclasta—Canada) is approved by the FDA for the treatment (5 mg by intravenous infusion over at least 15 minutes once yearly) and prevention (an infusion administered every 2 years is now approved in the United States) of osteoporosis in postmenopausal women. Zoledronic acid reduces the incidence of vertebral fractures by about 70%, hip fractures by about 41%, and nonvertebral fractures by about 25% over 3 years. Zoledronic acid is also indicated for the prevention of new clinical fractures in patients who have recently had a hip fracture. Prior to administration, patients must have two blood tests: One is for creatinine to confirm that kidney function is normal; the other test is for calcium to confirm that the serum calcium level is within normal limits (Dawson-Hughes et al., 2008; NAMS, 2010b; Pinkerton & Dalkin, 2009).

CALCITONIN

Salmon calcitonin (Miacalcin, Fortical) is FDA approved for the treatment of osteoporosis in women who are at least 5 years postmenopausal. It is delivered as a single daily intranasal spray that provides 200 IU of the drug. Subcutaneous administration by injection also is available; side effects associated with this administration route include local inflammation and flushing of the face or hands. Intranasal calcitonin is generally considered safe although some patients experience rhinitis and, rarely, epistaxis. Oral calcitonin has been approved by the FDA for the treatment

of osteoporosis. However, because calcitonin is a less effective agent than other pharmacological therapies for osteoporosis, it is reserved as an alternative for women who cannot or choose not to take one of the other osteoporosis agents (ACOG, 2004; Dawson-Hughes et al., 2008; NAMS, 2010b; Sherman, 2009b).

ESTROGEN/HORMONE THERAPY (ET/HT)

Estrogen therapy (Climara, Estrace, Estraderm, Estratab, Ogen, Ortho-Est, Premarin, Vivelle) and hormone therapy (Activella, Femhrt, Premphase, Prempro, etc.) are approved by the FDA for the prevention of osteoporosis and relief of vasomotor symptoms and vulvovaginal atrophy associated with menopause. Women who have not had a hysterectomy require HT, which contains a progestin to protect the uterine lining. The Woman's Health Initiative (WHI) found that 5 years of HT (Prempro) reduced the risk of clinical vertebral fractures and hip fractures by 34% and other osteoporotic fractures by 23% (Dawson-Hughes et al., 2008).

The WHI reported increased risks of myocardial infarction, stroke, invasive breast cancer, pulmonary emboli, and deep vein phlebitis during 5 years of treatment with conjugated equine estrogen and medroxyprogesterone (Prempro). Subsequent analysis of these data showed no increase in cardiovascular disease in women who started treatment within 10 years of menopause. In the estrogen-only arm of WHI, no increase in breast cancer incidence was noted over 7.1 years of treatment. Other doses and combinations of estrogen and progestins were not studied. Because of the risks, ET/HT should be used in the lowest effective doses for the shortest duration to meet treatment goals. When ET/HT use is considered solely for the prevention of osteoporosis, the FDA recommends that approved nonestrogen treatments should first be carefully considered (Dawson-Hughes et al., 2008).

ESTROGEN AGONIST/ANTAGONIST

Formerly known as a selective estrogen-receptor modulator (SERM), the drug raloxifene (Evista) is approved by the FDA for both prevention and treatment of osteoporosis in postmenopausal women. Raloxifene reduces the risk of vertebral fractures by about 30% in patients with a prior vertebral fracture and by about 55% in patients without a prior vertebral fracture over 3 years. Bone loss often resumes when raloxifene therapy is stopped. Raloxifene is indicated for the reduction in risk of invasive breast cancer in postmenopausal women with osteoporosis. This medication increases the risk of deep vein thrombosis to a degree similar to that observed with estrogen, and it also increases the frequency of night sweats and hot flashes (ACOG, 2004; Dawson-Hughes et al., 2008; NAMS, 2010b).

PARATHYROID HORMONE (PTH)

Teriparatide (recombinant human PTH 1-34, marketed as Forteo) is approved by the FDA for the treatment of osteoporosis in postmenopausal women at high risk for fracture. It is a bone-building (anabolic) agent that directly stimulates osteoblastic bone formation, resulting in substantial increases in trabecular bone density and connectivity. This mechanism of action is very different from that of antiresorptive agents such as estrogen and bisphosphonates, which reduce bone resorption. It is administered by daily subcutaneous injection. Teriparatide in a dose of 20 mcg daily has been shown to decrease the risk of vertebral fractures by 65% and nonvertebral fractures by 53% in patients with osteoporosis, after an average of 18 months of therapy. This medication should only be used for a maximum of 2 years, and it is contraindicated in patients with an increased risk of osteosarcoma and those having prior radiation of the skeleton, bone metastases, hypercalcemia, or a history of skeletal malignancy. Teriparatide is also indicated for the treatment of glucocorticoid-induced osteoporosis and male osteoporosis (Dawson-Hughes et al., 2008; NAMS, 2010b).

Matuszewski, Freeman, Quan, Lasseter, Mucklow, & Porras, 1995; Kaunitz, 2008; Pinkerton & Dalton, 2009; Sunyecz & Derman, 2007; Wysowski, 2009).

There have been rare reports of osteonecrosis (death of the bone cells or tissue) of the jaw with bisphosphonate medications. Nearly all of these cases occurred in cancer patients receiving an intravenous bisphosphonate. Although unusual, there are also reports of osteonecrosis of the jaw in patients being treated with the bisphosphonate tablets alendronate (Fosamax), ibandronate (Boniva), and risedronate (Actonel) for osteoporosis prevention or treatment. Although the risk for this complication in healthy women is estimated as less than 1 in 100,000 treatment years, dental evaluation is recommended prior to the initiation of bisphosphonate therapy. Also, there have been rare reports of esophageal cancer in women taking oral bisphosphonates. Owing to this potential complication, patients with Barrett's esophagus (a premalignant condition caused by an abnormal change in the cells of the distal portion of the esophagus) should not use oral bisphosphonates. An essential component of health teaching for all women who take oral bisphosphonate tablets includes the warning that side effects such as chest pain, new or worsening heartburn, or difficult or painful swallowing must be immediately reported to the health-care provider (ACOG, 2004; Cole, 2009; Dawson-Hughes et al., 2008; Pinkerton & Dalton, 2009; Wysowski, 2009).

Because bisphosphonates are associated with esophageal irritation, it is important to provide detailed dosing information when counseling women about the use of these medications. Alendronate and risedronate tablets should be taken first thing in the morning with 8 ounces of plain water. Patients using the liquid formulation of alendronate should swallow one bottle (75 mL) and follow with at least 2 ounces of plain water. After taking these medications, patients must wait at least 30 minutes before eating, drinking, or taking any other medication. Patients should remain upright (sitting or standing) during this interval (Dawson-Hughes et al., 2008).

Oral ibandronate tablets should be taken on an empty stomach, the first thing in the morning, with 8 ounces of plain water (no other liquid). After taking this medication, patients should be instructed to wait at least 60 minutes before eating, drinking, or taking any other medication. Patients must remain upright for at least 1 hour after taking the medication. Ibandronate, 3 mg per 3 mL prefilled syringe, is given by intravenous injection over 15 to 30 seconds, once every 3 months. Patients should be advised that serum calcium and creatinine levels will be checked before each injection (Bachmann, 2009; Dawson-Hughes et al., 2008; Pinkerton & Dalton, 2009).

❝ What to say ❞ — *Preparing patients for zoledronic acid infusion*

Nurses can help prepare patients who will be treated with an intravenous infusion of zoledronic acid (Reclast) by offering the following information:

- Eat normally and drink at least 2 glasses of fluids before the treatment.
- Your treatment will take at least 15 minutes.

- You may resume your normal activities immediately after the treatment.
- After the first treatment, common side effects may include flu-like symptoms such as fever, muscle or joint pain, and headache.
- You may receive acetaminophen (Tylenol) prior to the infusion to reduce the risk of developing these symptoms; after the treatment, you may continue to use a mild pain reliever as needed for discomfort.
- Side effects are much less common after successive treatments.

(Bachmann, 2008; Dawson-Hughes et al., 2008).

NOF recommends BMD testing every 2 years. For women undergoing pharmacological therapy for osteoporosis, a repeat C-DEXA scan should be performed 2 years after the initiation of treatment and at subsequent 2-year intervals (Dawson-Hughes, 2008; Simon, 2008).

 Optimizing Outcomes— **Educating women about osteoporosis resources for consumers**

- *Know My Bones* is a new educational program for women diagnosed with postmenopausal osteoporosis. The program, available at http://www.knowmybones.com, offers women new insights in understanding the science of bone health, healthful high-calcium recipes, helpful lifestyle tips, and more. The Know My Bones Council, formed to enhance educational efforts about postmenopausal osteoporosis, includes members such as Amgen, Inc. (an international biotechnology company), the National Osteoporosis Foundation, the National Association of Nurse Practitioners in Women's Health, and the Society for Women's Health Research.
- The U.S. Department of Health & Human Services (DHHS) Agency for Healthcare Research and Quality (AHRQ)'s Effective Health Care summary guides have produced *Osteoporosis Treatments That Help Prevent Broken Bones: A Guide for Women After Menopause*, a resource for consumers. The guide is based on a government-funded review of research reports about osteoporosis treatments to prevent broken bones and is available at http://effectivehealthcare.ahrq.gov/index.cfm/search-for-guides-reviews-and-reports/?pageaction=displayproduct&productID=92&returnpage=.

 Optimizing Outcomes— **With professional resources to guide clinical care**

Several clinical and governmental organizations have published guidelines to assist clinicians in informing and guiding women toward appropriate treatments that will help to relieve their menopausal symptoms without placing their health in undue jeopardy. These organizations include the American College of Obstetricians and Gynecologists (ACOG); the North American Menopause Society (NAMS); the National Association of Nurse Practitioners in Women's Health (NPWH); the National Osteoporosis Foundation (NOF); the International Osteoporosis Foundation (IOF); the Association of Women's Health, Obstetric, and

Neonatal Nurses (AWHONN); the U.S. Food and Drug Administration (FDA), and the U.S. Preventive Services Task Force (USPSTF). Nurses can use these recommendations to discuss options with their patients and provide current, evidence-based care (Alexander, 2007).

Now Can You—— Discuss certain aspects of osteoporosis?

1. Explain why menopausal women are at increased risk for osteoporosis and how to conduct a risk assessment for the condition?
2. Counsel a woman about preparing for a C-DEXA examination?
3. Develop an osteoporosis educational program that includes strategies for reducing risk and tips for optimizing bone health?
4. Counsel a woman about the safe use of medications for the prevention and/or treatment of osteoporosis?

---

summary points

◆ Today, American women can expect to live to be 80 years old and spend close to one-third of their lives as menopausal women.

◆ Nurses can empower midlife women with factual, evidence-based information about menopause, the normal aging process, and strategies to optimize cardiovascular and skeletal health.

◆ Complementary and alternative medicine approaches such as stress management, guided imagery, biofeedback, yoga, and massage therapy may be useful in minimizing various menopausal symptoms.

◆ An important role for nurses centers on counseling women to become informed about any herbal preparations they are considering and to consult with their health-care providers before using any of them.

◆ Estrogen-containing drugs for menopausal use are divided into two categories: estrogen therapy (ET) and combined estrogen-progestogen therapy (EPT).

◆ The number-one killer of older American women is cardiovascular disease, which includes coronary heart disease, stroke, congestive heart failure, hypertension, and other diseases of the heart and vascular system.

◆ Educating women about strategies to control the five cardiovascular risk factors (smoking, hyperlipidemia, diabetes mellitus, hypertension, obesity) can empower them to make changes that can greatly reduce their lifetime risk for cardiovascular disease.

◆ Bone health promotion includes strategies such as optimizing calcium intake, preventing the loss of calcium and other minerals from the bone, maintaining the soft tissue components around the bone, and promoting the efficiency of bone repair.

◆ An essential role for nurses who care for women who take prescribed osteoporosis medications centers on education and counseling about potential risks and side effects as well as the importance of adhering to specific dosing recommendations for the bisphosphonates.

review questions

Multiple Choice

1. Normal physiological changes that accompany menopause include:
   a. Vaginal lengthening with an increased production of cervical mucus
   b. An increase in muscle mass
   c. Less elastic skin with decreased melanin
   d. Increased levels of estrogen and progesterone

2. Nurses can teach women about self-care strategies to help reduce menopausal symptoms, such as:
   a. Dressing in layers
   b. Consuming foods and beverages that contain caffeine
   c. Reducing physical activity
   d. Consuming foods that are highly seasoned

3. According to recommendations from the North American Menopause Society, recommendations for hormone therapy use include:
   a. Prevention of diabetes mellitus
   b. Short-term treatment for severe vasomotor symptoms
   c. Prevention of coronary heart disease
   d. Prevention of dementia

4. Risk factors for cardiovascular disease include:
   a. Normal body weight
   b. Parkinson's disease
   c. Psychological stress
   d. Regular dietary consumption of fiber, fruits, and vegetables

5. Risk factors for osteoporosis include:
   a. Excessive sun exposure
   b. Large body build
   c. Late menopause
   d. Caucasian ethnicity

REFERENCES

Alexander, I.M.(2006). Bioidentical hormones for menopause therapy: Separating the myths from the reality. *Women's Health Care, 5*(1), 7–17.

Alexander, I.M. (2007). Overview of current HT recommendations using evidence-based decision making. *American Journal for Nurse Practitioners, 11*(10), 29–41.

Alexander, I.M. (2009). Harnessing the hot flash: More choices for midlife women. *Advance for Nurse Practitioners, 17*(7), 31–34.

Allmen, T., & Moore, A. (2010). Attention and intervention: Responding to vaginal changes of menopause. *Women's Health Care: A Practical Journal for Nurse Practitioners, 9*(5), 38–51.

Altman, A.M. (2008). Postmenopausal hormone therapy—updates. *Women's Health Care, 7*(10), 7–15.

Altman, A. (2009). Transdermal hormone therapy compared to oral hormone therapy: The impact of the first-pass effect. *Contemporary OB/GYN (Supplement), 22*(1), S8–S12.

Altman, A.M., Moore, A., Speroff, L., & Wysocki, S. (2009). Tackling the tricky issue of bioidentical hormones. *Women's Health Care: A Practical Journal for Nurse Practitioners, 8*(7), 7–15.

American College of Obstetricians and Gynecologists (ACOG). (2001). *Use of botanicals for management of menopausal symptoms.* (Practice Bulletin Number 28), 1–10. Washington, DC: Author.

American College of Obstetricians and Gynecologists (ACOG). (2004a). *Osteoporosis.* (Practice Bulletin Number 50), 1170–1183. Washington, DC: Author.

American College of Obstetricians and Gynecologists (ACOG). (2004b). Hormone therapy: Cognition and dementia. *Obstetrics and Gynecology, 104*(Suppl), 25S–40S.

American College of Obstetricians and Gynecologists (ACOG). (2005). *Compounded bioidentical hormones.* (Committee Opinion Number 322), 298–299. Washington, DC: Author.

American College of Obstetricians and Gynecologists (ACOG). (2007). *Women's health care: A Resource manual* (3rd ed.). Washington, DC: Author.

American College of Obstetricians and Gynecologists (ACOG). (2008a). *Hormone therapy and heart disease.* (Committee Opinion Number 420), 115–118. Washington, DC: Author.

American College of Obstetricians and Gynecologists (ACOG). (2008b). *Low bone mass (osteopenia) and fracture risk.* (Committee Opinion Number 407), 102–104. Washington, DC: Author.

American Diabetes Association (ADA). (2006). *The cardiometabolic risk initiative: Moving beyond the metabolic syndrome.* Retrieved June 5, 2010, from http://professional.diabetes.org/ResourcesForProfessionals.aspx?cid=60379

American Heart Association (AHA). (2002). National Cholesterol Education Program (NCEP) Expert Panel on Detection, Evaluation, and Treatment of High Blood Cholesterol in Adults (Adult Treatment Panel III). Third report of the National Cholesterol Education Program (NCEP) Expert Panel on Detection, Evaluation, and Treatment of High Blood Cholesterol in Adults (Adult Treatment Panel III) Final Report. *Circulation, 106*(25), 3143–3421.

American Heart Association (AHA). (2010). *Heart disease & stroke statistics: 2010 update.* Retrieved May 18, 2010, from http://www.americanheart.org/downloadable/heart/1265665152970DS-3241HeartStrokeUpdate_2010.pdf

American Heart Association (AHA). (2010). *Facts about women and cardiovascular diseases.* Retrieved May 18, 2010, from http://www.americanheart.org/presenter.jhtml?identifier=1200011

Bachmann, G.A. (2008). A menopausal hormone therapy update. *The Female Patient, 34*(3), 24–25.

Bachmann, G.A. (2008). The utilization of intravenous bisphosphonates. *The Female Patient (Supplement), 33*(11), S9–12.

Berga, S.L. (2009). Putting hormones and aging into perspective: State of hormone therapy for vasomotor symptoms. *Contemporary OB/GYN (Supplement), 22*(1), S3–S7.

Bergfeld, W.F., & Harrison, S. (2009). Treating osteoporosis and postmenopausal hair loss. *Contemporary OB/GYN, 54*(5), 32–33.

Blumenthal, R.S., Michos, E.D., & Nasir, K. (2007). Further improvements in CHD risk prediction for Women. *Journal of the American Medical Association, 297*(6), 641–643.

Burdette, L. (2009). Managing the vaginal and urinary symptoms of postmenopausal urogenital atrophy: A case-based approach. *Women's Health Care: A Practical Journal for Nurse Practitioners, 8*(9), 12–21.

Burdette, L., Moore, A., Speroff, L., & Wysocki, S. (2009). Hormone therapy in menopause: Applying research findings to optimal patient care and education. *Women's Health Care: A Practical Journal for Nurse Practitioners, 8*(5), 10–21.

Burkman, R.T. (2009). Are your patients asking for bioidentical hormones? *The Female Patient, 34*(6), 15–16.

Cadarette, S.M., Katz, J.N., Brookhart, M.A., Levin, R., Stedman, M.R., Choudhry, N.K., & Solomon, D.H. (2008). Trends in drug prescribing for osteoporosis after hip fracture, 1995–2004. *Journal of Rheumatology, 35*(2), 319–326.

Christian, A.H., Rosamond, W., White, A.R., & Mosca, L. (2007). Nine-year trends and racial and ethnic disparities in women's awareness of heart disease and stroke: An American Heart Association national study. *Journal of Women's Health, 16*(1), 68–81.

Cole, R.E. (2009). A new drug in a new class for postmenopausal osteoporosis. *The Female Patient, 34*(11), 20–24.

Costantino, D., & Guaraldi, C. (2008). Effectiveness and safety of vaginal suppositories for the treatment of the vaginal atrophy in postmenopausal women: An open, non-controlled clinical trial. *European Review for Medical and Pharmacological Sciences, 12*(6), 411–416.

Dawson-Hughes, B., Lindsay, R., Khosla, S., Melton, L.J., III, Tosteson, A.N.A., Favus, M., & Baim, S. (2008). *Clinician's guide to prevention and treatment of osteoporosis.* National Osteoporosis Foundation: Washington, DC.

Dranov, P. (2007). Homone therapy is making a comeback. *The Clinical Advisor, 10*(5), 72–83.

Edelman, J. (2010). Managing the menopausal patient. *The Clinical Advisor, 55*(1), 84.

Ettinger, B., & Ettinger, K.M. (2009). FRAX: Using the new fracture risk assessment tool. *Contemporary OB/GYN, 54*(7), 22–28.

Flores, V., & Taylor, H.S. (2010). Current and future SERMs: An update. *The Female Patient, 35*(5), 21–24.

Freeman, R. (2009). Changes in hair growth patterns in postmenopausal women. *The Female Patient, 34*(10), 47–48.

Freeman, S.B. (2009). Micronized progesterone: An important option for oral hormone therapy. *Women's Health Care: A Practical Journal for Nurse Practitioners, 8*(12), 7–13.

Geller, S.E., & Studee, L. (2008). Botanical and dietary supplements for menopause. *The Female Patient, 33*(6), 19–24.

Gersh, F.L. (2009).Estradiol gel 0.1% clinical data. *Contemporary OB/GYN (Supplement). 22*(1), S16–S19.

Gertz, B.J., Holland, S.D., Kline, W.F., Matuszewski, B.K., Freeman, A., Quan, H., Lasseter, K.C., Mucklow, J.C., & Porras, A.G. (1995). Studies of the oral bioavailability of alendronate. *Clinical Pharmacology & Therapeutics, 58*(3), 288–298.

Gies, C., & Lessick, M. (2009). Alzheimer disease in women: A clinical and genetics perspective. *Nursing for Women's Health, 13*(4), 314–324.

Giovannucci, E. (2009).Vitamin D and cancer incidence in the Harvard cohorts. *Annals of Epidemiology, 19*(4), 84–88.

Goldstein, S.R. (2008). Osteoporosis: Screening and diagnosis in clinical practice. *The Female Patient (Supplement), 33*(11), S1–4.

Goldstein, L., & Alexander, J.L. (2005). Practical aspects in the management of vaginal atrophy and sexual dysfunction in perimenopausal and postmenopausal women. *Journal of Sexual Medicine, 2*(Suppl. 3), 154–165.

Greenblum, C., Greenblum, J., & Neff, D. (2009). Vaginal estrogen use in menopause: Is it safe? *The American Journal for Nurse Practitioners, 13*(9), 26–35.

Hellwig, J.P. (2009). Economics of exercise: Community-based physical activity programs are cost effective. *Nursing for Women's Health, 13*(1), 16.

Helmrich, G. (2010). NAMS position on hormone therapy. *Menopause, 19*(4), 34–36.

Henderson, V.W. (2009). Estrogen-containing hormone therapy and cognition: Consensus and controversy. *The Female Patient, 34*(5), 25–27.

Hess, H., London, A., Moore, A., & Simon, J. (2009). Pharmacologic treatment options for menopausal symptoms. *The Female Patient (Supplement), 34*(5), S1–S8.

Hsia, J., Langer, R.D., Manson, J.E., Kuller, J., Johnson, K.C., & Hendrix, S.L., et al. (2006). Conjugated equine estrogens and coronary heart disease: The Women's Health Initiative. *Archives of Internal Medicine, 166*(3), 357–365.

Jones, K.A., Bryson, E., & Harmanli, O. (2010). Successful pelvic floor rehabilitation practice for the obstetrician/gynecologist. *The Female Patient, 35*(5), 41–43.

Kagan, R. (2009). Charting a course for postmenopausal women after hormone therapy. *Contemporary OB/GYN, 54*(11), 22–24.

Kapustin, J. (2010). Chronic disease prevention across the lifespan. *The Journal for Nurse Practitioners, 6*(1), 16–24.

Kaunitz, A.M. (2008). Counseling patients on the management of osteoporosis. *The Female Patient (Supplement), 33*(11), S13–16.

Kellogg-Spadt, S. (2010). Vulvovaginal atrophy: Who benefits most from estrogen therapy? *Advance for Nurse Practitioners, 18*(4), 31–36.

Kessenich, C.R. (2009). Fracture risk assessment in osteoporosis management. *The American Journal for Nurse Practitioners, 13*(9), 36–42.

Kupferer, E.M., Dormire, S.L., & Becker, H. (2009). Complementary and alternative medicine use for vasomotor symptoms among women who have discontinued hormone therapy. *Journal of Obstetric, Gynecologic, and Neonatal Nurses, 38*(1), 50–59.

LaCroix, A.Z. (2005). Estrogen with and without progestin: Benefits and risks of short-term use. *American Journal of Medicine, 118*(12 Suppl. 2), 79–87.

Lake, K. (2007). Beware of bioidentical hormones! *The Clinical Advisor, 10*(9), 121.

Lichtenstein, A.H., Appel, L.J., Brands, M., et al. (2006). Diet and lifestyle recommendations revision 2006: A scientific statement from the American Heart Association nutrition committee. *Circulation, 114*(1), 82–96.

Liu, J.H. (2007). Progestins in hormone therapy: What are the options? *Female Patient, 32*(2), 33–39.

Loprinzi, C.L., Levitt, R., Barton, D., Sloan, J.A., Dakhil, S.R., Nikcevich, D.A., et al. (2006). Phase III comparison of depomedroxyprogesterone acetate to vanlafaxine for managing hot flashes: North Central

Cancer Treatment Group Trial N99C7. *Journal of Clinical Oncology, 24*(9), 1409–1414.

Madala, M.C., Franklin, B.A., Chen, A.Y., & Berman, A.D., et al. (2008). Obesity and age of first non-ST segment elevation myocardial infarction. *Journal of the American College of Cardiology, 52*(12), 979–985.

Malone, R.W., & Kessenich, C. (2008). Vitamin D deficiency: Implications across the lifespan. *The Journal for Nurse Practitioners, 4*(6), 448–454.

Manson, J.E. (2009). Expert advice on aspirin, MI, and stroke. *Contemporary OB-GYN, 54*(9), 66–67.

Margolis, M. (2010). How drug delivery and pharmacokinetics impact estrogen therapy. *The Female Patient (Supplement), 35*(5), S1–S8.

Mayhew, M.S. (2009). Vitamin D deficiency and treatment. *The Journal for Nurse Practitioners, 5*(10), 773–774.

McKee, J., & Warber, S.L. (2005). Integrative therapies for menopause. *Southern Medical Journal, 98*(3), 319–326.

McNeal, C.J., & Birchem, J. (2009a). Cardiovascular disease in women, part 1: Identification of women at risk. *The Female Patient, 34*(6), 43–48.

McNeal, C.J., & Birchem, J. (2009b). Cardiovascular disease in women, part 2: The therapeutic spectrum. *The Female Patient, 34*(7), 44–50.

Mehta, A., & Bachmann, G. (2008). Vulvovaginal complaints. *Clinical Obstetrics and Gynecology, 51*(3), 549–555.

Miller, P.D. (2009). Treating osteoporosis and postmenopausal hair loss. *Contemporary OB/GYN, 54*(5), 31–32.

Minarik, P.A. (2009). Sleep disturbance in midlife women. *Journal of Obstetric, Gynecologic, and Neonatal Nurses, 38*(3), 333–343.

Minkin, M.J. (2010). Transdermal estrogen therapy: Personalized treatment approaches. *The Female Patient, 35*(6), 16–18.

Moore, A. (2010). Bioidentical hormone therapy: What practitioners need to know now. *Women's Health care: A Practical Journal for Nurse Practitioners, 9*(5), 10–18.

Mosca, L., Banka, C.L., Benjamin, E.J., Berra, K., Bushnell, C., Dolor, R.J., et al. (2007). Evidence-based guidelines for cardiovascular disease prevention in women: 2007 update. *Circulation, 115*(11), 1481–1501.

Mosca, L., Ferris, A., Fabunmi, R., & Robertson, R.M. (2004).Tracking women's awareness of heart disease: An American Heart Association national study. *Circulation, 109*(5), 573–579.

Mosca, L., Mochari, H., Christian, A., Berra, K., Taubert, K., Mills, T., Burdick, K.A., & Simpson, S.L. (2006). National study of women's awareness, preventive action, and barriers to cardiovascular health. *Circulation, 113*(4), 525–534.

Nachtigall, L.E. (2009). Understanding the pathophysiology of estrogen clotting issues: Oral vs transdermal routes. *Contemporary OB/GYN (Supplement), 22*(10), S12–S16.

Nachtigall, L.E., Baber, R.J., Barentsen, R., Durand, N., Panay, N., & Pitkin, J., et al. (2006). Complementary and hormonal therapy for vasomotor symptom relief: A conservative clinical approach. *Journal of Obstetrics and Gynaecology Canada, 28*(4), 279–289.

National Institutes of Health. (2005). National Institutes of Health state-of the science conference statement: Management of menopause-related symptoms. *Annals of Internal Medicine, 142*(12 Part 1), 1003–1013.

National Institutes of Health. (2009). *Dietary supplement fact sheet: Calcium.* Retrieved May 30, 2010, from http://ods.od.nih.gov/factsheets/calcium.asp

National Osteoporosis Foundation (NOF). (2008a). *Medications to prevent & treat osteoporosis.* Retrieved May 18, 2010, from http://www.nof.org/patientinfo/medications.htm

National Osteoporosis Foundation (NOF). (2008b). *Fast facts on osteoporosis.* Retrieved May 25, 2010, from http://www.nof.org/osteoporosis/diseasefacts.htm

National Osteoporosis Foundation (NOF). (2008c). *Prevention: Calcium.* Retrieved May 30, 2010, from http://www.nof.org/prevention/calcium2.htm

National Osteoporosis Foundation (NOF). (2008d).*Prevention: Exercise for healthy bones.* Retrieved May 28, 2010, from http://www.nof.org/prevention/exercise.htm

National Women's Health Network. (2000). *Taking hormones and women's health: Choices, Risks, and benefits* (5th ed.). Washington, DC: Author.

Nelson, A.L. (2009). Fracture risk reduction: How to use FRAX in your practice. *The Female Patient, 34*(2), 22–24.

Nelson, A.L., & Stewart, F.H. (2008). Menopause and perimenopausal health. In R. Hatcher, J. Trussell, A. Nelson, W. Cates, Jr., F. Stewart, & D. Kowal (Eds.), *Contraceptive technology,* (19th ed., pp. 699–745). New York: Thomson Reuters.

Nelson, H.D., Haney, E., Humphrey, L., Miller, J., Nedrow, A., Nicolaidis, C., Vesco, K., Walker, M., Bougatsos, C., & Nygren, P. (2005). Management of menopause-related symptoms. Summary, Evidence Report/Technology Assessment: Number 120. *AHRQ Publication No. 05-E016-1.* Retrieved June 8, 2010, from http://www.ahrq.gov/clinic/epcsums/menosum.htm

Nelson, H.D., Vesco, K.K., Haney, E., Fu, R., Nedrow, A., & Miller, J., et al. (2006). Non-hormonal therapies for menopausal hot flashes: Systematic review and meta-analysis. *Journal of the American Medical Association, 295*(17), 2057–2071.

Palacios, S. (2009). Managing urogenital atrophy. *Maturitas, 63*(4), 315–318.

Patel, P., & Nunley, J.R. (2010). Lichen sclerosis et atrophicus. *The Clinical Advisor, 35*(2), 59–60.

Pinkerton, J.V., & Dalkin, A.C. (2007). Combination therapy for treatment of osteoporosis: A review. *American Journal of Obstetrics and Gynecology, 197*(6), 559–565.

Pinkerton J.V., & Dalkin, A.C. (2009). Approaches to the treatment of osteoporosis. *The Female Patient, 34*(6), 30–33.

Pugliese, J.M., Morey, A.F., & Peterson, A.C. (2007). Lichen sclerosus: Review of the literature and current recommendations for management. *The Journal of Urology, 178*(6), 2268–2276.

Reeve, K., & Bailes, B. (2010). Insomnia in adults: Etiology and management. *The Journal for Nurse Practitioners, 6*(1), 53–60.

Reiter, S. (2009). Sexual dysfunction and vaginal atrophy in menopausal women: An approach to effective communication and management. *Women's Health Care: A Practical Journal for Nurse Practitioners, 8*(9), 22–33.

Ridker, P.M., Buring, J.E., Rifai, N., & Cook, N.R. (2007). Development and validation of improved algorithms for the assessment of global cardiovascular risk in women: The Reynolds Risk Score. *Journal of the American Medical Association, 297*(6), 611–619.

Rosenthal, M.S. (2008). Ethical problems with bioidentical hormones. *International Journal of Impotence Research, 20*(1), 45–52.

Rosenthal, M.S. (2009). Bioidentical hormones: Ethics and misinformed consent. *The Female Patient, 34*(8), 28–31.

Ruhl, C. (2009). Cardiometabolic health: Connecting the dots. *Nursing for Women's Health, 13*(1), 78–82.

Ruhl, C. (2010). Sleep is a vital sign: Why assessing sleep is an important part of women's health care. *Nursing for Women's Health, 14*(3), 243–247.

Rutecki, G.W. (2009). May the sun shine half day long: Balancing the risks and benefits of sun exposure. *Consultant, 49*(8), 509.

Scott, A. (2009). FDA approves new drug indication for Forteo. *Drug Topics E-News.* Retrieved May 30, 2010, from http://drugtopics.modernmedicine.com/drugtopics/Community+Practice/FDA-approves-new-drug-indication-for-Forteo/ArticleStandard/Article/detail/614527

Secor, R.M., & Simon, J.A. (2006). New options for treating the symptoms of menopause. *Women's Health in Primary Care, 6*(4), 44–52.

Sego, S. (2009). Olive oil. *The Clinical Advisor, 12*(9), 71–72.

Sherman, C. (2009a). Hormone therapy following menopause. *The Clinical Advisor, 12*(11), 29–35.

Sherman, C. (2009b). Osteoporosis: No gender gap for therapy. *The Clinical Advisor, 12*(6), 16–20.

Shulman, L.P. (2008). Advances in treating vasomotor symptoms in postmenopausal women. *The Female Patient (Supplement), 33*(6), S27–31.

Simon, J.A. (2008). Pharmacologic prevention and treatment of osteoporosis. *The Female Patient (Supplement), 33*(11), S5–8.

Slentz, C.A., Duscha, B.D., & Johnson, J.L., et al. (2004). Effects of the amount of exercise on body weight, body composition, and measures of central obesity: STRRIDE—a randomized controlled study. *Archives of Internal Medicine, 164*(1), 31–39.

Smith, S.C., Jr., Allen, J., Blair, S.N., & Bonow, R.O., et al. (2006). ACC guidelines for secondary prevention for patients with coronary and other atherosclerotic vascular disease: 2006 update: Endorsed by the National Heart, Lung, and Blood Institute. *Circulation, 113*(19), 2363–2372.

Speroff, L., & Fritz, M.A. (2005). *Clinical gynecologic endocrinology and infertility* (7th ed.). Philadelphia: Lippincott Williams & Wilkins.

Syroney, L., & Franjesevic, A. (2010). Vitamin D deficiency: Screening and treatment in primary care. *Advance for Nurse Practitioners, 18*(5), 37–40.

Thanavaro, J.L. (2005). Barriers to coronary heart disease risk modification in women without prior history of coronary heart disease. *Journal of the American Academy of Nurse Practitioners, 17*(11), 487–493.

Theroux, R. (2008). Postmenopausal hormone use: What does the latest evidence show? *Nursing for Women's Health, 12*(1), 56–61.

The North American Menopause Society (NAMS). (2007). *Menopause practice: A clinician's guide* (3rd ed.). Cleveland, OH: Author.

The North American Menopause Society (NAMS). (2010a). *Estrogen and progestogen use in postmenopausal women: 2010 position statement of The North American Menopause Society, 17*(2), 242–255.

The North American Menopause Society (NAMS). (2010b). *Osteoporosis in postmenopausal women: 2010 position statement.* Retrieved June 1, 2010, from http://www.medscape.com/viewarticle/714984_2

U.S. Preventive Services Task Force (USPSTF). (2002). *Osteoporosis screening.* Retrieved May 25, 2010, from http://www.ahrq.gov/clinic/3rduspstf/osteoporosis/

U.S. Preventive Services Task Force (USPSTF). (2009). *Guide to clinical preventive health services, 2009: Recommendations of the U.S. Preventive Services Task Force* (AHRQ Publication No. 09-IP006). Available from http://www.ahrq.gov

Utian, W.H. (2008). The practical clinical application of the NAMS 2008 position statement on estrogen and progestogen use in postmenopausal women. *Women's Health Care: A Practical Journal for Nurse Practitioners, 7*(8), 50–59.

Utian, W.H., Archer, D.F., Bachmann, G.A., et al; North American Menopause Society. (2008). Estrogen andprogestogen use in postmenopausal women: July 2008 position statement of The North American Menopause Society. *Menopause, 15*(4, pt 1), 584–602.

Valerio, T.D. (2009). Much more than a nuisance: Health consequences of sleep disorders. *Advance for Nurse Practitioners, 17*(9), 57–60.

Vassar, K.A. (2009). Promoting cardiovascular health in women. *Women's Health Care: A Practical Journal for Nurse Practitioners, 8*(12), 28–33.

Venes, D. (2010). *Taber's cyclopedic medical dictionary* (21st ed.). Philadelphia: F.A. Davis Company.

Watts, N.B., Ettinger, B., & LeBoff, M.S. (2009). FRAX facts. *Journal of Bone and Mineral Research, 24*(3), 975–979.

Weed, S. (2002). *New menopausal years, the wise woman way: Alternative approaches for Women.* Woodstock, NY: Ash Tree.

Weil, E. (2009). Bioidentical hormones: Examining the debate. *Advance for Nurse Practitioners, 17*(9), 37–41.

Wenger, N.K. (2007). Cardiovascular risk assessment and intervention strategies in women. *Women's Health in Primary Care, Supplement,* September, 2007, S1–S11.

Williams, J. K., & Brownlee, J. (2010). The dietary clinical trials of the Women's Health Initiative: Part 2. *The Female Patient, 35*(4), 39–41.

Writing Group for the Women's Health Initiative Investigators. (2002). Risks and benefits of estrogen plus progestin in healthy postmenopausal women. *Journal of the American Medical Association, 288* (7), 321–333.

Wysocki, S. (2008). Etiology, consequences, and management of vaginal atrophy. *The American Journal for Nurse Practitioners, 12*(11/12), 36–46.

Wysocki, S. (2009a). Local estrogen therapy—Preferred treatment for symptoms of menopausal vulvovaginal atrophy. *Women's Health Care: A Practical Journal for Nurse Practitioners, 8*(11), 8–16.

Wysocki, S. (2009b). Targeting the urogenital health of postmenopausal women: A spotlight on vaginal atrophy. *Women's Health Care: A Practical Journal for Nurse Practitioners, 9*(9), 10–11.

Wysowski, D.K. (2009). Reports of esophageal cancer with oral bisphosphonate use. *New England Journal of Medicine, 360*(1), 89–90.

Index